SO-AJO-338

ABNORMAL PSYCHOLOGY 98/99

Third Edition

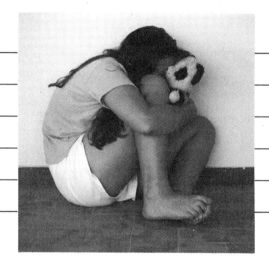

Editor

Dr. Joseph J. Palladino
University of Southern Indiana

Joseph J. Palladino, a professor at the University of Southern Indiana in Evansville, Indiana, received all his degrees from Fordham University, including his Ph.D. in 1982. Dr. Palladino has taught abnormal psychology for more than two decades.

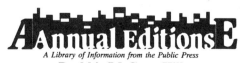
Annual Editions
A Library of Information from the Public Press
Dushkin/McGraw·Hill
Sluice Dock, Guilford, Connecticut 06437

*Visit us on the Internet—*http://www.dushkin.com/annualeditions

The Annual Editions Series

ANNUAL EDITIONS, including GLOBAL STUDIES, consist of over 70 volumes designed to provide the reader with convenient, low-cost access to a wide range of current, carefully selected articles from some of the most important magazines, newspapers, and journals published today. ANNUAL EDITIONS are updated on an annual basis through a continuous monitoring of over 300 periodical sources. All ANNUAL EDITIONS have a number of features that are designed to make them particularly useful, including topic guides, annotated tables of contents, unit overviews, and indexes. For the teacher using ANNUAL EDITIONS in the classroom, an Instructor's Resource Guide with test questions is available for each volume. GLOBAL STUDIES titles provide comprehensive background information and selected world press articles on the regions and countries of the world.

VOLUMES AVAILABLE

ANNUAL EDITIONS
Abnormal Psychology
Accounting
Adolescent Psychology
Aging
American Foreign Policy
American Government
American History,
    Pre-Civil War
American History,
    Post-Civil War
American Public Policy
Anthropology
Archaeology
Astronomy
Biopsychology
Business Ethics
Canadian Politics
Child Growth and Development
Comparative Politics
Computers in Education
Computers in Society
Criminal Justice
Criminology
Developing World
Deviant Behavior

Drugs, Society, and Behavior
Dying, Death, and Bereavement
Early Childhood Education
Economics
Educating Exceptional Children
Education
Educational Psychology
Environment
Geography
Geology
Global Issues
Health
Human Development
Human Resources
Human Sexuality
International Business
Macroeconomics
Management
Marketing
Marriage and Family
Mass Media
Microeconomics
Multicultural Education
Nutrition
Personal Growth and Behavior
Physical Anthropology
Psychology

Public Administration
Race and Ethnic Relations
Social Problems
Social Psychology
Sociology
State and Local Government
Teaching English as a Second
    Language
Urban Society
Violence and Terrorism
Western Civilization,
    Pre-Reformation
Western Civilization,
    Post-Reformation
Women's Health
World History, Pre-Modern
World History, Modern
World Politics

GLOBAL STUDIES
Africa
China
India and South Asia
Japan and the Pacific Rim
Latin America
Middle East
Russia, the Eurasian Republics,
    and Central/Eastern Europe

Cataloging in Publication Data
Main entry under title: Annual Editions: Abnormal Psychology. 1998/99.
    1. Mental illness—Periodicals. 2. Psychology, Pathological—Periodicals. I. Palladino, Joseph, comp.
II. Title: Abnormal psychology.
ISBN 0–697–39126–4   362.2'05   ISSN 1094–2599

© 1998 by Dushkin/McGraw-Hill, Guilford, CT 06437, A Division of The McGraw-Hill Companies.

Copyright law prohibits the reproduction, storage, or transmission in any form by any means of any portion of this publication without the express written permission of Dushkin/McGraw-Hill, and of the copyright holder (if different) of the part of the publication to be reproduced. The Guidelines for Classroom Copying endorsed by Congress explicitly state that unauthorized copying may not be used to create, to replace, or to substitute for anthologies, compilations, or collective works.

Annual Editions® is a Registered Trademark of Dushkin/McGraw-Hill, A Division of The McGraw-Hill Companies.

Third Edition

Cover image © 1998 PhotoDisc, Inc.

Printed in the United States of America

Printed on Recycled Paper

75
973

Editors/Advisory Board

Members of the Advisory Board are instrumental in the final selection of articles for each edition of ANNUAL EDITIONS. Their review of articles for content, level, currentness, and appropriateness provides critical direction to the editor and staff. We think that you will find their careful consideration well reflected in this volume.

LIFE Pacific College
Alumni Library
1100 West Covina Blvd.
San Dimas, CA 91773

EDITOR

Dr. Joseph J. Palladino
University of Southern Indiana

ADVISORY BOARD

Linda S. Bosmajian
Hood College

Edward G. Boyd
Mater Dei College

Ellen Cash
Green River Community College

Keith Corodimas
*Philadelphia College of Textiles
& Science*

Linda K. Davis
Mt. Hood Community College

Joan F. DiGiovanni
Western New England College

Karen L. Freiberg
*University of Maryland
Baltimore County*

Richard P. Halgin
*University of Massachusetts
Amherst*

Jacqueline B. Horn
*University of California
Davis*

Kevin C. Krycka
Seattle University

Bette Levine
*University of South Carolina
Salkehatchie*

James E. Maddux
George Mason University

Larry L. Mullins
Oklahoma State University

Les Parrott
Seattle Pacific University

Mary Procidano
Fordham University

Kathy Sexton-Radek
Elmhurst College

Sandra Solomon
University of Vermont

Ann Stearns
Essex Community College

Timothy P. Tomczak
Genesee Community College

Staff

Ian A. Nielsen, Publisher

EDITORIAL STAFF

Roberta Monaco, Developmental Editor
Dorothy Fink, Associate Developmental Editor
Addie Raucci, Senior Administrative Editor
Cheryl Greenleaf, Permissions Editor
Deanna Herrschaft, Permissions Assistant
Diane Barker, Proofreader
Lisa Holmes-Doebrick, Program Coordinator

PRODUCTION STAFF

Brenda S. Filley, Production Manager
Charles Vitelli, Designer
Lara M. Johnson, Design/Advertising Coordinator
Shawn Callahan, Graphics
Laura Levine, Graphics
Mike Campbell, Graphics
Joseph Offredi, Graphics
Juliana Arbo, Typesetting Supervisor
Jane Jaegersen, Typesetter
Marie Lazauskas, Word Processor
Kathleen D'Amico, Word Processor
Larry Killian, Copier Coordinator

048000

To the Reader

In publishing ANNUAL EDITIONS we recognize the enormous role played by the magazines, newspapers, and journals of the *public press* in providing current, first-rate educational information in a broad spectrum of interest areas. Many of these articles are appropriate for students, researchers, and professionals seeking accurate, current material to help bridge the gap between principles and theories and the real world. These articles, however, become more useful for study when those of lasting value are carefully *collected, organized, indexed,* and *reproduced* in a *low-cost format,* which provides easy and permanent access when the material is needed. That is the role played by ANNUAL EDITIONS. Under the direction of each volume's *academic editor,* who is an expert in the subject area, and with the guidance of an *Advisory Board,* each year we seek to provide in each ANNUAL EDITION a current, well-balanced, carefully selected collection of the best of the public press for your study and enjoyment. We think that you will find this volume useful, and we hope that you will take a moment to let us know what you think.

If you pick up your television remote control and start scanning the channels, you are likely to find talk shows where individuals freely describe the symptoms of some psychological disorders that have dramatically affected their lives. If you pick up the newspaper, you may read about a new drug that is being touted as the cure for an increasing array of maladies. As you listen and read, you may stop to think: Who decides what is normal and what is abnormal? How do such decisions affect individuals? If you have some distressing symptoms and decide to seek treatment, what types of treatment would be appropriate, how long would the treatment last, and what is the possible benefit?

As you continue scanning the television channels, you may find a program focusing on recent advances in neuroimaging and genetics. You listen to reports of breakthroughs in the search for causes of well-known disorders. Neuroimaging studies can tell us about abnormalities in the brain that may be significant in understanding some disorders, and more research is directed to finding how genetic factors can influence disorders.

What we perceive as abnormal fascinates us because we recognize some of the signs and symptoms in ourselves. The anxiety experienced by a person with a panic disorder may be similar to the experience you had while preparing to give a speech. All of us have, at one time or another, experienced muted versions of the ups and downs that occur in mood disorders. Who has heard a sound that others did not hear or heard a voice when there was no possible source? This recognition of similarity leads us to wonder how symptoms develop and how they can be treated. We sometimes find that possible answers to our questions accumulate at a furious pace. The rapid pace of advances in understanding and treating

abnormal behavior also leads to controversy. For example, we wonder if the influence of genetic factors is being overstated.

The articles in *Annual Editions: Abnormal Psychology 98/99* were selected to allow students to explore recent findings that touch on some of the exciting and controversial issues in abnormal psychology. Many of the articles were written by journalists for respected magazines; others were drawn from professional sources.

As you peruse the *table of contents,* you will find that readings address familiar topics such as panic disorder and schizophrenia as well as less familiar but intriguing disorders such as Munchausen by proxy. This collection not only supplements the material that is being covered in your class, but also covers topics that are not typically included in class. I hope that this anthology will inform you and also encourage you to ask additional questions about what you are reading.

New to this edition of *Annual Editions: Abnormal Psychology* are *World Wide Web* sites that can be used to further explore the topics. These sites are cross-referenced by number in the *topic guide.*

As the title *Annual Editions* indicates, this book will undergo continual review and revision. Thus, we welcome and encourage your comments and suggestions for future editions of *Annual Editions: Abnormal Psychology.* Please fill out and return the postage-paid article rating form at the end of this book.

Joseph J. Palladino
Editor

Contents

UNIT 1

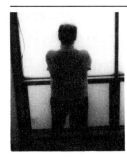

Perspectives on the Causes and Diagnosis of Abnormal Behavior

Six articles discuss how abnormal behavior is defined and diagnosed.

The concepts in bold italics are developed in the article. For further expansion please refer to the Topic Guide and the Index.

UNIT 2

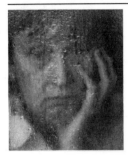

Anxiety Disorders, Mood Disorders, and Suicide

Eight selections examine how trauma, obsessive-compulsive emotions, and feelings of panic impact on the physical and psychological well-being of an individual.

The concepts in bold italics are developed in the article. For further expansion please refer to the Topic Guide and the Index.

UNIT 3

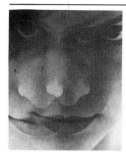

Schizophrenia

Six articles look at various aspects of the common psychological disorder of schizophrenia.

The concepts in bold italics are developed in the article. For further expansion please refer to the Topic Guide and the Index.

UNIT 4

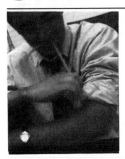

Drug/Alcohol Abuse and Violence

Five selections examine the extent to which drug and alcohol usage can contribute to the psychological imbalance of an individual.

UNIT 5

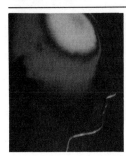

Dissociative Disorders and Memory

Five selections discuss repression and forms of mental abuse that can contribute to psychological disorders.

UNIT 6

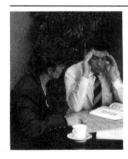

Physical Symptoms

Four articles examine the extent to which stress, anger, and ambition impact on the psychological health of an individual.

The concepts in bold italics are developed in the article. For further expansion please refer to the Topic Guide and the Index.

UNIT 7

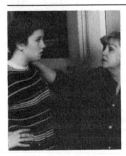

Therapy: Psychological Approaches

Five selections discuss psychological therapy as an approach to correcting abnormal disorders.

UNIT 8

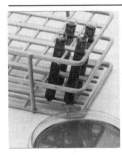

Biological Therapies

The five articles in this section examine the effects of biological therapies to correct mental disorders.

The concepts in bold italics are developed in the article. For further expansion please refer to the Topic Guide and the Index.

The concepts in bold italics are developed in the article. For further expansion please refer to the Topic Guide and the Index.

Topic Guide

This topic guide suggests how the selections in this book relate to topics of traditional concern to psychology students and professionals It is useful for locating interrelated articles for reading and research. The guide is arranged alphabetically according to topic. Articles may, of course, treat topics that do not appear in the topic guide. In turn, entries in the topic guide do not necessarily constitute a comprehensive listing of all the contents of each selection. **In addition, relevant Web sites, which are annotated on pages 4 and 5, are noted in bold italics under the topic articles.**

TOPIC AREA	TREATED IN	TOPIC AREA	TREATED IN
Addiction	23. Addicted *(16, 17, 18)*	**Depression**	4. Is Mental Illness Catching? 8. Making Sense of Mania and Depression 11. Dysthymic Disorder 12. Undate on Major Depression 14. Suicide—Part 1 31. Hearts and Minds—Part 1 39. Cognitive-Behavioral Therapy Today 43. Pharmacotherapy for the Treatment of Depression *(9, 13, 23)*
Alcohol	22. Health and Behavioral Consequences of Binge Drinking in College *(17, 18)*		
Alzheimer's Disease	30. Is It Normal Aging—or Alzheimer's? *(23)*		
Anorexia Nervosa	33. Dying to Win *(2, 4, 8)*	**Diagnosis**	3. Out of the Shadows *(2, 4, 5, 6, 8, 27)*
Antisocial Personality Disorder	25. Predators *(4, 5, 6)*	**Drug Abuse**	24. Fear of Heroin Is Shooting Up *(16, 17, 18, 31)*
Attention Deficit Hyperactivity Disorder	42. Mother's Little Helper *(7, 8)*	**Drug Treatment**	40. One Pill Makes You Larger, and One Pill Makes You Small 41. Prescriptions for Happiness? 42. Mother's Little Helper 43. Pharmacotherapy for the Treatment of Depression *(17, 18, 31)*
Behavioral Medicine	32. Behavioral Medicine, Clinical Health Psychology, and Cost Offset *(8, 25)*		
Biological Factors	1. Major Disorders of Mind and Brain 3. Out of the Shadows 4. Is Mental Illness Catching? 18. Release of the Mentally Ill from Institutions 19. Schizophrenia 20. Thalamic Abnormalities in Schizophrenia 23. Addicted *(3, 8, 16, 17)*	**Economic Costs**	32. Behavioral Medicine, Clinical Health Psychology, and Cost Offset *(1, 2, 3, 25, 26)*
		Effectiveness of Psychotherapy	35. Mental Health: Does Psychotherapy Help? 37. Patterns of Symptomatic Recovery in Psychotherapy *(2, 8, 23, 29, 32)*
Deinstitution-alization	18. Release of the Mentally Ill from Institutions *(5, 15)*	**Health Psychology**	32. Behavioral Medicine, Clinical Health Psychology, and Cost Offset *(1, 2, 3, 30, 32)*
		Insanity	6. Insanity Pleas Fail a Lot of Defendants as Fear of Crime Rises *(2, 4, 5)*

Selected World Wide Web Sites for
Annual Editions: Abnormal Psychology

All of these Web sites are hot-linked through the *Annual Editions* home page:
http://www.dushkin.com/annualeditions (just click on a book). In addition, these sites are referenced
by number and appear where relevant in the Topic Guide on the previous two pages.

Some Web sites are continually changing their structure and content, so the information listed may not always be available.

General Sources

1. Psychology Associations—*http://foyt.iupui.edu/subjectareas/ psychology/assoc.html*—This site is very useful for its links to journals, directors, handbooks, and manuals related to psychology and to some of the most prominent professional associations. These sites, in turn, provide a wealth of information in many different topics of interest to psychologists and psychiatrists.

2. Resources for Psychology and Cognitive Sciences—*http://www.ke. shinshu-u.ac.jp/psych/index.html*—This frequently updated site of resources for psychology and cognitive science on the Internet provides many links of value. There are directories of college and university psychology-related committees and departments, news, lists of conferences, online library information, electronic journals, and more.

3. National Institutes of Health (NIH)—*http://www.nih.gov/*—Consult this site for links to extensive health information and scientific resources. Comprised of 24 separate institutes, centers, and divisions—including the Institute of Mental Health—the NIH is one of eight health agencies of the Public Health Service, which, in turn, is part of the U.S. Department of Health and Human Services.

Perspectives on the Causes and Diagnosis of Abnormal Behavior

4. AACAP Facts for Families—*http://www.aacap.org/web/aacap/ factsFam/*—This American Academy of Child & Adolescent Psychiatry site, which focuses on psychiatric disorders in children and adolescents, addresses such issues as possible connections between mental disorders and violence.

5. Relationship Between Schizophrenics, Crime, and Rehospitalization—*http://academic.uofs.edu/student/jam1/post.html*—This site of a research abstract by a University of Scranton student also lists some articles and reports that will be of interest to others who are researching possible relationships between psychiatric disorders and violent crime.

6. David Willshire's Forensic Psychology & Psychiatry Links—*http:// www.ozemail.com.au/~dwillsh/*—This site offers an enormous number of links to professional journals and associations. It is a valuable resource for study into possible connections between violence and mental disorders. Topics include serial killers, sex offending, and trauma.

7. National Attention Deficit Disorder Information—*http://www.add. org/*—This site of the NADD association, some of which is under construction, will lead you to information about ADD/ADHD. It has links to self-help and support groups, outlines behaviors and diagnostics, answers FAQs, and suggests books and other resources.

8. The National Academy for Child Development Home Page—*http://www.nacd.org/*—The NACD, an international organization, is dedicated to helping children and adults reach their full potential. Its home page presents links to various programs, research, and resources into such topics as ADD.

Anxiety Disorders, Mood Disorders, and Suicide

9. Dr. Ivan's Depression Central—*http://www.psycom.net/depression. central.html*—This extensive site describes itself as the "Internet's central clearinghouse for information on all types of depressive disorders and on the most effective treatments" for these disorders—and it lives up to the billing. Students of psychology and psychiatry are likely to turn to this site and its numerous links again and again.

10. Obsessive-Compulsive Foundation—*http://pages.prodigy.com/ alwillen/ocf.html*—This OCF site on obsessive-compulsive disorder offers a forum for online discussion and learning about OCD. It provides a complete listing of U.S. and international OCD support groups. Related Web sites and areas of interest are also noted.

11. National Center for Research amd Education on Post-Traumatic Stress Disorder (PTSD)—*http://www.dartmouth.edu/dms/ptsd/*—Review the material available through this site provided by the National Center for PTSD, part of the U.S. Department of Veterans Affairs, to learn about research and education on Post-Traumatic Stress Disorder. An electronic index to the worldwide literature on traumatic stress is included.

12. Anxiety-Panic Internet Resource—*http://www.algy.com/anxiety/ panic.html*—This page provides information on the symptoms and causes of various anxiety and panic disorders. It provides links to many related articles and addresses psychopharmacology and other issues. The *DSM-IV* entry on Panic Disorders is reproduced.

13. Suicide and Suicide Prevention/Depression Central—*http://www. psycom.net/depression.central.suicide.html*—This site is part of Dr. Ivan's Depression Central but merits separate mention here because of its far-reaching links to sensitive information about suicide, insight into people who commit—or who may commit—suicide, and help for friends and families of people who have killed themselves.

Schizophrenia

14. Doctors Guide to Schizophrenia Information & Resources—*http:// www.pslgroup.com/SCHIZOPHR.HTM*—The material available through this page, "Schizophrenia Information and Resources," discusses such issues related to the understanding of schizophrenia as age of onset and gender. The site lists medical news and alerts and provides links to discussion groups and newsgroups.

15. National Mental Health Association—*http://www.nmha.org/index. html*—The NMHA is a citizen volunteer advocacy organization that works to improve the mental health of all individuals. Consult this site for information on institutionalization and deinstitutionalization.

Drug/Alcohol Abuse and Violence

16. Drug Dependence Research Center—*http://itsa.ucsf.edu/~ddrc/about.html*—The Drug Dependence Research Center at the University of California at San Francisco studies the pharmacology, physiology, and psychology of commonly abused drugs in humans. This site provides information on the DDRC's profile of medical marijuana users, its research into the cardiac effects of cocaine, and other topics.

17. Biological Components of Substance Abuse and Addiction—*http://www.norml.org/research/aa/aaota_cont.html*—National Organization for the Reform of Marijuana Laws (NORML), which works to legalize marijuana, offers this material about the biological components of substance abuse and addiction. It describes drug action, genetic factors that may be involved in substance abuse and addiction, and more.

18. National Institute on Drug Abuse—*http://165.112.78.61/*—Use this site index of the National Institute on Drug Abuse for NIDA publications and communications, information on drugs of abuse, and links to other related Web sites.

19. Simcoe County Mental Health Education—*http://www.mhcva.on.ca/mhcpen1.htm*—This site, which reproduces articles from the hospital newsletter *Entre Nous*, contains many items of interest in the study of abnormal psychology. People interested in information about psychopaths will find useful information here.

20. Crime Times—*http://www.crime-times.org/titles.htm*—This interesting site lists research reviews and other information regarding biological causes of criminal, violent, and psychopathic behavior. It consists of many articles, listed by title. It is provided by the nonprofit Wacker Foundation, publisher of *Crime Times*.

Dissociative Disorders and Memory

21. Memory, Repressed Memory, and False Memory—*http://wheel.ucdavis.edu/~btcarrol/skeptic/memory.html*—Access this University of California at Davis site to consult *The Skeptic's Dictionary* and to read material about memory, repressed memory, and false memory. It asks, "How accurate and reliable is memory?"

22. Ottawa Recovered Memory Page—*http://www.carleton.ca/~whovdest/and.s.macdonald.ormp.html*—This page provides links to articles about recovered memories of childhood abuse and the recovered memory debate. Summaries of articles and books are included, as well as useful bibliographies.

23. Mental Health Net: Disorders and Treatment Index—*http://www.cmhc.com/selfhelp.htm*—This site and its many links are geared to providing information on mental disorders, with an emphasis on self-help. Aging and Alzheimer's and many other topics, from cancer to depression, are described here.

24. GROHOL Mental Health Page: Dissociative Identity Disorder—*http://www.unc.edu/~juliette/did.html*—Consult this site for links to articles, quizzes, and other information about and perspectives on dissociative disorders and repressed or false memories. Causes, social perceptions, and treatments are among the topics addressed.

Physical Symptoms

25. Behavioral Medicine Resources—*http://socbehmed.org/sbm/sisterorg.htm*—This site of the Society of Behavioral Medicine provides listings of major, general health institutes and organizations as well as discipline-specific links and resources in medicine, psychology, nursing, and public health.

26. Internet Mental Health—*http://www.mentalhealth.com/p13.html*—This huge site announces that it "lists only those English-language Web sites providing more than 10 pages of free, scientifically sound mental health information." It has everything from links to information about anxiety, mood, and sleep disorders to information about journals and associations.

Therapy: Psychological Approaches

27. The American Psychoanalytic Association—*http://apsa.org/*—The home page of this professional organization of psychoanalysts presents links that provide information about psychoanalysis in general, a literature search, meeting dates and places, and partial access to *The American Psychoanalyst*.

28. Online Dictionary of Mental Health—*http://www.shef.ac.uk/~psysc/psychotherapy/*—This site gives you access to *The Online Dictionary of Mental Health*, described here as "a global information resource and research tool" covering all of the disciplines contributing to an understanding of mental health. The site provides information about psychotherapy.

29. American Journal of Psychotherapy—*http://www.ajp.org/*—The *AJP* is "devoted to the advancement of psychotherapy and to the continuation of discussions, scientific writings, clinical impressions, and articles of special interest to psychotherapists." Find articles here as well as Web links to other useful sites.

Biological Therapies

30. U.S. National Library of Medicine (NLM)—*http://www.nlm.nih.gov/*—This huge site permits you to search a number of databases and electronic information sources such as MEDLINE, learn about research projects and programs, keep up on recent medical news, and peruse the national network of medical libraries.

31. Dr. Bob's Psychopharmacology Tips—*http://uhs.bsd.uchicago.edu/~bhsiung/tips/tips.html*—Open this site to gain access to a wide variety of information related to psychopharmacology, with its links to specific drug sites and to specific disorders.

32. Clinical Psychology Resources—*http://www.psychologie.uni-bonn.de/kap/links_20.htm*—This page from Germany's University of Bonn Department of Clinical and Applied Psychology contains Web resources for clinical and abnormal psychology, behavioral medicine, and mental health. There are links to journals, organizations, psychotherapy topics, and discussions of specific disorders.

We highly recommend that you review our Web site for expanded information and our other product lines. We are continually updating and adding links to our Web site in order to offer you the most usable and useful information that will support and expand the value of your Annual Editions. You can reach us at: *http://www. dushkin.com/annualeditions/.*

Perspectives on the Causes and Diagnosis of Abnormal Behavior

The field of abnormal psychology changes quite rapidly; the pace of new information makes it difficult to keep track of the changes. However, concerns about two major issues seem to have been constant: diagnosis and etiology. How do we recognize abnormal behavior? When we recognize it, what should we call it? What are the possible causes of the abnormalities that we identify? The answers to these questions influence how we try to alleviate the symptoms of a disorder. Those answers can also determine whether or not an individual's freedom is denied, as when someone suffering from a mental disorder is involuntarily committed to an institution. Some of us can remember, for example, how such decisions were influenced by political considerations in the former Soviet Union. Because there are no clear-cut guidelines for differentiating normal from abnormal behaviors, it will always be a matter for debate and controversy.

The public exhibits a widespread fear of individuals who suffer with mental disorders. These individuals are viewed as violence-prone. The media play a significant role in spreading this fear; the typical media report about former mental patients involves murder. Are individuals who are diagnosed with serious mental disorders more likely to be arrested? This question is difficult to answer because it requires a longitudinal design, which is costly and time-consuming. Researchers would have to identify individuals who have a diagnosis of mental illness and then determine at a later time whether they had been arrested. The result of this kind of research has implications for the ways in which we deal with individuals diagnosed with serious disorders.

There is growing interest in biological causes of mental disorders. Researchers are finding that heredity has a much stronger role to play in several disorders than previously thought. For example, schizophrenia and manic-depressive illness (bipolar disorder) appear to be related to both structural and biochemical changes that may have a genetic basis. Although the search continues, the specific genes responsible for these disorders have not yet been located. Some experts believe that those genes may be located before the turn of the century.

Researchers are also focusing on other potential biological factors that may be responsible for several mental disorders; among these factors are infections. The focus on biological factors has led some observers to suggest that what may be termed "normal craziness" may be the result of biological factors. Various difficulties in interpersonal behaviors or unusual but not incapacitating symptoms may be mild cases of full-blown disorders that have a common biological origin. At the same time, researchers are focusing on personality variables that may make some of us more likely to develop psychological disorders. Personality variables that can make us vulnerable may have a genetic basis, whereas other characteristics that increase our vulnerability result from interpersonal and cognitive influences.

Insanity is one of most controversial issues related to psychological disorders; it is also one of the most difficult issues for the general public to understand. Although insanity is a legal decision—rendered by a judge or a jury—mental health professionals typically offer their opinions in court. Following John Hinckley's attempted assassination of President Ronald Reagan and the jury's judgment that he was "not guilty by reason of insanity," most states revised their insanity laws. The toughening of laws governing insanity pleas continues today, and most defendants find it increasingly difficult to be judged "not guilty by reason of insanity."

Looking Ahead: Challenge Questions

How do cultural factors affect the determination of what is normal and what is abnormal?

How might the media help to educate the public concerning the actual risk of violent behavior among individuals with mental disorders?

How might the focus on biological factors in mental disorders affect efforts to reduce the incidence of certain disorders?

How might personality variables influence the probability that someone might develop a mental disorder? Discuss whether or not these personality variables can be altered to reduce their influence on mental disorders.

UNIT 1

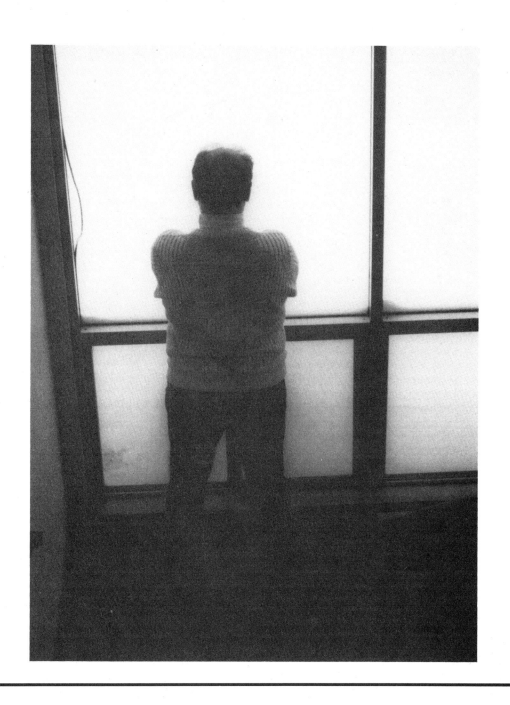

Major Disorders of Mind and Brain

Schizophrenia and manic-depressive illness are shaped by heredity and marked by structural and biochemical changes in the brain. The predisposing genes remain unknown

Elliot S. Gershon and Ronald O. Rieder

Elliott S. Gershon and Ronald O. Rieder began collaborating on the study of mental illness at the Intramural Research Program of the National Institute of Mental Health. Gershon heads the program's Clinical Neurogenetics Branch and specializes in the population genetics and molecular genetics of normal and abnormal behavior. He graduated from Harvard Medical School in 1965, trained in psychiatry at the Massachusetts Mental Health Center and moved to the NIMH in 1969. Rieder graduated from Harvard Medical School in 1968 and trained in psychiatry at Albert Einstein College of Medicine. At the NIMH he conducted research on schizophrenia. Now he directs research and psychiatric residency training at Columbia University.

Madness was understood for centuries by religion and poetry as an affliction of the spirit and by medicine as a disorder of various humors and organs of the body. In the past century, physicians have recognized the most common forms of psychosis (our current word for madness) as two chronic disorders—schizophrenia and mania—and have begun to understand the abnormalities in brain structure and function that accompany them. Each affects about 1 percent of the population. Both flare episodically, although schizophrenia follows a deteriorating course, whereas patients with bipolar manic-depressive illness, who have episodes of mania and depression, are usually mentally normal between episodes.

The anatomic, biochemical and hereditary bases of these disorders are now emerging. Some research has already shaped the development of new treatments. These subject form the focus of our article. First, however, it is useful to consider what these disorders are like for the people who have them.

When Mrs. T. was 16 years old, she began to experience her first symptom of schizophrenia: a profound feeling that people were staring at her. These bouts of self-consciousness soon forced her to end her public piano performances. Her self-consciousness led to withdrawal, then to fearful delusions that others were speaking of her and finally to suspicions that they were plotting to harm her. At first Mrs. T.'s illness was intermittent, and the return of her intelligence, warmth and ambition between episodes allowed her to complete several years of college, to marry and to rear three children. She had to enter a hospital for the first time at 28, after the birth of her third child, when she began to hallucinate.

Now, at 45, Mrs. T. is never entirely well. She has seen dinosaurs on the street and live animals in her refrigerator. While hallucinating, she speaks and writes in an incoherent, but almost poetic, way. At other times, she is more lucid, but even then her voices sometimes lead her to do dangerous things, such as driving very fast down the highway in the middle of the night, dressed only in a nightgown. As an episode winds down, Mrs. T. usually becomes deeply depressed and hopeless about her condition. Often she sits in her car with the engine running and contemplates committing suicide.

Over the past five years she has taken antipsychotic medications, such as haloperidol, that suppress the hallucinations and help her stay out of the hospital. Stress, however, can bring the hallucinations and delusions back for days or weeks, as happened after her recent separation from her husband and the subsequent sale of her home. At such times, her voices shout terrible criticisms. After her daughter left for college, they shouted, "You'll never see her again, you have been a bad mother, she'll die." At other times and without any apparent stimulus, Mrs. T. has bizarre visual hallucinations. For example, she saw cherubs in the grocery store. These experiences leave her preoccupied, confused and frightened, unable to perform such everyday tasks as cooking or playing the piano. When feeling well, however, she does volunteer work at church.

The mood disorders, which are distinct from schizophrenia, are called unipolar when the patient has episodes of depression alone and bipolar when there are episodes of both mania and depression. (The term "manic-depressive ill-

Reprinted with permission from *Scientific American*, September 1992, pp. 127-133. © 1992 by Scientific American, Inc. All rights reserved.

ness" encompasses both the unipolar and the bipolar form; the term "bipolar" is also used for the rare cases in which mania occurs without depression.) The depressions are quite severe, and suicide is an all too frequent outcome. Mania, a state of excitement usually characterized by impulsive behavior, can, when untreated, ultimately ruin marriages, careers and fortunes.

Mania can develop suddenly and shockingly, as illustrated in a case cited by a group led by Robert L. Spitzer of Columbia University. Daryl, a 25-year-old dancer, was cast in a part for a Broadway show. He began to come home at the end of rehearsal making disparaging remarks about the sessions and the director. A week later a fellow performer called Daryl's wife to complain that her husband had been trying to take over the rehearsals, giving unsolicited advice to the director and the other performers. At this point, his wife realized that Daryl's usually easygoing demeanor has turned tense and irritable. He began making nasty comments about his wife's figure and their recent sex life. Three days later he began shouting obscenities at other performers and was ejected from the theater. At home, he talked "a mile a minute" and paced incessantly, dressed only in his underwear. He felt no need to eat or sleep. The next day he skipped work to make a number of extravagant purchases.

At this time, two weeks after he had displayed his first symptoms, Daryl accepted hospitalization. He received one dose of a tranquilizer yet spent most of the night disrupting the ward. Then he signed out, against medical advice, in the morning. Eventually he responded well to lithium carbonate. Daryl's father has had a similar but more prolonged history, losing many jobs over 20 years after episodes of excited confrontations with his bosses. Over the past five years, however, he too has responded well to lithium.

Although schizophrenia and manic-depression can devastate patients' lives, the disorders do not preclude the performance of highly creative work. Schizophrenic patients confined in institutions have occasionally produced extraordinary works of graphic art. Manic-depressive illness often occurs in conjunction with extraordinary talent, even genius, in politics and military leadership, as well as in literature and music and the other performing arts. Among those thought to have had the disorder are William Blake, Lord Byron, Virginia Woolf, Robert Schumann, Oliver Cromwell and Winston Churchill. Many observers have suggested that extremes of mood and changes in outlook may spur creativity; they also speculate that the energy and facility of thought that typify the milder stages of mania can be a source of creativity.

Even though schizophrenia and severe mood disorders manifest themselves as intangible mental experiences, they are biologically determined to a major degree. (Only a few of the biological discoveries can be discussed in this brief article.) The first evidence of determinants came early in this century, when genetic studies showed that both schizophrenia and manic-depressive illness ran in families. Most workers discounted these correlations, however, on the grounds that families share environment as well as genes. To consider the two factors in isolation, researchers turned to adoptees, who, once adopted, have environmental families that are different from their genetic families.

In the best-known study, begun in the 1960s, Seymour S. Kety and his colleagues at the National Institute of Mental Health and at a psychological institute in Scandinavia identified schizophrenics adopted in infancy and traced their biological relatives through the adoption register. The study indicated that biological relatives had an increased risk of developing the illnesses but adoptive relatives did not. The control group—biological relatives of nonpsychotic adoptees—faced no excess risk of schizophrenia or of any mental illness resembling it.

Twin studies are also revealing because different types of twins vary widely in their genetic relatedness. When schizophrenia or bipolar disease develops in one twin, the chance that it will develop in the other is much greater in identical twins, who share all their genes, than in fraternal twins, who share only about half. Moreover, although about half of the identical twins of schizophrenics never develop the illness, the children of even the well twins are at increased risk. These correlations imply two things. The risk of illness rises with increasing genetic similarity, but even a perfect identity of genes does not produce a perfect correspondence. Some environmental factor, or interaction of genes with the environment, must therefore push susceptible people over the threshold of illness. Studies have already implicated one possible factor: prenatal exposure to the influenza virus.

Mood disorders also stem from the interaction of genes with some aspect of the environment. Rates of major depression in every age group have steadily increased in several of the developed countries since the 1940s. This trend was first spotted some 10 years ago in an epidemiological study in Sweden. A similar increase in suicide over the same four decades occurred in Alberta, Canada. These findings have been firmly established as birth-cohort effects: suicide rates among 15- to 19-year-olds, for instance, were 10 times higher for those born in the late 1950s than for those born in the early 1930s. Similar birth-cohort increases appeared, over these decades, in suicide and unipolar disorder in the U.S., in bipolar disorder in the U.S. and Switzerland, and in alcoholism in males in the U.S. [see *illustration on page 11*].

Rates of depression, mania and suicide continue to rise as each new birth cohort ages, a pattern that harbors ominous public health consequences. Such birth-cohort effects are even more pronounced in the relatives of patients than in the general population—in other words, at comparable ages, the children of patients are far more susceptible to these disorders than are their ill parents' siblings. This relation clearly implies an interaction between genes and some environmental factor, which must have been changing continuously over the past few decades. The factor remains a mystery.

The biological abnormalities that genes and environment somehow put into motion were quite mysterious until the 1970s, when new imaging technologies allowed physicians to visualize the living brain in great detail.

One imaging technique, computerized tomography (CT scanning), was first applied to the brains of schizophrenic patients in 1978 by Eve C. Johnstone and her colleagues at the Clinical Research Centre in Middlesex, England. They observed that the lateral cerebral ventricles were much larger than in normal subjects. If the ventricles or the spaces between convolutions are enlarged, one can conclude there has been a failure of development or a loss of brain tissue. Other x-ray evidence confirmed this conclusion by showing less tissue and more fluid-filled spaces around the convolutions in the cerebral cortex.

Another technique, magnetic resonance imaging (MRI), confirmed the ventricular enlargement. Daniel R. Weinberger's group at the National Institute of Mental Health used MRI to compare identical twins in which one twin had schizophrenia and the other did not. In 12 of 15 sets of such twins, the schizophrenic one had the larger cerebral ventricles. Relative diminution of specific brain structures has been demonstrated, too, in autop-

Medicines for Mental Disorders

Drugs may act on several points in the synapse. Antidepressants that affect the presynaptic cell include those that block the cell's reuptake of monoamines (a). These drugs include tricyclic antidepressants, such as imipramine, which block reuptake of several monoamines, and more specific blockers, such as fluoxetine, for serotonin, and buproprion, for dopamine. Other antidepressants known as monoamine oxidase inhibitors (b) prevent the presynaptic cell from metabolizing monoamines. Drugs that affect the postsynaptic cell include agents that either block monoamine receptors or stimulate their ability to respond (c). Haloperidol, an antipsychotic, is a dopamine receptor blocker. Finally, some drugs affect the second messenger (d) that is normally produced after a receptor has been activated. For example, lithium carbonate, an antidepressant and antimanic agent, works by inhibiting the synthesis of phosphatidyl inositol. Here a postsynaptic receptor is shown coupled to a stimulatory G protein; this is its activated state, which causes more second-messenger chemicals to be synthesized, triggering molecular cascades that determine how the postsynaptic cell will respond.

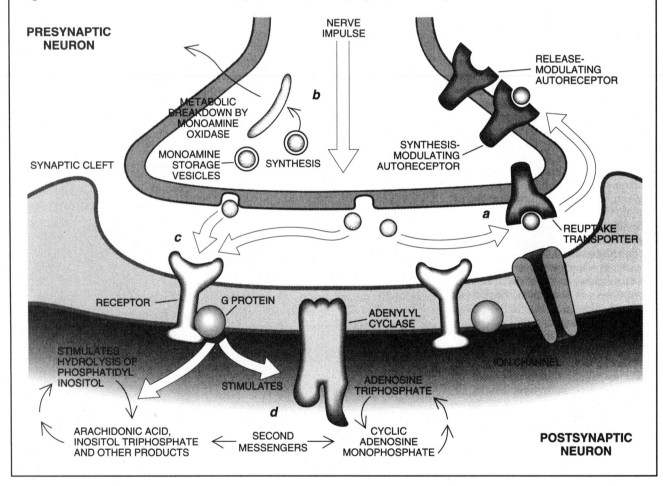

sies and by MRI scans of schizophrenic patients. The most striking examples of such diminution appear in the hippocampal region, part of the limbic system in the temporal lobe of the cerebrum, which modulates emotional response, memory and other functions.

The new imaging devices also showed functional abnormalities for the first time. In 1974 David H. Ingvar of University Hospital in Lund, Sweden, found reduced blood flow in the frontal cerebrum of schizophrenic patients, imply-ing decreased neuronal activity there. This finding has since been corroborated many times.

Weinberger's group presents evidence linking both structural and functional abnormalities in the brain to a schizophrenic cognitive trait. They found that normal subjects show increased blood flow in the prefrontal cerebral cortex while taking the Wisconsin Card Sort, a test of working memory and abstract thinking, whereas schizophrenic subjects show less of an increase in flow and do worse on the test. Moreover, those schizophrenic patients whose hippocampal structures are the smallest show the greatest deficit in prefrontal blood flow. The hippocampus connects to the prefrontal cortex, which manages working memory in primates [see "Working Memory and the Mind," by Patricia S. Goldman-Rakic, SCIENTIFIC AMERICAN, September 1992.]

Postmortem studies of schizophrenic patients have also uncovered abnormalities in the number of brain cells and in their organization, particularly in the temporal lobe. Yet the tissue shows none of the scarring one would expect from an infection, nor do the abnormalities progress over time. Some researchers therefore speculate that the abnormalities stem from a developmental disorder, perhaps a failure of the growth of neurons and the development of their connections, or from a disturbance in the "pruning" of neurons that normally occurs between the ages of three and 15 [see "The Developing Brain," by Carla J. Shatz, SCIENTIFIC AMERICAN, September 1992.]

How might such abnormalities cause the symptoms of schizophrenia? While conducting surgery on nonschizophrenic patients, Wilder G. Penfield of the Montreal Neurological Institute discovered that certain structures in the brain are related to hallucinations. (Such patients are often kept awake so that they can help ascertain the functions of brain tissues near the field in which the surgeon is operating.) Penfield found that when he touched his diagnostic electrode to the temporal lobe he often elicited in his patients sights and sounds resembling hallucinations.

Further research showed that the frontal parts of the temporal cortex receive highly processed and filtered sensory information from other parts of the cortex. That information eventually reaches the limbic system and other structures that mediate emotional response, or affect. Perhaps, then, some overactivation of the temporal cortex or abnormalities in the filtering process produce the common experiences of schizophrenic patients: auditory hallucinations and a sense of being overwhelmed by all the senses.

The first effective medications for schizophrenia and depression were discovered serendipitously, without any knowledge of their effects on brain chemistry. Chlorpromazine was developed in the 1950s as a surgical anesthetic but turned out to alleviate the symptoms of both schizophrenia and mania. It thus became the first widely used antipsychotic drug. Scientists then used it as a model for the synthesis of imipramine, which they expected would also serve as an antipsychotic agent. Instead it turned out to be very effective in the treatment of depression. Lithium was introduced into the treatment of manic-depressive illness after John Cade, an Australian psychiatrist, noted in 1949 that lithium salts sedated rodents in his laboratory.

Insight into the way antidepressant agents act began with the study of reserpine, a drug derived from the plant *Rau-wolfia serpentina*, used in traditional medicine in India. Reserpine was one of the first effective medications for high blood pressure. Physicians noted, however, that the drug sometimes brought on severe depression in patients—a few even committed suicide.

Biochemists discovered that reserpine depletes certain neurotransmitters classed as monoamines, among them norepinephrine, dopamine and serotonin. All the antidepressant drugs known in the mid-1960s effectively concentrated these monoamines in the synapse, either by inhibiting their metabolic breakdown or by preventing cells from reabsorbing them from the synaptic space (a process known as reuptake).

This pattern led Joseph J. Schildkraut, then at the National Institute of Mental Health, to propose in 1965 that depression was associated with a reduction in synaptic availability of catecholamines (norepinephrine and dopamine), particularly dopamine, and mania with an increase of catecholamines. Nevertheless, there are antidepressant drugs, such as iprindole, that are associated with no observable change in norepinephrine reuptake or metabolism.

Biochemical pharmacologists therefore looked beyond the neurotransmitters to the synaptic receptor molecules that bind with them. The workers knew that norepinephrine has several pharmacologically distinct receptors, called adrenoceptors, but their experiments in binding various antidepressant drugs to the receptors produced no consistent change.

Then, in 1975, Fridolin Sulser's laboratory at Vanderbilt University found an answer by looking not at binding itself but at the intracellular response that one type of binding elicits. They studied how norepinephrine stimulates beta-receptors, a class of adrenoceptors that mediates the release of cyclic adenosine monophosphate inside the nerve cell. This molecule then serves as a second chemical messenger. But after long-term administration of certain antidepressants, including iprindole, this secondary response consistently decreases. Virtually all antidepressants, including those discovered after the finding was published, produce this result. So does electroconvulsive therapy, a very effective treatment for depression in which shocks are administered to the cerebrum to induce artificial seizures.

A number of receptors for each of the monoamines exist, and new receptors continue to be discovered. With each discovery, workers learn more about how antidepressants alter these receptors and their second-messenger systems. It turns out that many, but not all, antidepressants produce dysregulations in other receptors, including postsynaptic and presynaptic adrenoceptors and certain subclasses of the dopamine and serotonin receptors.

These multiple actions of therapeutic drugs suggest that many kinds of biological defects may play a part in manic-depressive illness. Possible defects in neurotransmission include abnormalities in receptors and related molecules; various components of the second-messenger pathways; various proteins that modulate ion transport and indirectly increase or decrease activity in second-messenger systems; and various G proteins, which couple to receptors and stimulate or inhibit intracellular second

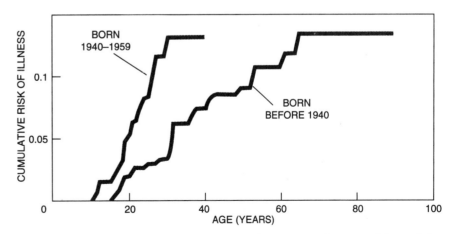

ALARMING GENERATIONAL TREND suggests that some environmental factor is increasing the incidence of mood disorders in people who are genetically susceptible to it. These graphs compare two groups of relatives of bipolar patients—one born before 1940, the other born later. At each age at which a comparison is possible, the later cohort is at far higher risk of developing bipolar illness or related psychosis.

messengers [see "G Proteins," by Maurine E. Linder and Alfred G. Gilman; SCIENTIFIC AMERICAN, July 1992. So far, however, no one has found direct evidence of any such molecular abnormality in patients.]

Episodes of illness gradually become more frequent and more severe in many manic-depressive patients. This pattern of deterioration suggested to Robert M. Post of the National Institute of Mental Health an analogy with an experimental process known as kindling. Scientists kindle convulsions in rodents by stimulating the animals' brains with electricity to induce seizures. Each repetition of the experiment lowers the electrical threshold for the next seizure, leading finally to spontaneous seizures.

Post proposed that manic-depressive illness progresses in a similar fashion, each episode facilitating the next one. This mechanism would account for both the progression of the illness and the deleterious effects of interrupting treatment with lithium or anticonvulsant medication. After such an interruption, patients may fail to respond to a resumption of the medication, even if it had been effective earlier.

One can also infer aspects of the biology of schizophrenia from the biochemical action of the therapeutic neuroleptic drugs, which include chlorpromazine. Arvid Carlsson of the University of Göteborg sought to explain why these drugs cause animals to produce increased quantities of breakdown products of dopamine. He suggested the effect was a compensatory response of the presynaptic neuron to a postsynaptic blockade [see illustration on page 10].

As the different molecular and pharmacologic forms of dopamine receptors became known, the D$_2$ dopamine receptor emerged as the principal site of action of antipsychotic medications. Some of the drugs seem to work by means of interactions with other neuro-

BRAIN STRESS SYSTEM extends from the hindbrain and hypothalamus to cerebral destinations inside and outside the limbic system (A). It includes neurons containing norepinephrine (B), CRH (C) and dopamine (D). When activated, the system affects mood, thought and, indirectly, the secretion of cortisol by the adrenal glands. Deactivation normally begins when cortisol binds to hypothalamic receptors. But in depression this shutdown fails, producing chronic activation.

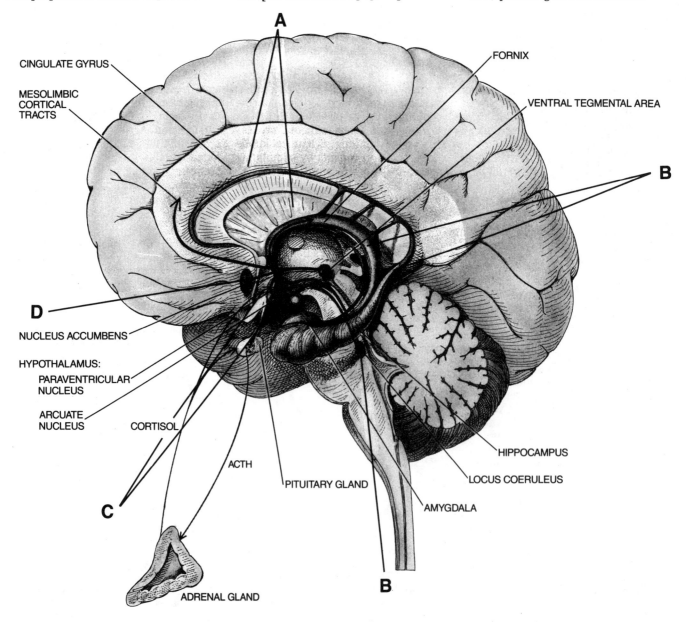

transmitter systems: among these interactions are the balance between the neural pathways containing the D_1 and the D_2 dopamine receptors and the balance between pathways containing certain serotonin receptors ($5HT_2$) and the D_2 dopamine receptors.

Maria and Arvid Carlsson recently proposed that schizophrenia is characterized by the disruption of a balance between dopamine neurons originating in the midbrain and glutamate neurons originating in the cerebral cortex. The imbalance could be an excess of dopamine or a deficit of glutamate, or both. A reduction in glutamate neurons would be consistent with the apparent cortical atrophy seen in schizophrenia. This theory fits with the effects of known psychosis-producing drugs of abuse: PCP, a hallucinogen, blocks glutamate receptors, whereas amphetamine, which can produce psychosis with chronic use, stimulates dopamine release.

Studies of the biochemical action of these drugs and related clinical research have brought us to an era of rationally based design of medications. Once neuropharmacologists understood that chlorpromazine works by blocking dopamine receptors, they were able to synthesize haloperidol, which strongly blocks dopamine receptors but has little effect on other receptors. Similarly, after scientists found that the antidepressant imipramine blocks reuptake of the neurotransmitter serotonin, they were able to design fluoxetine, which specifically blocks serotonin reuptake but has very little effect on the reuptake of other monoamines.

Pharmacology and neurobiology continue to feed off each other. Over the past few years, clinical trials have shown that clozapine helps about 30 percent of those schizophrenic patients who do not respond to other antipsychotic medications or who develop intolerable side effects. This drug's unusual properties, such as its specific interaction with certain dopamine and serotonin receptors (D_4 and $5HT_2$), may help in the effort to understand schizophrenia itself.

Depression turns out to involve hormonal systems of a much wider scope than had been realized. Cortisol, a hormone secreted by the adrenal glands, constitutes the main circulating steroid associated with stress in humans. Many severely depressed patients show persistently elevated blood cortisol, implying a malfunction in the system that normally governs it.

George P. Chrousos of the National Institute of Child Health and Development and Philip W. Gold of the National Institute of Mental Health interpret this failure as the result of a prolonged activation of the brain's stress system. This system—a complex of neuronal, hormonal and immunologic responses—comes into play when some stress provokes the brain, causing its hypothalamic centers to secrete corticotropin-releasing hormone (CRH). This factor in turn stimulates the pituitary gland—just under the brain—to produce the hormone adrenocorticotropin, which circulates to the adrenal glands and stimulates their release of cortisol. This process normally turns itself off when the excess cortisol reaches its receptors (glucocorticoid receptors) in the brain and suppresses CRH production there. In depressed patients, however, Gold found that production of CRH is excessive and that this suppression fails.

The CRH-producing neurons of the hypothalamus are principally regulated by neurons containing norepinephrine, which originate in the hindbrain. These CRH and norepinephrine neurons serve the stress system as central stations. Each set of neurons stimulates the other. In addition, each responds similarly to many neurotransmitters and peptide modulators of neurotransmission. Because many antidepressant drugs affect these neurotransmitters, they must also influence the regulation of the stress system.

The stress system of the brain sets the level of arousal and the emotional tone, alters the ease with which various kinds of information can be retrieved and analyzed, and aids in the initiation of specific actions. All these functions are disordered in depressed patients, and as a result they become sad, have trouble concentrating and become incapable of making decisions.

The anatomy of the stress system starts with the locus coeruleus in the hindbrain (the major source of norepinephrine-producing neurons) and the paraventricular nucleus of the hypothalamus (the brain's major CRH-producing region). From there the connections reach into the cerebrum; these connections include dopamine-producing neurons that project into the mesolimbic dopamine tract, which helps to control motivation, reward and reinforcement. A connection of CRH neurons to the amygdala and hippocampus is important for memory retrieval and emotional analysis of information pertinent to the environmental events that induced the stress.

The general concepts of stress system dysregulation apply to many psychiatric and other diseases, and it will require a considerable amount of basic and clinical research to determine whether a causal relation exists between mood disorders and this kind of stress response dysregulation.

Molecular genetics can test hypotheses on the biology of these diseases because the predisposition to them is almost certainly inherited. The task is made difficult, however, by the complexity of inheritance in schizophrenia and manic-depression. Neither illness is inherited through one dominant or recessive gene. Analysts must take into account that illness might result from coordinated actions of several genes at several different locations (loci) or, alternatively, from genetic heterogeneity (in which the same illness can be caused by a mutation at any one of several loci).

There are two major strategies for finding pathogenic genes. One can systematically search each chromosome, or one can investigate a candidate gene—such as that for a given receptor—which is known to code for proteins related to the disease.

DNA markers now exist for nearly every segment of every chromosome. In any family, each parent contributes to the child a single segment from either one or the other chromosome in a given pair of chromosomes. The illness is linked to a marker location on the genetic map if, and only if, one ancestral chromosome segment is consistently inherited with illness throughout a pedigree. Whenever there is a linkage to the marker, one can be sure that a gene for the illness resides somewhere on that chromosome segment.

Such mapping has consistently shown that a proportion of the families of Alzheimer's patients have illness linked to markers on the long arm of chromosome 21. No such linkages have been demonstrated conclusively for manic-depressive illness or schizophrenia. One widely publicized study of a large Amish pedigree linked manic-depressive illness to markers on chromosome 11; another study of a series of pedigrees in Iceland and England linked schizophrenia to markers on chromosome 5. But later analyses led the investigators to withdraw their conclusions, and no other researchers have confirmed the findings.

Linkage to manic-depressive illness has been reported more than once at the tip of the long arm of the X chromosome, but the linkage remains controversial. One can expect more definitive results from several large-scale international efforts, now under way, to scan the entire gene map of families touched by either schizophrenia or manic-depressive illness.

Many genes encoding the molecules involved in neurotransmission are candidates for the defects underlying manic-depressive illness or schizophrenia. A study of several such candidates for manic-depressive illness was performed on a series of 20 pedigrees at the National Institute of Mental Health by Margret R. Hoehe, Sevilla D. Detera-Wadleigh, Wade H. Berrettini, Pablo V. Gejman and one of us (Gershon). The group tested structural genes for many of the receptors we have described, including norepinephrine (three alpha-receptor genes and two beta-receptor genes), dopamine (D_2 and D_4) and corticosteroid receptors, and the gene of a G protein subunit ($G_{s\alpha}$). Other investigators have studied the D_2 dopamine receptor in schizophrenia pedigrees. Linkage was strongly excluded for each of these genes.

When linkage of a candidate gene to illness can be ruled out, one can conclude that no mutation in the candidate gene determines inheritance of the susceptibility to the illness. The only qualification to this general rule is the statistical and technical limits on our power to detect or rule out linkage. Methods other than linkage can also scan for mutations in candidate genes, and many genes remain to be examined.

We expect our understanding of the biology of schizophrenia and mood disorders to expand dramatically, fueled by the impressive advances in neurobiology, cognitive neuroscience and genetics. Precise diagnostic tests for persons at risk for illness, treatments based on knowledge of molecular alterations that lead to illness, understanding of how environmental events interact with the brain to produce illness and, eventually, the development of gene therapy are all goals that may be achieved.

FURTHER READING

INTERACTIONS BETWEEN GLUTAMATERGIC AND MONOAMINERGIC SYSTEMS WITHIN THE BASAL GANGLIA—IMPLICATIONS FOR SCHIZOPHRENIA AND PARKINSON'S DISEASE. M. Carlsson and A. Carlsson in *Trends in Neurosciences,* Vol. 13, No. 7, pages 272–276; July 1990.

GENETIC MAPPING OF COMMON DISEASES: THE CHALLENGES OF MANIC-DEPRESSIVE ILLNESS AND SCHIZOPHRENIA. E. S. Gershon, M. Martinez, L. R. Goldin and P. V. Gejman in *Trends in Genetics,* Vol. 6, No. 9, pages 282–287; September 1990.

MANIC-DEPRESSIVE ILLNESS. Frederick K. Goodwin and Kay Redfield Jamison. Oxford University Press, 1990.

THE BIOCHEMICAL BASIS OF NEUROPHARMACOLOGY. Jack R. Cooper, Floyd E. Bloom and Robert H. Roth. Oxford University Press, 1991.

THE CONCEPTS OF STRESS AND STRESS SYSTEM DISORDERS: OVERVIEW OF PHYSICAL AND BEHAVIORAL HOMEOSTASIS. George P. Chrousos and Philip W. Gold in *Journal of the American Medical Association,* Vol. 267, No. 9, pages 1244–1252; March 4, 1992.

Does Psychiatric Disorder Predict Violent Crime Among Released Jail Detainees?

A Six-Year Longitudinal Study

Linda A. Teplin, Karen M. Abram, and Gary M. McClelland

The authors examined whether jail detainees with schizo-phrenia, major affective disorders, alcohol or drug use disorders, or psychotic symptoms (hallucinations and delusions) are arrested more often for violent crimes six years after release than detainees with no disorders. Trained interviewers assessed 728 randomly selected male jail detainees using the National Institute of Mental Health Diagnostic Interview Schedule and then obtained follow-up arrest data for six years. Neither severe mental disorder nor substance abuse or dependence predicted the probability of arrest or the number of arrests for violent crime. Persons with symptoms of both hallucinations and delusions had a slightly higher number of arrests for violent crime, but not significantly so. These findings held even after controlling for prior violence and age. The findings do not support the stereotype that mentally ill criminals invariably commit violent crimes after they are released. Future directions for research are suggested.

There is a long-standing stereotype that persons with mental illnesses are prone to violence (Monahan, 1992; Steadman & Cocozza, 1978), an image reinforced by the news and entertainment media (Gerbner, Gross, Morgan, & Signorielli, 1981; Mayer & Barry, 1992; Wahl, 1992). Empirical research, however, provides less than definitive support for this stereotype. Some studies have found a relationship between mental disorder and violence (Lindquist & Allebeck, 1990; Schuerman & Kobrin, 1984; Sosowsky, 1978, 1980; Swanson, 1994; Swanson, Holzer, Ganju, & Jono, 1990). Others have found that, after controlling for demographic variables, the relationship disappears (Steadman, Cocozza, & Melick, 1978; Steadman & Ribner, 1980; Teplin, 1985). Even studies that found an association, however, concluded that mental disorder is a relatively small risk factor for violence (Link, Andrews, & Cullen, 1992; Monahan, 1992; Swanson et al., 1990) and that mentally ill persons do not pose a high risk in "absolute terms" (Swanson, 1994).

Yet, the stereotype persists. Perhaps the most feared group is mentally ill persons charged with or convicted of crimes (Shah, 1990; Steadman & Cocozza, 1978). Perlin (1992) suggested that the public views such persons as the most dangerous potential offenders. No study has yet determined, however, whether this stereotype is true: We do not know whether mentally disordered offenders are more likely than nondisordered offenders to commit violent crimes after they are released from jail or prison.

This question is particularly timely because of the burgeoning of jail and prison populations. Jails in the United States are so crowded (U.S. Department of Justice, 1993) that more arrestees are being released into the community than ever before (U.S. Department of Justice, 1988). Many of those being released have mental disorders (Bland, Newman, Dyck, & Orn, 1990; Lamb & Grant, 1982; Monahan & McDonough, 1980; Nielsen, 1979; Petrich, 1976; Schuckit, Herrman, & Schuckit, 1977; Swank & Winer, 1976; Teplin, 1990b, 1994). Irrespective of their psychiatric status, all released jail detainees are at risk for committing violent crimes (U.S. Department of Justice, 1991b). The critical question is whether mental

Editor's note. Articles based on APA award addresses that appear in the *American Psychologist* are scholarly articles by distinguished contributors to the field. As such, they are given special consideration in the *American Psychologist*'s editorial selection process.

This article was originally presented as part of a Distinguished Contribution to Research in Public Policy award address by Linda A. Teplin at the 101st Annual Convention of the American Psychological Association in Toronto, Ontario, Canada, in August 1993. Dr. Teplin dedicated her award address to the memory of Dr. Saleem Shah.

Authors' note. Linda A. Teplin, Karen M. Abram, and Gary M. McClelland, Northwestern University Medical School, Psycho-Legal Studies Program, Department of Psychiatry and Behavioral Sciences.

This work was supported by National Institute of Mental Health Grant #1R01MH37988 and National Institute of Alcohol Abuse and Alcoholism Grant #1R01AA05884. We are grateful to James Beck, Mary Durham, Virginia Hiday, John Monahan, Henry Steadman, Ecford Voit, and Christopher Winship for their constructive suggestions. We also wish to acknowledge the editorial advice of Laura Coats.

Correspondence concerning this article should be addressed to Linda A. Teplin, Northwestern University Medical School, 303 East Chicago Avenue, Suite 9-200, Chicago, IL 60611.

From *American Psychologist*, April 1994, pp. 335-342. © 1994 by the American Psychological Association. Reprinted by permission.

disorder increases the likelihood of violent criminal recidivism after release from jail.

There have been, however, few studies of jails. Most studies of mental disorder and violence have studied prison populations—sentenced offenders in long-term facilities—rather than jails. With few exceptions (Cirincione, Steadman, Robbins, and Monahan, in press), most have been retrospective, collecting only current charge or criminal history data. This literature yields equivocal findings: Some studies have found a relationship between mental disorder and violence (Ashford, 1989; Langevin, Ben-Aron, Wortzman, Dickey, & Handy 1987; Packard & Rosner, 1985; Roman & Gerbring, 1989; Rosner, Wiederlight, & Wieczorek, 1985; Taylor & Gunn, 1984), whereas others have not (Cirincione et al., in press; Hodgins & Cote, 1993; Phillips, Wolf, & Coons, 1988). Still others have found that it depends on the disorder (Collins & Bailey, 1990).

The reason for the disparities may be methodological: Most studies have not randomly sampled the full range of offenders. Studies have described specific populations, such as sex offenders (Packard & Rosner, 1985) or forensic patients (Phillips et al., 1988; Roman & Gerbring, 1989; Rosner et al., 1985), without comparing them to a control group. Taylor and Gunn (1984) focused on detainees charged with violent crimes or referred for mental health treatment. Others have studied the effect of only a few disorders (Collins & Bailey, 1990) or limited their subjects to specific criminal charges (Langevin et al., 1987). Many studies have used treatment samples (e.g., Ashford, 1989; Lamb & Grant, 1982) rather than random samples. Finally, current charge is an imperfect predictor of violence after release because it is only one sample from the subject's universe of arrests. Criminal history data are also an imperfect indicator unless the data are corrected for the time at risk—that is, the time the subject is not in jail, prison, or hospital and is thus free to engage in crime. In sum, no study has used an unbiased sample of jail detainees, an appropriate control group, reliable diagnostic measures of mental disorder, and, most important, prospective, longitudinal data on violent crime controlling for time at risk.

In this article, we examine the following question: Are jail detainees with severe mental disorders (schizophrenia or major affective disorders), substance use disorders (alcohol and drug), or psychotic symptoms (hallucinations and delusions) rearrested more often for violent crimes six years after release than are nondisordered detainees? We examine the effect of both psychiatric disorder and psychotic symptoms because recent research has suggested that psychotic symptoms may be more predictive of violence than is disorder per se (Link et al., 1992; Link & Stueve, 1994).

Our data are part of a larger project investigating the prevalence and treatment of mental disorder among jail detainees (Abram & Teplin, 1991; Teplin, 1990a, 1990b, 1994). For that epidemiologic study, we administered psychiatric interviews during jail intake to a random sample of 728 arrestees. The extensive diagnostic information we collected provides an opportunity to compare the criminal careers of mentally ill and nonill jail detainees. Here we present six-year longitudinal arrest data to examine whether arrest rates for violent crime differed as a function of psychiatric disorder.

Method

Subjects

Diagnostic data were collected between November 1983 and November 1984 at the Cook County Department of Corrections (CCDC) in Chicago, Illinois. Like most jails, CCDC is used solely for pretrial detention and for offenders sentenced on misdemeanor charges for less than one year.

Subjects were 728 male arrestees detained at CCDC and were randomly selected after pretrial arraignment. To include a sufficient number of detainees accused of serious crimes, we stratified subjects by arrest charge (one half misdemeanants, one half felons). Persons charged with both misdemeanors and felonies were categorized as felons. Data were then weighted to reflect the jail's actual misdemeanor–felony distribution.

All detainees, excluding persons with gunshot wounds or other traumatic injuries, were part of the sampling pool. Jail personnel referred all potential subjects regardless of their mental state, potential for violence, or fitness to stand trial. Because no detainee was a priori ruled ineligible, the sample was unbiased in relation to the larger jail population.

Subjects ranged in age from 16 to 68 years, with mean and median ages of 26.3 and 25, respectively. The majority were Black (80.8%), 12% were White, and 6.5% were Hispanic. Most of the remaining (0.8%) subjects were either Asian or American Indian. Fewer than one half of the detainees were employed at the time of their arrest (42.6%). Education level ranged from 2 to 16 years, with mean and median being 10.6 and 11.0 years, respectively. These demographic characteristics are similar to those found in many large urban jails nationwide, such as in Detroit, Philadelphia, and Cleveland (U.S. Department of Justice, 1991a).

Procedure

Interviewers were three clinical psychologists, extensively trained in interviewing techniques, psychopathology, and the data collection instrument. Persons targeted by the random sampling procedure were approached by the interviewer during the routine jail intake process. Detainees who agreed to participate signed a consent form and were paid five dollars for taking part. Persons who declined to participate proceeded through intake.

Of 767 detainees approached, only 35 (4.6%) declined to participate. The low refusal rate was probably because the detainees viewed the interview as a way to avoid the crowded and dismal conditions of the regular intake area. Two subjects were excluded because the interviewer felt they were inventing their responses. Two others were duplicate subjects; they were rearrested some time after their initial interview and randomly reselected. The final sample was 728.

Subjects were interviewed in a soundproof, private glass booth in the central intake area. Diagnostic assessments were made using the National Institute of Mental Health Diagnostic Interview Schedule (NIMH-DIS; Robins, Helzer, Croughan, Williams, & Spitzer, 1981). Empirical tests have documented the reliability of the NIMH-DIS in both institutionalized samples and the general population (Burke, 1986; Helzer et al., 1985; Robins, Helzer, Croughan, & Ratcliff, 1981; Robins, Helzer, Ratcliff, & Seyfried, 1982; in contrast, see Anthony et al., 1985).

The NIMH-DIS provides diagnostic categories rather than global psychopathology scores. Because of subject variance over time and the rarity of many disorders, it is difficult to assess the reliability and validity of psychiatric instruments (Robins, 1985). Nevertheless, a test–retest consistency check yielded results that compare favorably with other studies (Robins, 1985): 93% agreement across all diagnoses and 95% agreement for the severe disorders. Two independent interviewers gave nearly identical profiles for 85% of the cases. Interviewer consistency was maintained after the initial three-month training period using mock interviews with live subjects, spot checks, and videotape training.

We collected subjects' arrest data ("rap sheets") from Chicago Police Department records. We matched subjects to their rap sheets using the Identification Record (IR) Number, a unique number that the county assigns to each detainee. We confirmed the accuracy of the match using name, alias(es), birth date, social security number, race and ethnicity, and other key demographic information. Charges incurred outside the county or state are routinely transcribed from Federal Bureau of Investigation (FBI) and Illinois Bureau of Investigation (IBI) records. For each subject, we obtained data on arrests six years after the interview.

Psychiatric variables. To meet criteria for a disorder, the subject had to attain the *definite* or *severe* category (whichever was applicable); all *possible* or *mild* diagnoses were scored as absent. In no case did the presence of one disorder preclude the diagnosis of another disorder through exclusionary criteria (Boyd et al., 1984). Because most serious disorders tend to recur, we used lifetime diagnosis for all analyses. Subjects were scored as having hallucinations or delusions if they scored positively on any of the DIS items in these areas. We counted hallucinations and delusions as positive only if the subject reported that they were not due to drugs, alcohol, or physical illness.

Final sample size. We omitted subjects who met criteria for severe cognitive impairment ($n = 2$) because there were too few cases to analyze. The six-year follow-up data were unavailable for 38 subjects either because they had died with no known date of death ($n = 3$) or because their rap sheets were missing ($n = 35$). These 38 missing cases were similar to the entire sample on diagnosis and current charge (Teplin, 1990b, 1994): None

had lifetime schizophrenia or manic episode, 3 (7.9%) had major depressive episode, 12 (31.6%) had drug use disorders, and 22 (57.9%) had alcohol use disorder. Another 24 subjects were omitted because they were incarcerated for the entire six years. Interestingly, all 24 were in jails or prisons but never in mental hospitals. Mental disorder was not overrepresented in this subsample (Teplin, 1990b, 1994): None had schizophrenia, 2 (8.3%) had lifetime manic episode, none had major depressive episode, 4 (16.7%) had a drug use disorder, and 12 (50.0%) had alcohol use disorder. Our final sample size was 664 ($728 - 2 - 38 - 24 = 664$).

Units of analysis. Because subjects can have more than one disorder, we analyzed the data in two complementary ways:

1. Disorder as the unit of analysis. These analyses show the effect of each disorder on the dependent variable. Because many subjects have more than one disorder, the total of all the categories added together is more than the whole sample.

2. Subject as the unit of analysis. These analyses demonstrate what proportion of the sample was arrested for violent crimes. Irrespective of their comorbidity, each subject was assigned to only one diagnostic group. Because we are interested in the relationship between severe disorders and violence, we developed the following hierarchy to categorize subjects: schizophrenia, schizophreniform disorders or manic episode, major depressive episode, drug and alcohol use disorder, drug use disorder only, alcohol use disorder only, and no disorder. Persons are categorized only by the highest disorder in the hierarchy. For example, a person categorized as schizophrenic may possibly have another disorder. Likewise, a person with depression would not have a higher diagnosis but might have an alcohol use disorder. We did not categorize subjects with multiple disorders into more specific groups because the sample was not large enough to analyze the effect of comorbidity. Because our findings were the same irrespective of the unit of analysis, we present only the results based on diagnosis. (Hierarchical tables are available from the authors.)

Defining and measuring violent crime. We measured violent crime using arrest rates rather than self-reports for two reasons. First, tracking 664 released jail detainees is not feasible. Second, although self-reports have been used successfully in such populations as mental patients (Steadman et al., 1993), such data are more problematic in criminal populations because offenders often distort their criminal careers (Gottfredson & Hirschi, 1990; Hindelang, Hirschi, & Weis, 1981). Although self-reports are reliable and valid for relatively minor offenses, more serious offenses are more efficiently revealed (and with fairly little bias) by official data (Hindelang et al., 1981; Widom, 1989). For our purposes, official arrest records are the best way to collect violence data because they are reasonably complete, provide detailed information on date of arrest, and do not suffer from the biases of nonresponse or intentional misrepresentation associated with self-reports (Blumstein & Cohen, 1987).

Table 1
Probability of Being Arrested for any Violent Crime and Major Violent Crime One or More Times During Six-Year Follow-Up Period by Diagnosis, Adjusted for Time at Risk, With 95% Confidence Intervals

	Any violent crime			Major violent crime			
Psychiatric disorder	Six-year probability of arrest	Lower 95% confidence interval	Upper 95% confidence interval	Six-year probability of arrest	Lower 95% confidence interval	Upper 95% confidence interval	n
Severe disorder	.438	.346	.518	.180	.071	.277	61
Schizophrenia/mania	.453	.342	.547	.152	.026	.262	36
Depression	.430	.307	.531	.182	.039	.304	36
Any substance abuse or dependence disorder	.462	.427	.495	.174	.138	.209	405
Drug and alcohol	.441	.374	.501	.168	.106	.227	147
Drug	.451	.407	.491	.169	.115	.221	220
Alcohol	.460	.424	.494	.175	.128	.220	332
No disorder	.481	.432	.526	.196	.139	.250	255
Total	.468	.443	.493	.182	.155	.209	664

Note. There were no significant differences between the no disorder group and each diagnostic group.

We categorized the following arrest charges as violent: assault, aggravated assault, battery, aggravated battery, murder, attempted murder, manslaughter, robbery, unlawful restraint, armed violence, cruelty to children, criminal sexual assault, rape, deviant sexual assault, aggravated criminal sexual assault, and kidnapping. Nonviolent crime, the residual category, included theft, burglary, drug crimes, arson, traffic offenses, probation and parole violations, and crimes against order and morals (pimping, disorderly conduct, etc.).

A common problem in longitudinal crime research is controlling for time at risk (Blumstein & Cohen, 1979; Blumstein, Cohen, Roth, & Visher, 1986). For example, a detainee who was in jail for two of the six follow-up years would have less opportunity to commit violent crime than a person who was free the entire six years. We used data from four sources to adjust our violence variables for time at risk: CCDC, the Chicago Police Department (rap sheets), the Cook County Medical Examiner's Office (deaths), and the Illinois Department of Mental Health (hospitalizations).

Results

We analyzed the data using an epidemiologic framework because it best fit our question. Epidemiologic tables allow us to assess the relative risk of violent crime between the nondisordered and disordered groups.

For each diagnostic group, we calculated four dependent variables of recidivism: (a) probability of arrest for any violent crime listed above (misdemeanor or felony); (b) probability of arrest for major violent crime (all felonious violent crimes excluding robbery); (c) the number of arrests for any violent crime; and, (d) the number of arrests for major violent crime. Our overall hypothesis is that the psychiatric disorder groups will have higher rates of violent arrest than the no disorder group. All tests are one-tailed.

Probability of Arrest for Violent Crime During Six-Year Follow-Up

Controlling for time at risk, we calculated the probability of being arrested for a violent crime for each diagnostic group by dividing the number of persons in each group who had a rearrest for a violent crime by time at risk:

$$1 - \left(1 - \frac{\text{Number of Subjects Arrested}}{\text{Time at Risk}}\right)^{72}$$

This probability represents the chance of being arrested for a violent crime during the six-year (72-month) follow-up period (Mendenhall, 1985). Except where noted otherwise, we estimated the variances and confidence intervals reported in this article with bootstrap techniques with $n = N$ and iterations = 100 (Efron & Tibshirani 1986).

Any violent crime. Table 1 reports the probability of arrest for any violent crime by diagnostic group. As noted above, the ns in all tables sum to more than 100% because many subjects have more than one disorder. This jail sample is highly recidivistic. Subjects had a nearly even chance (.468) of being arrested for a violent crime within six years of the interview. Using t tests, we tested whether any of the diagnostic groups had a higher probability of arrest than the no disorder group. There were no significant differences at the .05 level.

Major violent crime. The probability of being arrested for a major violent crime within six years of release was fairly high for the entire sample (.182). Table 1 shows that none of the diagnostic groups had a significantly higher probability of being arrested than the no disorder group at the .05 level.

Number of Arrests for Violent Crime

For each group, we calculated the ratio of the total number of arrests for violent crime to time at risk:

Number of Arrests

Time at Risk

We first estimated variances and standard errors with the Poisson approximation. Because we found evidence of overdispersion for the any violent crime variable, we estimated variances and confidence intervals with bootstrap techniques with $n = N$ and iterations = 100 (Efron & Tibshirani, 1986). Table 2 shows the ratio of the total number of arrests for violent crime to time at risk for each diagnostic group.

Any violent crime. Using t tests, we tested whether any of the disorder groups had a higher number of arrests for any violent crime than the no disorder group. Table 2 shows that there were no significant differences.

Major violent crime. Because the Poisson approximation fit these data well, reported variances and standard errors are derived from the Poisson distribution. Table 2 shows that none of the diagnostic groups had a significantly higher number of arrests for major violent crime than the no disorder group.

Effect of Psychotic Symptoms

We also performed the analyses shown in Tables 1 and 2 using psychotic symptoms—hallucinations or delusions—as the independent variable. Persons with either hallucinations or delusions did not have a significantly higher probability of being arrested for a violent crime after release. However, persons with both hallucinations and delusions ($n = 31$) had a slightly, but not significantly, higher number of arrests for violent crime (2.01) than persons with no symptoms (1.41). A post hoc power analysis showed that this difference would have been significant at the .05 level had the same difference been obtained with a larger sample ($n = 49$). There were no significant differences on major violent crime. (Tables are available from the authors.)

Controlling for Prior Violent Crime

We did not control for prior violent crime in our initial analyses because there were not enough subjects to control simultaneously for type of severe disorder (schizophrenia-manic episode vs. depression) and prior violence. In Table 3, the severe disorders are collapsed so that we can control for prior violent crime. Here, we check if interactions between prior violent crime and diagnosis masked true differences between the diagnostic groups on violent crime. Not surprisingly, a large proportion (70.0%) of these jail detainees had a history of arrest for violent crime. The disordered groups had slightly (albeit not significantly) higher rates of prior violent arrest (72%–76%) than the no disorder group (62.7%), probably because they are older (Teplin, 1990b, 1994) and have had more time to develop an arrest history.

Table 3 shows that in every diagnostic category, persons with a prior arrest for a violent crime were about twice as likely to be arrested for a violent crime during the six-year follow-up period than persons with no violent arrest record. However, the effect of prior violent crime was the same across diagnostic groups. Even after controlling for prior arrest for violent crime, none of the disordered groups had significantly higher rates than the no disorder group. We conducted the same analysis using the major violent crime variable. The results were the same. (The major violent crime table is available from the authors.)

Controlling for Age

On average, our disordered subjects were slightly older than subjects with no disorder (Teplin, 1990b, 1994). Because violent crime decreases with age (Maguire & Flanagan, 1991), we checked to see whether the effect of age masked true differences between the diagnostic groups. We modeled the reported probabilities and counts using the generalized linear model with logistic and Poisson

---

Table 2

Number of Arrests for Violent Crimes and Major Violent Crimes Per Six-Year Period by Diagnosis, Adjusted for Time at Risk, With 95% Confidence Intervals

Psychiatric disorder	All violent crimes			Major violent crimes			
	Six-year number of arrests	Lower 95% confidence interval	Upper 95% confidence interval	Six-year number of arrests	Lower 95% confidence interval	Upper 95% confidence interval	n
Severe disorder	1.43	0.95	1.91	0.24	0.11	0.36	61
Schizophrenia/mania	1.56	0.97	2.16	0.19	0.05	0.33	36
Depression	1.31	0.63	1.99	0.24	0.08	0.40	36
Any substance abuse or dependence disorder	1.52	1.27	1.76	0.23	0.18	0.27	405
Drug and alcohol	1.49	1.07	1.92	0.23	0.15	0.31	147
Drug	1.40	1.10	1.69	0.22	0.16	0.28	220
Alcohol	1.58	1.28	1.89	0.23	0.18	0.28	332
No disorder	1.27	1.08	1.47	0.26	0.20	0.32	255
Total	1.43	1.26	1.59	0.24	0.20	0.28	664

Note. There were no significant differences between the no disorder group and each diagnostic group.

Table 3

Probability of Being Arrested for any Violent Crime One or More Times During Six-Year Follow-Up Period by Diagnosis and Prior Violence, Adjusted for Time at Risk, With 95% Confidence Intervals

Psychiatric disorder	No prior violence				Prior violence				% with prior violence	n
	Six-year probability of arrest	Lower 95% confidence interval	Upper 95% confidence interval	n	Six-year probability of arrest	Lower 95% confidence interval	Upper 95% confidence interval	n		
Severe disorder	.221	.019	.381	17	.504	.412	.582	44	72.1	61
Any substance abuse or dependence disorder	.283	.209	.350	103	.518	.485	.549	302	74.6	405
Drug and alcohol	.205	.090	.305	37	.510	.451	.562	110	74.8	147
Drug	.307	.195	.404	60	.502	.445	.553	160	72.7	220
Alcohol	.229	.136	.312	80	.524	.487	.558	252	75.9	332
No disorder	.329	.254	.396	95	.574	.526	.617	160	62.7	255
Total	.307	.255	.355	199	.529	.504	.553	465	70.0	664

Note. There were no significant differences between each disorder group and the no disorder group within each prior violence category.

specifications (Agresti, 1990). Our reported findings could not be accounted for by age differences between the comparison groups. (Tables are available from the authors.)

Discussion

Our sample of jail detainees was highly recidivistic: Nearly one half were arrested for a violent crime during the six-year follow-up period. In this extremely recidivistic population, however, psychiatric disorder did not increase the probability of being arrested for violent crimes after release. This finding still obtained even after controlling for age and prior violence.

A history of both hallucinations and delusions increased the number of arrests for violent crimes after release, but not significantly. This finding might have been stronger if we had had data on the recency of the psychotic symptoms. Nevertheless, this pattern corroborates prior studies (Link et al., 1992; Link & Stueve, 1994) and suggests that psychotic symptoms may be more powerful predictors of violent crime than diagnoses per se (Link et al., 1992; Link & Stueve, 1994).

One potential threat to validity should be highlighted: Perhaps serious mental disorder failed to predict the probability of arrest for violent crime because the mentally ill subjects were hospitalized instead of arrested when they were violent (Klassen & O'Connor, 1988). This is unlikely. In Illinois, mentally ill persons suspected of a felony must be arrested and then treated at the jail. In practice, even mentally ill misdemeanants are usually arrested before being treated (Teplin, 1984). Because of their arrest history, former jail detainees may be more likely to be rearrested than hospitalized when they are violent.

Several limitations of this study should be kept in mind. First, the dependent variable—violence—incorporated only detected crime. Many crimes are not detected or do not culminate in an arrest. Thus, our arrest data can be used only to compare the mentally ill groups with the no disorder group. We cannot use arrest data to infer the overall prevalence of violent crime among released mentally ill jail detainees. Second, because our sample was random, the number of subjects with severe mental disorders was relatively small and did not allow us to control for potentially important variables such as psychiatric comorbidity.

Because our sample included only jail detainees, our data cannot be used to draw inferences about the relationship between mental disorder and violence in the general population. Nevertheless, our major finding—that psychiatric disorder was irrelevant to the probability of arrest for violent crime after release—has important public policy implications for judicial decision making. Mental disorder alone is not a meaningful variable when deciding who should be released before trial or given probation. Our data do confirm, however, that irrespective of psychiatric disorder, one of the best predictors of future violent crime is prior violent crime (Monahan & Steadman, 1983).

We suggest several directions for future research:

1. Explore the role of specific symptoms of mental disorder in violence. It is possible that mental disorder is too heterogeneous a phenomenon to reliably predict violence. For example, certain symptoms, their duration, and age of onset may vary between two people who meet criteria for the same disorder. These aspects of a disorder may be more meaningful predictors of violence than diagnosis per se. Recent research has focused on the role of psychotic symptoms in predicting violence (Link et al., 1992; Link & Stueve, 1994). This work merits further study in view of Link et al's work and the findings of this study.

2. Comorbidity. Many detainees with schizophrenia or major affective disorders also have substance abuse or antisocial personality disorder (Abram & Teplin, 1991). Despite the prevalence of comorbidity, its impact on violent crime has yet to be determined. Alcohol intoxication and antisocial personality disorder have been linked to

violence (Collins, 1993; Pernanen, 1991). The effect of drug use disorders on violence is still being debated (cf. Abram, 1989; Gandossy, Williams, Cohen, & Harwood, 1980; Swanson, 1994). Robins (1993) suggested that severe psychopathology is much less important in predicting crime than are the disorders that often co-occur with severe disorders—antisocial personality and substance abuse. Clearly, further research is necessary to disentangle the effects of the various disorders on violent crime.

3. Actuarial methods. Predictions can be improved by using actuarial techniques to better identify those mentally ill who are at risk for repeated violence (Monahan, 1981, 1984). Such studies require extremely large samples. A new research study designed to improve violence predictions holds great promise (Steadman et al., 1993). Ideally, actuarial techniques would allow us to discriminate between mentally ill persons who are not likely to commit violent acts after release from those who might (Harris, Rice, & Quinsey, 1993).

Further research is needed to critically examine the stereotypes of mentally ill persons portrayed in the media (Hyler, Gabbard, & Schneider, 1991; Mayer & Barry, 1992; Signorelli, 1989; Wahl, 1992). Research is also vital to help mental health professionals make better decisions concerning the violence potential of mentally ill persons (Lidz, Mulvey, & Gardner, 1993). By learning to predict violence more accurately, we will balance our responsibility to treat mentally disordered offenders with our obligation to protect the safety and welfare of the public.

REFERENCES

Abram, K. M. (1989). The effect of co-occurring disorders on criminal careers: Interaction of antisocial personality, alcoholism, and drug disorders. *International Journal of Law and Psychiatry, 12,* 133–148.

Abram, K. M., & Teplin, L. A. (1991). Co-occurring disorders among mentally ill jail detainees: Implications for public policy. *American Psychologist, 46,* 1036–1045.

Agresti, A. (1990). *Categorical data analysis.* New York: Wiley.

Anthony, J. C., Folstein, M., Romanoski, A. J., Von Korff, M. R., Nestadt, G. R., Cahal, R., Merchant, A., Brown, H., Shapiro, S., Kramer, M., & Gruenberg, E. M. (1985). Comparison of the lay Diagnostic Interview Schedule and a standardized psychiatric diagnosis. *Archives of General Psychiatry, 42,* 667–675.

Ashford, J. B. (1989). Offense comparisons between mentally disordered and non-mentally disordered inmates. *Canadian Journal of Criminology, 31,* 35–48.

Bland, R. C., Newman, S. C., Dyck, R. J., & Orn, H. (1990). Prevalence of psychiatric disorders and suicide attempts in a prison population. *Canadian Journal of Psychiatry, 35,* 407–413.

Blumstein, A., & Cohen, J. (1979). Estimation of individual crime rates from arrest records. *Journal of Criminal Law and Criminology, 70,* 561–585.

Blumstein, A., & Cohen, J. (1987). Characterizing criminal careers. *Science, 237,* 985–991.

Blumstein, A., Cohen, J., Roth, J., & Visher, C. (1986). *Criminal careers and "career criminals"* (Vol. 1). Washington, DC: National Academy Press.

Boyd, J. H., Burke, J. D., Gruenberg, E., Holzer, C. E., Rae, D. S., George, L. K., Karno, M., Stoltzman, R., McEvoy, L., & Nestadt, G. (1984). Exclusion criteria of *DSM–III. Archives of General Psychiatry, 41,* 983–989.

Burke, J. D. (1986). Diagnostic categorization by the Diagnostic Interview Schedule (DIS): A comparison with other methods of assessment. In J. Barret & R. Rose (Eds.), *Mental disorders in the community* (pp.255–285). New York: Guilford Press.

Cirincione, C., Steadman, H. J., Robbins, P. C., & Monahan, J. (in press). Mental illness as a factor in criminality: A study of prisoners and mental patients. *Criminal Behaviour and Mental Health.*

Collins, J. J. (1993). *Drinking and violence: An individual offender focus* (Unpublished revision of a paper presented at the conference of Interdisciplinary Research on Alcohol and Violence, sponsored by the National Institute on Alcohol Abuse and Alcoholism, Washington, DC, May 14–15, 1992).

Collins, J. J., & Bailey, S. L. (1990). Relationship of mood disorders to violence. *The Journal of Nervous and Mental Disease, 178,* 44–47.

Efron, B., & Tibshirani, R. (1986). Bootstrap methods for standard errors, confidence intervals, and other measures of statistical accuracy. *Statistical Science, 1,* 54–77,

Gandossy, R. P., Williams, J. R., Cohen J., & Harwood, H. J. (1980). *Drugs and crime: A survey and analysis of the literature.* Washington, DC: National Institute of Justice.

Gerbner, G., Gross, L., Morgan, M., & Signorielli, N. (1981). Health and medicine on television. *New England Journal of Medicine, 305,* 901–904.

Gottfredson, M. R., & Hirschi, T. (1990). *A general theory of crime.* Stanford, CA: Stanford University Press.

Harris, G. T., Rice, M. E., & Quinsey, V. L. (1993). Violent recidivism of mentally disordered offenders: The development of a statistical prediction instrument. *Criminal Justice and Behavior, 20,* 315–335.

Helzer, J. E., Robins, L. N., McEvoy, L. T., Spiptznagel, E. L., Stoltzman, R. K., Farmer, A., & Brockington, I. F. (1985). A comparison of clinical and Diagnostic Interview Schedule diagnoses. *Archives of General Psychiatry, 42,* 657–666.

Hindelang, M. J., Hirschi, T., & Weis, J. G. (1981). *Measuring delinquency.* Beverly Hills, CA: Sage.

Hodgins, S., & Cote, G. (1993). The criminality of mentally disordered offenders. *Criminal Justice and Behavior, 20,* 115–129.

Hyler, S. E., Gabbard, G. O., & Schneider, I. (1991). Homicidal maniacs and narcissistic parasites: Stigmatization of mentally ill persons in the movies. *Hospital and Community Psychiatry, 42,* 1044–1048.

Klassen, D., & O'Connor, W. A. (1988). Crime, inpatient admissions, and violence among male mental patients. *International Journal of Law and Psychiatry, 11,* 305–312.

Lamb, R., & Grant, R. W. (1982). The mentally ill in an urban county jail. *Archives of General Psychiatry, 39,* 17–22.

Langevin, R., Ben-Aron, M., Wortzman, G., Dickey, R., & Handy, L. (1987). Brain damage, diagnosis, and substance abuse among violent offenders. *Behavioral Sciences and the Law, 5,* 77–94.

Lidz, C. W., Mulvey, E. P., & Gardner, W. (1993). The accuracy of prediction of violence to others. *Journal of the American Medical Association, 269,* 1007–1011.

Lindquist, P., & Allebeck, P. (1990). Schizophrenia and crime: A longitudinal follow-up of 644 schizophrenics in Stockholm. *British Journal of Psychiatry, 157,* 345–350.

Link, B. G., Andrews, H., & Cullen, F. T. (1992). The violent and illegal behavior of mental patients reconsidered. *American Sociological Review, 57,* 275–292.

Link, B., & Stueve, A. (1994). Psychotic symptoms and the violent/illegal behavior of mental patients compared to community controls. In J. Monahan & H. Steadman (Eds.), *Violence and mental disorder: Developments in risk assessment* (pp. 137–159). Chicago: University of Chicago Press.

Maguire, K., & Flanagan, T. J. (Eds.) (1991). *Sourcebook of criminal justice statistics—1990.* Washington, DC: U. S. Department of Justice.

Mayer, A., & Barry, D. D. (1992). Working with the media to destigmatize mental illness. *Hospital and Community Psychiatry, 43,* 77–78.

Mendenhall, W. (1985). *Introduction to probability and statistics* (7th ed.). Boston: PWS-Kent.

Monahan, J. (1981). *Predicting violent behavior: An assessment of clinical techniques.* Beverly Hills, CA: Sage.

Monahan, J. (1984). The prediction of violent behavior: Toward a second generation of theory and policy. *American Journal of Psychiatry, 141,* 10–15.

Monahan, J. (1992). Mental disorder and violent behavior: Perceptions and evidence. *American Psychologist, 47,* 511–521.

Monahan, J., & McDonough, L. B. (1980). Delivering community mental health services to a county jail population: A research note. *Bulletin of the American Academy of Psychiatry and Law, 8,* 28–32.

Monahan, J., & Steadman, H. (1983). Crime and mental disorders: An epidemiological approach. In N. Morris & M. Tonry (Eds.), *Crime and justice: An annual review of research* (pp. 145–189). Chicago: University of Chicago Press.

Nielsen, E. D. (1979). Community mental health services in the community jail. *Community Mental Health Journal, 15,* 27–32.

Packard, W. S., & Rosner, R. (1985). Psychiatric evaluations of sexual offenders. *Journal of Forensic Science, 30,* 715–720.

Perlin, M. L. (1992). On "sanism." *Southern Methodist Univeristy Law Review, 46,* 373–407.

Pernanen, K. (1991). *Alcohol in human violence.* New York: Guilford Press.

Petrich, J. (1976). Rate of psychiatric morbidity in a metropolitan county jail population. *American Journal of Psychiatry, 133,* 1439–1444.

Phillips, M. R., Wolf, A. S., & Coons, D. J. (1988). Psychiatry and the criminal justice system: Testing the myths. *American Journal of Psychiatry, 145,* 605–610.

Robins, L. N. (1985). Epidemiology: Reflections on testing the validity of psychiatric interviews. *Archives of General Psychiatry, 42,* 918–924.

Robins, L. N. (1993). Childhood conduct problems, adult psychopathology, and crime. In S. Hodgins (Ed.), *Mental disorder and crime* (pp. 173–193). Newbury Park, CA: Sage.

Robins, L. N., Helzer, J. E., Croughan, J., & Ratcliff, K. (1981). National Institute of Mental Health Diagnostic Interview Schedule: Its history, characteristics, and validity . *Archives of General Psychiatry, 38,* 381–389.

Robins, L. N., Helzer, J. E., Croughan, J., Williams, J., & Spitzer, R. L. (1981). *NIMH Diagnostic Interview Schedule: Version III.* Rockville, MD: National Institute of Mental Health.

Robins, L. N., Helzer, J. E., Ratcliff, K. S., & Seyfried, W. (1982). Validity of the Diagnostic Interview Schedule, Version II: *DSM-III* diagnoses. *Psychological Medicine, 12,* 855–870.

Roman, D. D., & Gerbring, D. W. (1989). The mentally disordered criminal offender: A description based on demographic, clinical, and MMPI data. *Journal of Clinical Psychology, 45,* 983–990.

Rosner, R., Wiederlight, M., Wieczorek, R. R. (1985). Forensic psychiatric evaluations of women accused of felonies: A three-year descriptive study. *Journal of Forensic Sciences, 30,* 721–729.

Schuerman, L. A., & Kobrin, S. (1984). Exposure of community mental health clients to the criminal justice system: Client/criminal or patient/prisoner. In L. A. Teplin (Ed.), *Mental health and criminal justice* (pp. 87–118). Beverly Hills, CA: Sage.

Schuckit, M. A., Herrman, G., & Schuckit, J. (1977). The importance of psychiatric illness in newly arrested prisoners. *Journal of Nervous and Mental Disease, 165,* 118–125.

Shah, S. (1990). The mentally disordered offenders: Some issues of policy and planning. In E. H. Cox-Feith & B. N. W. de Smit (Eds.), *Innovations in mental health legislation and government policy: A European perspective.* The Hague: The Netherlands Ministry of Justice.

Signorielli, N. (1989). The stigma of mental illness on television. *Journal of Broadcasting and Electronic Media, 33,* 325–331.

Sosowsky, L. (1978). Crime and violence among mental patients reconsidered in view of the new legal relationship between the state and the mentally ill. *American Journal of Psychiatry, 135,* 33–42.

Sosowsky, L. (1980). Explaining the increased arrest rate among mental patients: A cautionary note. *American Journal of Psychiatry, 137,* 1602–1605.

Steadman, H., & Cocozza, J. (1978). Selective reporting and the public's misconceptions of the criminally insane. *Public Opinion Quarterly, 41,* 523–533.

Steadman, H. J., Cocozza, J. J., & Melick, M. E. (1978). Explaining the increased arrest rate among mental patients: The changing clientele of state hospitals. *American Journal of Psychiatry, 135,* 816–820.

Steadman, H. J., Monahan, J., Robbins, P. C., Appclbaum, P., Grisso, T., Klassen, D., Mulvey, E. P., & Roth, L. (1993). From dangerousness to risk assessment: Implications for appropriate research strategies. In S. Hodgins (Ed.), *Mental disorder and crime* (pp. 39–62). Newbury Park, CA: Sage.

Steadman, H. J., & Ribner, S. A. (1980). Changing perceptions of the mental health needs of inmates in local jails. *American Journal of Psychiatry, 137,* 1115–1116.

Swank, G. E., & Winer, D. (1976). Occurrence of psychiatric disorder in a county jail population. *American Journal of Psychiatry, 133,* 1331–1333.

Swanson, J. W. (1994). Mental disorder, substance abuse, and community violence: An epidemiological approach. In J. Monahan & H. Steadman (Eds.), *Violence and mental disorder: Developments in risk assessment* (pp. 101–136). Chicago: University of Chicago Press.

Swanson, J. W., Holzer, C. E., Ganju, V. K., & Jono, R. T. (1990). Violence and psychiatric disorder in the community: Evidence from the Epidemiologic Catchment Area surveys. *Hospital and Community Psychiatry, 41,* 761–770.

Taylor, P., & Gunn, J. (1984). Violence and psychosis I—Risk of violence among psychotic men. *British Medical Journal, 288,* 1945—1949.

Teplin, L. A. (1984). Criminalizing mental disorder: The comparative arrest rate of the mentally ill. *American Psychologist, 39,* 794–803.

Teplin, L. A. (1985). The criminality of the mentally ill: A dangerous misconception. *American Journal of Psychiatry, 142,* 593–599.

Teplin, L. A. (1990a). Detecting disorder: The treatment of mental illness among jail detainees. *Journal of Consulting and Clinical Psychology, 58,* 233–236.

Teplin, L. A. (1990b). The prevalence of severe mental disorder among male urban jail detainees: Comparison with the Epidemiologic Catchment Area program. *American Journal of Public Health, 80,* 663–669.

Teplin, L. A. (1994). Psychiatric and substance abuse disorders among male urban jail detainees. *American Journal of Public Health, 84,* 290–293.

U.S. Department of Justice. (1988). *Our crowded jails: A national plight* (NCJ-111846). Washington, DC: Bureau of Justice Statistics.

U.S. Department of Justice. (1991a). *Drug use forecasting: Drugs and crime 1990 annual report.* Washington, DC: National Institute of Justice.

U.S. Department of Justice. (1991b). *Profile of jail inmates, 1989* (NCJ-129097). Washington, DC: Bureau of Justice Statistics.

U.S. Department of Justice. (1993). *Jail inmates 1992* (NCJ-143284). Washington, DC: Bureau of Justice Statistics.

Wahl, O. F. (1992). Mass media images of mental illness: A review of the literature. *Journal of Community Psychology, 20,* 343–352.

Widom, C. S. (1989). The cycle of violence. *Science, 244,* 160–166.

*S*Out of the *Shadows*

A leading psychiatrist contends that many of the problems we've always blamed on character flaws may be due to mild versions of full-blown mental disorders like depression. Here's what you can do to keep your brain healthy.

By John Ratey, M.D., and Catherine Johnson, Ph.D.

Although the face Sandra presents to others is that of a relaxed and loyal friend, internally she is never at ease—she is driven to clean the house obsessively, or diet obsessively, or, most recently, to shop obsessively, having run up a debt of $15,000 within a few years' time. We might guess that Sandra comes from a dysfunctional family. Perhaps her parents were too demanding, or drank too much, or inflicted upon her their bad habits and character flaws. But neither we nor Sandra might suspect that there might be something biological going on.

Or take the case of Lou, a man who continually scans his body for signs of trouble, despite being in excellent condition for a man of 50. Lou not only worries obsessively about minor physical ailments, but compulsively questions his physician-wife about whether any of these troubles might be cancer. How do we explain Lou's behavior? Perhaps we see it as "normal craziness" similar to the obsessive neatness of the main character Jerry on the television show *Seinfeld*. Maybe we also view Lou as the victim of a bad childhood. What we don't think is that Lou, like Sandra, might be at the mercy of his own flawed brain chemistry.

But neuropsychiatry is now discovering that a great deal of "normal craziness" in fact is heavily influenced by the genetics, structure, and neurochemistry of the brain. Every troublesome personality likely has its roots in an unsuspected brain difference: the loner, the gifted person who cannot seem to live up to his or her potential, the needy neighbor you can't get off the telephone, the confirmed bachelor, the man who cannot talk about his feelings, or even

the husband who throws tantrums like a four year old. Neurologists and biopsychiatrists are now finding that the normal problems of normal people are gray and silver shadow versions of full-color mental illnesses. They're the same thing in outline, but indistinct in detail, and not easy to recognize for what they are. Just as shadows cast a pall across a day that might otherwise be sunny and clear, these "shadow syndromes" cast a shadow over the realms of work and love.

Life changes when we begin to realize that people can have subtle, hidden, or partial mental disorders. The impulse to blame people or their parents for their problems loses its power. The profound and corrosive sense of shame we feel over our own behavior begins to lift when we understand that it can be created by subtle differences in the brain. And the notion of the shadow syndrome helps us to see that talk therapy needs to address our biological selves as well as our psychological selves. Sandra, for example, sought out therapists and doctors to help her change her behaviors, but they focused on the fact that she was adopted—a fact that she had thought little about. However her childhood may be affecting her, Sandra faces challenges shaped by the facts of her biology as well, and she needs the help of her therapists in doing so.

This is not to dismiss our environments as a major source of who and what we are. A child with an innately anxious temperament who is born to an innately anxious mother may grow up to be a different person from the child with the anxious temperament whose mother does not share his difficulty. But the "new" biology can help us understand how environment and biol-

ogy work together to create the person—an understanding that we can use to make the changes we wish and hope to make.

Diagnosing Shadows

In order to understand "normal craziness," we can learn from "craziness" that is not so normal, such as schizophrenia or severe manic depression. Psychiatrists diagnose their patients with these and other disorders according to syndromes described in *DSM-IV*, the *Diagnostic and Statistical Manual*, Fourth Edition. A syndrome is a set of behaviors that consistently appear together, and which the patient, the doctor, or the patient's friends and family can observe and describe. However, real people often come into the doctor's office exhibiting only one or two symptoms of a particular syndrome, or may fit every aspect of a syndrome down to the smallest detail and yet be so mildly affected that even a good therapist might miss the diagnosis. In fact, most everyday people seem to have minor bits of this syndrome, small pieces of that.

Lou's hypochondriacal behavior can be seen as a mild version of obsessive-compulsive disorder (OCD), and Sandra has shown "streaks" of the syndromes on the anxiety spectrum. Other common shadow syndromes are mild but hidden depression; hypomania, a mildly manic state where a person possesses extraordinary energy and productivity and lacks ordinary self-doubt; mild rage problems, such as that of the tantruming husband; mild attention deficit

From *Psychology Today*, May/June 1997, pp. 47-48, 50, 78, 80. Excerpted from *Shadow Syndromes* by John Ratey and Catherine Johnson. © 1997 by John Ratey and Catherine Johnson. Reprinted by permission of Pantheon Books, a division of Random House, Inc.

A Conversation with John Ratey

PT: You're proposing that many of us have mild versions of familiar conditions like obsessive-compulsive disorder. It's odd that this idea hasn't been widely acknowledged before.

JR: For too many years we psychiatrists have been trying to put people into boxes and label them. We've refined our understanding of various disorders and made those boxes tighter in order to make our efforts seem more scientific. But this approach has been to the detriment of people who have two symptoms of a disorder instead of the five symptoms that you might need to be diagnosed with something like depression.

PT: Your perspective is a more compassionate one.

JR: For me it grew out of working with people with attention deficit disorder (ADD)—realizing how many people had it and how much they were blaming themselves for their foibles. Many creative, wonderful adults have a really poor self image because they have this brain difference. One of my patients had developed a company that IBM wanted to buy. He had all these people working for him, and he was just 32 years old. But the only thing he was focused on was going back to college to prove to himself that he was smart—he hadn't graduated because he failed math. Here he was blaming himself for this deficit, for not being good at math, instead of enjoying his accomplishments.

PT: The message of your book, *Shadow Syndromes,* is essentially "know thy brain."

JR: Absolutely. Get familiar with your brain and deal with it. Use the good qualities and acknowledge your deficits. This is not playing the excuse card at all—it's a call to responsibility. And to awareness.

PT: The brain scares people.

JR: Because it's so damn complicated. It's the black box nobody wants to open. The public still thinks of brain differences as differences in brain chemistry, of having a serotonin or dopamine imbalance. But often it's actual brain geography that's different. In dyslexia, autism, and even some people with OCD or ADD, brain structures are a bit altered, and that makes people see the world differently. They perceive things differently and react differently. So helping them may not simply be a matter of altering their brain's chemistry.

The other misconception people have is that if we focus on biology, there's nothing left for people to do in terms of their environment. But they can still benefit from psychotherapy. Or they can let the people they work with know that they need help in a certain area. You make trade offs—what I call "creative engineering."

PT: Could thinking about certain behaviors as shadow syndromes pathologize what we now think of as temperament?

JR: Calling something a shadow syndrome doesn't mean pathologizing it. We can't really draw a line between health and illness. A brain difference is pathological when it interferes with your life or prevents you from doing things you want to do.

PT: So if you're comfortable with your personality, your brain differences, there's no problem.

JR: Right. The other issue is whether it's affecting other people. In the book we write about a mildly depressive mother who was perfectly comfortable being who she was, but she was ruining her daughter's life because she was the ultimate killjoy—her temperament was making others miserable. That doesn't mean she has to run and take Prozac, but maybe she has to acknowledge that her temperament is somewhat depressive.

PT: What's been your most satisfying moment as a psychiatrist?

JR: Those moments of discovery with patients—helping them understand their biology. It's no magic bullet, but if you hit the target—man, does it change their life!

---

disorder (ADD), which does not unravel a life but may leave it disorganized; and autism-like social deficits that make a person incapable of relating well to others.

One of the most confusing issues is how many of the shadow syndromes normal people may fit. Sometimes depressed, sometimes impulsive, sometimes manic, sometimes obsessed: we may find aspects of ourselves, our families, and our friends in all of these categories. But there is one characteristic every shadow syndrome has in common: mental white noise. When we are mildly depressed, or mildly hyperactive, or mildly anything else, our brains cease to function as the quiet, reflective center of an ordered world. We become noisy on the inside.

What stress is to the body, noise is to the brain: the general response to the demands made upon it by difficult life circumstances or by flawed biology. The noisy brain cannot separate out stimuli or thoughts, either incoming or outgoing. For example, a person with mild ADD cannot filter stimuli from the environment; he or she will see everything out there, all at once.

A noisy brain invariably affects a person's capacity to deal with other people. Social skills occupy the very topmost level of the brain. Noise affects this top level, or cortex, causing the person afflicted to fall back to a more primitive, "lower" level of brain functioning that corresponds to the social strategies of the adolescent or child—or lower still, to the level of the "reptilian brain," where we respond reflexively instead of thoughtfully.

Brain Based Behavior

How do we know that this mental white noise is biologically based? In the case of obsessive-compulsive disorder, researchers have identified three specific brain structures that become locked together in a pattern and cause the behavior. Any damage to the primary brain structure, the caudate nucleus, whether from "bad genes," head injury, or even from the body's own immune system, can result in obsessive-compulsive disorder. In fact, OCD can develop in children as a result of a strep throat infection. The same antibody that attacks strep can also attack the caudate nucleus, causing a child to develop obsessive fears of contamination and to begin compulsively hand-washing. Treatment with blood plasma and antibiotics makes these symptoms decline noticeably.

But unlike obsessive-compulsive disorder, other shadow syndromes such as adult tantruming do not have their roots in a simple biological problem. In fact, many readers will be skeptical as to whether adult tantruming has a biological explanation at all. And yet anti-depressant medications have been shown to stop anger attacks altogether in 71 percent of a group of depressed patients, and reduce their incidence in the rest. This fact alone implies that for these patients, tantrums had a significant brain-based component.

It is also likely that temper tantrums in people who are not depressed are just as biologically based as anger attacks in depressed people. The experience of Gary, a man who averaged forty tantrums a month, provides evidence for this conclusion. By the time he went to see a psychiatrist, Gary had exhausted almost every available avenue to master his temper, except for medication. He had been a sober member of Alcoholics Anonymous for 10 years; he regularly attended a men's group to discuss feelings and relationships; he had been a runner for years; he had religiously practiced breathing, meditation, and relaxation exercises to calm himself. And none of it had worked. His second marriage was on the brink of collapse and his small daughter was terrified.

Gary went to see a psychiatrist because he had read about attention deficit disorder, and recognized symptoms in himself. The psychiatrist confirmed Gary's self-diagnosis, and prescribed a low dosage of the medication desipramine as treatment. Later, Gary self-consciously revealed a side-benefit from the medication: He had stopped having tantrums at home.

The fact that desipramine worked so well for Gary indicates that his tantrums very likely were the result of brain noise produced by random firings of the brain stem. An excess of mental noise from this lower region, which connects the brain with the spinal cord, can overwhelm the higher brain centers, the "seat of reason" found in the frontal lobes of the cortex, and allow the lower emotional brain to take over. In other words, emotion "hijacks" reason. Desipramine may act to reduce random, noisy brain-stem firings. By quieting those posterior areas, desipramine may then permit the frontal lobes to step in and stave off a rage attack.

A WHOLESOME SOLUTION

Gary's experience shows how a person can go about changing the way his or her brain works. First, the person must try to develop insight—to see himself as his loved ones see him. The person also needs to consult a doctor, and listen to what that doctor tells him or her about brain chemistry. Then, working with the doctor and loved ones, the person needs to create tools to short-circuit his or her biologically-based response to daily life. (Some examples are described below.) Finally, if these measures are not sufficient, he or she may have to take medication to restore brain functioning.

While relaxation exercises had not worked for Gary's rage attacks, insight and behavioral techniques alone have helped many people with shadow syndromes change. In a revolutionary UCLA study, obsessive-compulsive patients—those suffering from symptoms more severe than Sandra's or Lou's—were required to tell themselves that the obsession they were ex-

periencing was not real. Then they resisted performing the compulsion and instead forced themselves to do something wholesome and enjoyable—such as a hobby, volunteer work, or a good deed for a friend or a loved one—for at least 15 minutes. Twelve out of 18 patients in the study experienced striking reductions in their obsessive-compulsive symptoms. And, remarkably, the changes were reflected in before-and-after brain scans. In the "after" scans, several brain areas had begun to operate as they do in the normal brain. The UCLA researchers demonstrated the power of the mind to bend a malfunctioning brain to its will.

BOOSTING BRAIN PERFORMANCE

When it comes to making small changes in our lives and brains, the motto to embrace is: Everything matters. Exercise, food, sleep, the work we do, whom we marry—all of it affects our brains.

Perhaps the most important modest change any of us can make is to establish an exercise program, and stick to it. A growing body of evidence links aerobic exercise to sharpened memory, faster response times, elevated mood, and increased self-esteem. Most of these studies have been conducted on the elderly, but the results are so encouraging that many clinicians are convinced that even young children may benefit from a program of daily exercise.

Martial arts, forms of exercise that train the mind as well as the body, have helped a number of patients with shadow syndromes to make tremendous progress in their lives. Like meditation, which is also an excellent tool for soothing the noisy brain, martial arts train the body and brain to a achieve a state of relaxed readiness, which allows the trainee to react to any challenge without having to anticipate it.

We can also influence brain chemistry for the better through food, light, and sleep. Clear data indicate that light is good unless you are manic, and sleep is good unless you are depressed (when it may be bad). Food is a more complicated issue. For example, pure carbohydrates unaccompanied by fat may soothe anxiety, but decrease alertness at the same time. Whatever enters our bloodstream, from wheat germ to pork crackling, may affect the brain in a matter of seconds.

Beyond the common-sense tactic of striving to develop good habits in exercise and diet, we should hold ourselves open to the mysteries of the body and its brain. Solutions can come from places we would never look, and if we notice a positive effect in our own life, whether from food or

exercise or sleep or light or negative ions or simply the scent of autumn in the air, we should take it seriously.

Apart from these changes, the single most critical improvement anyone can make in brain function, and in character, is to find a mission in life. It is well known that idleness increases psychiatric and physical symptoms of all kinds. And almost any form of work, even work we do not particularly enjoy, can quiet the noisy brain. Work stimulates the cheer-seeking left side of the brain, taking us out of the stewing morass that is the right. An impassioned commitment to an activity pushes brain function in the direction of health, sanity, and well-being.

THE WINGS OF CHANGE

Perhaps the most useful theorem for anyone trying to change his brain is meteorologist Edward Lorenz's now famous "butterfly effect": a butterfly flapping its wings in Tokyo, he imagined, could set off a cascading chain of events that ended up as a hurricane over Texas. This theorem applies to mental fitness as well. The brain's interconnectivity tells us that small problems may cascade into large ones, so it can be important not to let even minor mental issues slide.

However, the good news is that complex systems such as the brain do not list in just one direction: Life is not inevitably a downhill proposition. A change as small as a new exercise program or a satisfying hobby might make all the difference in the world.

For most of us, the notion that a complex system may tip up as well as down is counterintuitive. As a culture, we have taken the second law of thermodynamics to heart: entropy rules. But we do possess some intuitive understanding of an anti-entropy force at work in life and love, when we speak of "things falling into place," or of being "on a roll," or when athletes hit "a winning streak." All of these experiences are, in a sense what we are hoping for when we think of changing our lives. We are hoping to reach that magic moment when life and love "self organize" into something splendid.

With greater knowledge of the brain's biology, people who struggle with shadow syndromes can move closer to that goal. We hope that the shame of having to live life as a flawed human being will eventually fade, and the potential to free the self from the bonds of biology will grow strong. We hope that it will help people to begin the journey out from the shadows and into the clear light of day.

Is Mental Illness Catching?

It may sound incredible, but there's evidence that psychological conditions such as depression, obsessive-compulsive disorder and schizophrenia can be caused by strep throat, the flu and other illnesses. Finally, startling proof that mental disorders are not all in the head.

By Lisa Collier Cool

Like many kids, Enid Rose of Tucker, GA, suffered recurrent strep throat infections. But neither her parents nor her doctors saw any reason to link these infections with the far more disabling symptoms that led to her being labeled "the weird kid in school," and that, when she grew up, limited her ability to work. "I've always had obsessive thoughts," says Rose, now age 30. "If I see a knife or anything sharp—even a pencil—I get scared it will somehow poke my eyes out or cut my Achilles tendons." Rose also has such a horror of dirt that she spends hours each day scouring her already immaculate kitchen and bathroom. She even vacuums her bed daily.

It wasn't until 1995 that she was diagnosed with obsessive-compulsive disorder, a condition that affects over 2% of Americans. Marked by the presence of persistent obsessive thoughts and worries, as well as compulsive rituals such as repeated handwashing or constantly checking that the stove is turned off, the illness was once thought to be brought on by destructive parenting practices, such as harsh toilet training. But recent, groundbreaking studies at the National Institute of Mental Health (NIMH) in Bethesda, MD, have revealed a surprising cause for OCD: an abnormal immune response to strep throat or flu-like infections.

The Infection Connection While the idea that you can "catch" a mental illness in the same way that you catch a cold may sound improbable, there's increasing evidence that psychological conditions such as depression, OCD and schizophrenia have biological roots. "What most people don't realize is that psychiatric disorders like OCD and schizophrenia are also true medical illnesses," says Susan Swedo, M.D., scien-

Is It All in Your Head?

Depression, anxiety and other emotional symptoms can, in some cases, be caused by a wide range of physical conditions. Consider your symptoms and the possible psychological and physical causes, then consult your doctor for a diagnosis.

Depression

Symptoms: Persistent sadness, fatigue, change in eating or sleeping patterns, loss of interest or pleasure in daily activities, suicidal thoughts, chronic body aches, memory problems
Other Conditions That Can Produce These Symptoms: Thyroid disease, stroke, chronic fatigue syndrome, lupus, mononucleosis, cancer, heart disease, diabetes

Obsessive-Compulsive Disorder

Symptoms: Repeated intrusive thoughts and worries; involuntary, senseless rituals or checking routines like compulsive cleaning or forever checking that a door is locked
Other Conditions That Can Produce These Symptoms: Irritable bowel disorder, adrenal gland disease, autoimmune disorders, brain injury or infection, neurological diseases

Schizophrenia

Symptoms: Delusional beliefs, lack of appropriate emotional responses or behavior, hallucinations, incoherent speech, paranoia
Other Conditions That Can Produce These Symptoms: Adrenal gland or thyroid disease, brain tumor, substance abuse (especially of LSD, PCP or cocaine), reaction to steroids

From *American Health for Women*, March 1997, pp. 72-75. © 1997 by Lisa Collier Cool. Reprinted by permission.

tific director of the NIMH and coauthor of *It's Not All in Your Head.* "Not only can a predisposition to mental illness run in a family, just as heart disease or breast cancer can, but it also may be sparked by the very same infections that trigger other diseases."

Dr. Swedo and her colleagues first suspected the connection among strep throat, OCD and Tourette's syndrome (a neurological disorder that causes vocal and physical tics), when earlier studies of patients with rheumatic fever (a strep throat complication that can damage the heart) showed that some also developed OCD-like obsessions and a movement disorder similar to Tourette's known as Sydenham's chorea. "So far," says Dr. Swedo, "we've

---

Old Think/New Think

Here are some of the more pervasive myths about common psychological disorders, along with a good dose of reality.

Obsessive-Compulsive Disorder Old Think: Caused by excessively harsh toilet training. **New Think:** Can result from an abnormal immune response to strep throat or a flu-like infection.

Schizophrenia Old Think: Caused by poor parenting. **New Think:** May result from biological and environmental factors, or when a fetus is exposed to its mother's illness in the womb.

Depression Old Think: People with depression can cheer up if they really want to. **New Think:** Results from chemical imbalances, such as abnormal levels of certain brain chemicals or thyroid dysfunction.

---

found 75 children whose parents told us that their perfectly well-adjusted kid woke up one morning after having an inadvertently untreated strep infection locked in obsessive-compulsive rituals, or that their child's mild OCD or Tourette's exploded in intensity after having had strep or a flu-like illness." So far, there's no evidence that strep infection triggers OCD in adults.

Though the NIMH study is small, it *is* revolutionary, and experts believe it could lead to fundamental changes in the treatment of mental disorders. For instance, researchers are now experimenting with giving penicillin on a continuing basis to kids with mild, strep-triggered OCD to prevent a recurrence of strep that could make their symptoms worse. They're also testing drugs that act on the immune system, based on the theory that when the immune system produces antibodies to fight strep, it also attacks a part of the brain that seems related to OCD. All the children in the NIMH study improved dramatically after such treatments, which suggests that their diseases are no more "psychological" than rheumatic fever is.

Of course, the vast majority of kids don't go on to develop OCD after a bout of strep throat, and more research is needed before penicillin and immune-altering therapies are routinely prescribed for OCD and Tourette's. But it's important to take your child to the doctor if you suspect she has strep (symptoms include fever, swollen glands, sore throat and pus on the tonsils).

A Flu in the Mind Until the late sixties, when the genetic link to schizophrenia was first discovered, parents took the rap for causing the disease, which affects about 1% of Americans and can cause delusions, paranoia and disordered thinking, among other symptoms. Mental health experts typically blamed the disorder on hostile mothers in particular, who supposedly warped their children's minds by constantly putting

them in stressful, no-win situations. Now there's evidence that a virus, *not* bad parenting, may play a role in triggering this devastating disease.

In a study of people born in the nine months after the 1957 Asian flu epidemic in Finland, University of Southern California psychology professor Sarnoff Mednick, Ph.D., found that the children whose mothers had the flu during their second trimester of pregnancy had a far higher than normal rate of schizophrenia later in life. This is the first time that schizophrenia, and perhaps any psychiatric disorder, has been connected to a maternal infection. Since then, studies suggest that prenatal exposure to other disorders, including toxoplasmosis (a parasitic infection), positive-negative blood incompatibility between a mother and her unborn baby, and even cold viruses may also increase a person's chances of developing schizophrenia.

Still, the exact role that viral infections play in causing schizophrenia remains unclear; most people who are exposed to viruses while in the womb don't go on to develop the disease. Like other mental illnesses, schizophrenia is thought to be caused by a variety of biological and environmental triggers. But there's no doubt that the damage to the brain that causes this illness occurs very early on. Babies who eventually develop schizophrenia (which typically occurs during adolescence) tend to sit up later and lag slightly behind other kids in speech and overall motor development, according to Kathryn Kotrla, M.D., assistant professor of psychiatry at Baylor College of Medicine in Houston. "It's clear," she says, "that these children are different from birth."

Depression: A Surprising Link After Debbie Harris, 42, of Fairborn, OH, was diagnosed with Graves' disease, a disorder of the thyroid gland, she found herself crying at the drop of a hat. She continued to feel extremely depressed after treatment with radioactive iodine and thyroid supplements and repeatedly asked her endocrinologist if her thyroid problems might be the cause. Each time he reassured her that, though her hormone levels were a bit low, they were within the normal range. Harris endured six years of misery before a psychiatrist advised her physician to increase her thyroid dose, which rapidly restored her former disposition.

According to preliminary findings by Robert Stern, Ph.D., associate professor of psychiatry and neurology at Brown University in Providence, RI, women who tested just slightly below normal in thyroid function seemed to be more susceptible to episodes of depression than women whose hormone levels were normal. There are other intriguing links between thyroid function and depression. "Lab tests reveal that 5% to 20% of people with depression have a slightly overactive thyroid, even though they show no thyroid symptoms," notes Dr. Stern. "And though we don't know why, some depressed patients with normal thyroid function don't respond to antidepressants unless they're also given thyroid hormones."

Scientists from the Free University of Berlin have found that the Borna disease virus, which causes horses and cats to act apathetic and listless, is also present in some depression patients. Since evidence of this virus appeared either during or before the time when these patients became depressed, it's possible that it triggers depression in people who are genetically predisposed to the disorder.

Shattering Stigmas As scientists focus on the organic rather than emotional underpinnings of these diseases, the 30 million to 45 million Americans with psychological ailments might finally feel free to step out of the shadows and get help. "One hundred years ago, the most common 'mental illnesses' were tuberculosis, epilepsy and syphilis," says James Hudson, M.D., an associate professor of psychiatry at Harvard Medical School in Boston. People with epilepsy, for instance, were sent to sanatoriums because they were considered to be too emotionally fragile to withstand the stress of industrial society—a theory that didn't die out until doctors discovered the characteristic brain-wave abnormalities for epilepsy in the mid-20th century. "Similarly," says Dr. Hudson, "we might one day find the idea that diseases like schizophrenia, depression, and OCD were ever viewed as 'emotional problems' just as laughable."

That would be a good thing, since 80% of people who currently suffer from psychological illnesses still don't get treatment. "There's so much shame surrounding mental illness that many people wait until they break down completely before they get help," says Victor Reus, M.D., a professor of psychiatry at the University of California at San Francisco School of Medicine. The truth is, mental illnesses are as real as any other disease, as the wealth of new findings makes clear. They're no different—and no more shameful—than having breast cancer or diabetes.

Lisa Collier Cool is a health writer living in Pelham, NY.

Where to Get Help

• **Depression** For information on mood disorders, send an SASE with $1.01 in postage to: National Foundation for Depressive Illness, P.O. Box 2257, New York, NY 10116; call 800-239-1293; or visit the NFDI's Website at http://www.depression.org.

• **OCD** For a list of doctors and support groups in your area and a newsletter, write to the Obsessive-Compulsive Foundation, P.O. Box 70, Milford, CT 06460; call 203-878-5669; or check out the group's Website at http://pages.prodigy.com/alwillen/ocf.html.

• **Schizophrenia** For brochures, treatment information and a newsletter on the latest research developments on the disease, contact: NARSAD Research, 60 Cutter Mill Road, Suite 404, Great Neck, NY 11021; call 800-829-8289; or visit its Website at http://www.mhsource.com.

Basic Behavioral Science Research for Mental Health

Vulnerability and Resilience

Basic Behavioral Science Task Force of the National Advisory Mental Health Council
Rockville, MD

Why do some people collapse under life stresses while others seem unscathed by traumatic circumstances such as severe illness, the death of loved ones, and extreme poverty, or even by major catastrophes such as natural disasters and war? Surprisingly large numbers of people mature into normal, successful adults despite stressful, disadvantaged, or even abusive childhoods. Yet other people are so emotionally vulnerable that seemingly minor losses and rebuffs can be devastating—sometimes even precipitating severe mental disorder. Most people's coping capacities lie somewhere between these extremes.

Basic behavioral science research on the nature of and variations in personality is illuminating the sources of these differences and revealing ways to bolster people's ability to deal with life's difficult and painful aspects. Studies to date suggest that there is no single source of resilience or vulnerability. Rather, many interacting factors come into play. They include not only individual genetic predispositions, which express themselves in enduring aspects of temperament, personality, and intelligence, but also qualities such as social skills and self-esteem. These, in turn, are shaped by a variety of environmental influences. For example, through their early experience and bonding with parents or other caregivers, children form expectations that shape later social experiences. These processes of social learning often influence self-esteem and behavior. Advances in behavioral science research are revealing sources of vulnerability and strength in several areas of investigation. Some key findings are described in this chapter.

Personality Psychology

Some people are shy, others extroverted; some are chronically anxious, others confident. These relatively stable personality traits set people apart as individuals and are the focus of fundamental questions being explored by personality researchers. Such questions include: How, and to what degree, are people psychologically different from one another? To what extent are those differences rooted in genetics, early experience, or current situational factors? What is the basic nature of those differences—that is, how do people differ in perceiving, constructing, and responding to their social environments? How do those differences affect mental health? How modifiable are per-

sonality traits? To what extent do these traits override the situation in determining a person's actions?

Personality, Psychopathology, and Resilience

Basic research on personality differences and their long-term behavioral expression is shedding light on important public health issues such as drug abuse and depression. One prospective longitudinal study, for example, revealed that some adolescent drug abusers had a distinctive personality pattern that often was identifiable in early childhood. In research more than a decade earlier, these troubled adolescents had been described as restless, fidgety, emotionally changeable, disobedient, nervous, domineering, immature under stress, and overreactive to frustration.

The same study revealed that the personalities of boys and girls who became severely depressed in late adolescence differed considerably during childhood. The boys had been described as undercontrolled, unsocialized, and aggressive; by contrast, the girls were seen as overcontrolled, oversocialized, shy, and introspective. Findings such as these suggest not only that depression has deep roots in early life, but that early personality patterns as-

Editor's note. This article is Chapter 2 of a report issued by the National Advisory Mental Health Council (NAMHC) in response to the request of the Senate Appropriations Committee for a national plan for behavioral science research. The report "Basic Behavioral Science Research for Mental Health: A National Investment," was written by the NIMH Basic Behavioral Science Task Force of the NAMHC, which consisted of 52 eminent behavioral and social scientists in the field and staff of the Division of Neuroscience and Behavioral Science of the National Institute of Mental Health (NIMH). The introductory and concluding sections of the report were printed in the July 1995 issue of the *American Psychologist*; an appendix listing the members of the task force and the NAMHC is attached to that article.

Chapters 3–7 of the report will appear serially in the *American Psychologist's* 1996 issues. Their titles are as follows: *3* Perception, Attention, Learning, and Memory; *4* Thought and Communication; *5* Social Influence and Social Cognition; *6* Family Processes and Social Networks; and *7* Sociocultural and Environmental Processes.

Author's note. To obtain the full report "Basic Behavioral Science Research for Mental Health: A National Investment," write to the Behavioral, Cognitive & Social Sciences Research Branch, National Institute of Mental Health, Room IIC-16, 5600 Fishers Lane, Rockville, MD 20857. Electronic mail should be addressed to BEHAVSCI@HELIX.NIMH.GOV.

sociated with later depression differ in important ways for males and females.

These differences may reflect the interaction of personality variables with the contrasting pressures society imposes upon males and females; it encourages males to be assertive risk takers but discourages such behavior in females. As a result, the undercontrolled young man and the overcontrolled young woman may be most at risk for later depression. When an already undercontrolled young man is encouraged to engage in risky behavior, his impulsivity may result in many negative experiences that contribute to depression. When an already overcontrolled young woman is cautioned to avoid risk, she may withdraw so much from the social world and its rewards that she, too, eventually experiences depression.

Understanding what can go wrong in personality development is essential; equally important is discovering what can go right—which personality traits contribute to psychological resilience. Research suggests, not surprisingly, that young girls who have been sexually abused usually suffer from lowered self-esteem, an impaired sense of control and competence, and increased negative emotions—all indicative of poor mental health. However, certain personality traits serve to lessen the ravages of abuse. An abused girl who can rationalize, explain, and comprehend what has happened to her and what she can do about it may thereby be able to maintain her feelings of competence. She may even take steps to end the abuse. While researchers continue to seek ways to understand and prevent child abuse, other research on "resilient" children is now focusing on ways to foster and strengthen those personality traits that help children grow up to be psychologically well adjusted, even after the severe trauma of rape.

An important conclusion from recent research is that personality patterns can change for the better under certain circumstances. For example, although patterns of antisocial, deviant, and even criminal behavior have been found to be remarkably stable from childhood through adult life, entering into a satisfying occupation and enriching personal relationships during early adulthood can break this pattern and greatly decrease the chances that deviant behavior will continue. Intervention programs are needed that build on these encouraging findings.

Personality research is helping us understand and prevent both physical and mental disorders. Increasingly, behavioral scientists are finding relationships between certain personality traits and particular diseases. The linkage between heart disease and the "Type A" personality—characterized by hostility, time urgency, impatience, anxiety, and a sense of stress—has received extensive study. One well-established finding is that people who are hostile (the "lethal" component of Type A behavior) are especially prone to develop heart disease. Most important, even when more conventional risk factors, such as heredity, obesity, diet, and smoking are accounted for, hostility is demonstrably a risk factor for heart disease.

Moreover, an additional link between hostility and heart disease seems to be through a behavioral pathway. Hostile people are particularly prone to behave in ways that jeopardize their health, such as smoking, drinking, and general risk taking.

However, results of an intervention study for Type A people recovering from a heart attack suggest that their destructive personality traits can be changed. In that study, the effects of standard cardiac counseling alone were compared with a combination of cardiac counseling and counseling focused on reducing hostility and other components of Type A behavior. Compared with the control group, those receiving the combined counseling showed reductions in Type A behavior and an almost 50% reduction in subsequent heart attacks during a 4½-year period.

Personality as Traits

Many researchers regard personality as a relatively stable collection of individual traits. In recent years, behavioral scientists have come to agree that most variation in personality across individuals can be accounted for by differences in five broad factors, sometimes called the "Big Five" personality traits:

- EXTRAVERSION: Gregarious, daring, and enthusiastic
- AGREEABLENESS: Affectionate, empathic, and cooperative
- CONSCIENTIOUSNESS: Organized, dependable, and prompt
- EMOTIONAL STABILITY (vs. NEUROTICISM): Unexcitable, without envy or nervousness
- INTELLECT: Intelligent, imaginative, and worldly

Research on personality shows that a given individual's overall profile on the Big Five traits is relatively stable, consistent, and predictable over many years. However, many individual characteristics change over time and social settings.

Emotional inhibition: Repression. One well-studied personality trait (the inverse of extraversion) is known as *emotional inhibition*. It includes both suppression (the conscious inhibition of emotion and thought) and repression (the unconscious inhibition of emotion and thought). At the turn of the century, Freud proposed that inappropriate repression was one of the most important contributors to mental illness. Only within the past 15 years have the measurement techniques become available to examine this phenomenon scientifically.

Through such advances, it is now possible to identify and study systematically the mental health of people who characteristically and unconsciously inhibit their emotions. These individuals, termed *repressors,* have been found to score low on personality test measures of distress but high on measures of defensiveness (i.e., unconscious self-protection). Although repressors do not seem anxious, their high defensiveness scores suggest that they experience distress but are either unaware of it or are denying it.

When repressors are exposed experimentally to a variety of emotion-producing situations, such as reading threatening phrases, they report feeling very little emotion, yet they display large physiological reactions, such as changes

Personality Processes

The Big Five personality taxonomy makes it possible to categorize people into a small number of types. It also helps to summarize broad differences among individuals in their overall behavioral tendencies. However, current personality research is also identifying the psychological factors that underlie distinctive individual characteristics. These factors include the concepts people use for interpreting their experiences and their enduring expectancies about what they can and cannot do effectively. Research is also clarifying how such factors influence not only what people experience and feel, but also the effectiveness and adaptiveness (or maladaptiveness) of their behavior as they try to cope with life tasks and stressors.

For example, research has clarified the mental strategies that underlie "will power"—regulating one's own behavior to achieve difficult long-term goals. These strategies are the basic components of a well-functioning personality. Even at age four, children differ appreciably in the strategies they use; some can delay gratification to reach a long-term goal, but others cannot. Following the development of these children into young adulthood shows that these early self-regulatory skills foreshadow other indices of coping and personal efficacy, such as school success and college entrance, years later.

in heart rate, blood pressure, and skin conductance. People who are not repressors have similar physiological responses when they are exposed to emotion-provoking situations and told to inhibit any overt display of emotion. Thus, the very act of suppressing overt emotional expression—whether done unconsciously or consciously—apparently causes a sharp rise in cardiac reactions.

Research clearly demonstrates that habitually inhibiting emotions can pose a threat to physical and mental health. For example, repressors have an increased risk for impaired immune system functioning and a wide variety of health problems, including atherosclerotic disease in men, cancer, and psychologically linked symptoms such as headaches and abdominal pain. Experimental studies have also shown that writing or talking about traumatic experiences and expressing one's emotional reactions may enhance physical health and immune function and lessen use of medical services.

Emotional inhibition: Shyness.
The roots of individual personality and physiological reactivity can be seen very early in development in the characteristic patterns of sociability, activity, and emotionality known as *temperament*. These patterns include being active and outgoing or shy and inhibited. Researchers have discovered that 15% to 20% of all infants are shy. When faced with novel or moderately challenging situations, these inhibited infants and children typically escape rapidly, cover, and hide. If forced to remain in the situation, they reveal higher levels of stress hormones and sympathetic nervous system activity than do uninhibited children.

Although some people who are shy as children spontaneously become less inhibited as they grow up (and others seek change through counseling), others seem to retain this temperamental trait throughout their life span. Most shy individuals appear to lead relatively normal lives, but severely inhibited children have an increased risk of developing various childhood and adolescent anxiety and depressive disorders. They are also more likely to have close relatives who have been diagnosed as clinically anxious or depressed, suggesting that there may be a familial basis for shyness.

Dramatic individual differences in temperament have been found among monkeys and apes as well as among humans; these differences may be a general characteristic of many animal species. Rhesus monkeys exhibit many of the physiological and behavioral patterns seen in humans, and as with human children, 15% to 20% of monkey infants are shy. These patterns, which are seen in the first weeks of life, appear to be relatively stable from infancy to old age.

Animal studies using selective breeding and biological parent/foster parent comparisons indicate that although shyness is partly heritable, it can be modified substantially by early social experiences. In monkeys, inadequate mothering, for example, seems to exaggerate both behavioral and physiological features of shyness. Rearing by especially nurturant "foster mothers" encourages the infants to overcome their natural shyness. Not only do they cope with the usual stressors more effectively than do inhibited peers raised by their own mothers (demonstrating more exploration away from their foster mothers and less behavioral disturbance during weaning), they even surpass their uninhibited peers! Moreover, inhibited female monkey infants who receive this increased nurturance later develop into especially nurturant mothers themselves.

Sources of Personality Variation
Behavioral Genetics

What is the source of individual differences in personality traits? Are they determined solely by genes, or are they molded solely by the environment? During the past two decades, behavioral genetics research on the heritability of personality traits has shown that neither extreme is correct. Studies of twins, adoptees, and ordinary families have demonstrated that genetic factors only moderately influence individual differences in most personality dimensions and that environmental factors are also important.

When the approaches of behavioral genetics and developmental psychology are combined, some novel findings emerge. For example, longitudinal studies of childhood temperament and early adult personality strongly suggest that personality stability over time stems more from genetic factors than from environmental constancy.

However, other studies suggest that genetic influences are dynamic—being activated at different times in life. For example, researchers have recently discovered that in newborns, individual differences in temperamental patterns such as activity level and irritability do not appear to be influenced by genes. Yet genes may influence these very same temperamental characteristics later in development. Scientists are now trying to understand how dynamic gene expression across the life span influences behavioral continuity and change.

Other issues currently under investigation concern genetic analyses of features of social life once considered to be "obviously" environmental in origin, such as divorce. Research suggests that many presumably social experiences can, in fact, be influenced by genes, which probably act indirectly through their influence on personality. Investigators have noted, for example, that pairs of identical twins are more likely to have the same divorce status than are pairs of fraternal twins, suggesting that genes may contribute to personality characteristics compatible with marriage.

To understand the mechanisms that link biology and behavior, more research is needed on the biological ties between genes and personality. Progress in this area will be helped by findings of the National Institutes of Health Human Genome Project, an ambitious attempt to map human chromosomes and to discover genes relevant to health and disease.

Experience and Environment

Ironically, studies in behavioral genetics provide strong evidence that the environment is influential in shaping behavior. Such research has shown, for example, that identical twins often have very different personalities, suggesting that environmental factors play a considerable role in personality differences.

Another important finding is that many key environmental influences on personality are experienced differently by the various members of a given family. For example, for siblings growing up in the same family, the shared family environment seems less important for some aspects of intelligence and personality than is the unshared part (e.g., a child's unique relationships with parents and peers). Thus, a fruitful research direction would be to assess directly how the psychological environment varies across time and across individuals within a family unit.

Psychologists have found that many behaviors, such as aggression and altruism, that are often attributed to people's personality traits are also influenced by situational and environmental factors. For example, children who observe aggressive behavior on television are more likely to behave aggressively toward others, especially when frustrated, than those who have not seen such models. In one long-term study, researchers found that—after controlling for baseline aggressiveness, intelligence, and socioeconomic status—the extent of viewing of TV violence at age 8 predicted the seriousness of criminal acts committed by age 30. This finding may have important implications for understanding and preventing the transmission of violence.

Attachment

Some of the most fruitful explorations of the close personal relationships moderating vulnerability and resilience involve studies of attachment, the special bond between infants and their caregivers. This relationship evolved both to meet the newborn infant's obvious physical needs and to provide security in the face of a complex and potentially dangerous environment.

When an attachment relationship is effective, the primary caregiver provides both a secure base for the infant's explorations and a safe haven the infant can return to when frightened, tired, or hungry. The more secure infants feel, the more willing they are to explore and interact with the physical and social world. As their physical and mental capabilities grow, infants increasingly direct their attention and activities away from their primary caregiver—as long as that person remains available in times of emotional need. When such emotional needs are not met, fear prevails and interferes with infants' exploration and interaction with others.

Consequences of Attachment Quality

Researchers have found that differences in infant attachment security, as measured on a brief behavioral test, can have long-term mental and emotional consequences. For example, children classified as securely attached to a caregiver during infancy will later approach problem-solving tasks more positively and with greater persistence than will children who are insecurely attached. Children with secure attachments also are likely to be more empathic, compliant, unconflicted, and generally competent in their relationships with adults and peers. Children with insecure attachments tend to have trouble relating to other people because their behavior is often either hostile and distant or overly dependent. These tendencies may extend into adolescence and adulthood, influencing significant social relationships as well as basic attitudes toward life.

Some researchers have hypothesized that the success or failure of an infant's early attachments establishes a cluster of expectations (internal working models) that set the stage for future social relationships. Some insecure and unhappy infants, for example, may have difficulty learning to deal with and trust others later in life.

An intriguing body of evidence from both human and animal studies suggests that early attachment relationships may be especially significant for later development of parenting skills. Some people who were neglected or abused as infants seem to have problems caring for their own children.

Other findings suggest a link between early attachment difficulties and risk for adolescent and adult mental health problems. Better understanding of the nature and extent of such links should aid in developing effective treatment and prevention programs for mental illness throughout the life span.

Researchers have been keenly interested in determining how differences in early attachment security arise. A key factor, according to the most widely accepted view, is the caregiver's sensitivity and responsiveness in interacting with the infant.

Building on such findings, one study found that, after a year of infant–parent psychotherapy, mothers of infants who had been anxiously attached showed greater empathy and were more interactive than untreated mothers of similar toddlers. The therapy focused on alleviating the mothers' psychological conflicts about their children and on providing individually tailored information about child development. While the therapeutic effects need further validation, in this study the children of the treated mothers became more sociable and less angry than the children of the untreated mothers.

Insecure Attachment and Psychopathology

How much does the quality of attachment in infancy contribute to later personality and mental illness? Answers should become much clearer in the next decade, as researchers piece together a developmental story that is still unfolding. Data are just now being collected on the psychological health of a group of adolescents and young adults whose attachment relationships were studied 15 to 20 years earlier during infancy.

There is already evidence that severely disordered early attachment relationships (as seen in cases of physical or sexual abuse and neglect) are significant risk factors for certain mental disorders, such as borderline personality disorder. Research suggests that insecure attachment in infancy predicts childhood problems such as difficulties in peer relationships. Compared with children who were insecurely attached to their mothers at 12 months, those with more secure attachments at that age were more resilient and cooperative, happier, and more likely to be leaders at three and six years.

The long-term mental health impact of various types of disturbed attachment has been examined through longitudinal studies of families affected by depression or maltreatment as well as families receiving therapy focused on low social support and certain behavior problems in children. Some major findings from these studies follow:

- Among children from low-income families, those who had been insecurely attached during infancy were, at ages 10 to 11 and 14 to 15, more dependent, less socially competent, and had lower self-esteem and resilience than those who had been securely attached. This study demonstrates striking consistency in individual adaptation between infancy and adolescence.
- Preschool children who had been maltreated by their parents were more likely than their peers to develop "fragmented attachments" in which, in a parent's presence, the child displays disorganized or disoriented behavior.
- Two-year-old children of mothers with major depression or manic–depressive illness had a higher proportion of insecure attachments than children of mothers with minor depression or no mood disorder. At five years of age, the children with disorganized attachment showed marked increases in hostility toward peers. Parental depression may contribute to children's insecure attachment through its influence on aspects of parent–child interaction and on broader aspects of the child-rearing environment, such as the psychological unavailability of the parent during periods of depression.

Self-Concept and Self-Esteem

Like the concept of attachment, the concept of self is central to our understanding of mental health and illness. In fact, attachment disturbances often contribute to poor self-concepts. Progress in several research areas (e.g., self-

regulation and perception of control, self-efficacy, and cultural influences on the self and identity) depends on understanding the factors and processes that regulate and occasionally distort people's self-concept. Research is clarifying how self-concept develops and functions normally, how the process can go awry, and what can be done to prevent or treat many forms of psychopathology (including borderline personality and sociopathy) that may be linked to disturbances of self-concept.

Researchers have concluded that, contrary to intuition, individuals have not one but several views of their selves, encompassing many domains of life, such as scholastic ability, physical appearance and romantic appeal, job competence, and adequacy as a provider. Further, self-esteem is often affected by social comparisons.

Studies in the academic domain have revealed, for example, that the self-esteem of African American students is higher in schools where they are numerically in the majority than where they are in the minority. The social comparison process that presumably contributes to these findings should be studied directly, however, since such research results have major implications for intervention. Other studies have revealed that, beginning in junior high school, many young girls reportedly feel inadequate in math, science, athletic ability, and physical appearance—a distressing set of findings that also deserves further exploration.

Researchers have discovered as well that, among a group of unpopular children, those deemed aggressive had relatively inflated self-esteem and overestimated their attributes and abilities in academics, appearance, athletics, and peer relations. By contrast, unpopular and withdrawn children had more negative—but accurate—conceptions of themselves, perhaps acknowledging their own deficiencies in social relationships. Children who are aggressive and unpopular are at increased risk for behavioral problems and juvenile delinquency, whereas withdrawn, unpopular children appear to sustain their low self-esteem through late childhood and are at increased risk for depression.

Pathways to Self-Esteem

Self-esteem begins to develop early in life; it has been studied in children as young as seven years of age. As children learn to describe aspects of themselves, such as their physical attributes, abilities, and preferences, they also begin to evaluate them. Becoming self-aware was once regarded as a uniformly positive step in development—a path to insight about one's own character. Recent research suggests that excessive self-awareness can interfere with concentration on important tasks in school, job, and social relationships and may undermine self-esteem. Indeed, overly harsh self-evaluation appears to be one cause of depression and suicidal behavior. Further study is needed of the boundaries between positive self-awareness, which can provide insights and promote healthy change, and negative self-consciousness, which can interfere with one's development.

Research findings have refuted the idea that a person's level of self-esteem is established in early childhood and remains stable throughout life. In many individuals, self-esteem changes dramatically over time. Long-term studies reveal that major transitions (e.g., marriage, parenthood, and job loss or promotion) are likely to provoke changes in self-esteem.

During the transition into junior high school, high school, or college, for example, the self-esteem of many students plummets. Some of them no longer feel competent scholastically (although they still value academic excellence), and others fail to gain the support of their new peer group. Still other students may respond to a school transition with enhanced self-esteem; they feel more competent in domains they value or they find themselves in a very supportive peer group.

The relationship of ethnicity and culture to self-esteem is complex. While one's ethnicity per se bears no natural relation to one's self-esteem, psychological factors associated with experience as a member of a particular ethnic or cultural group will influence self-esteem. However, across various ethnic populations, the same factors enhance children's self-esteem: their abilities in activities such as sports or academics that their culture values and the social support and approval of significant others.

Contributors to Low Self-Esteem

Low self-esteem plays an important role in mental illnesses. Research on self-esteem is beginning to explain interpersonal factors that lead people to devalue themselves, to become depressed, and even to consider suicide. Such factors include their assessments of their physical appearance, the behavior of parents and other caregivers, and the school environment.

Judgments of physical appearance. Beginning in preschool and continuing into middle age, people's evaluations of their physical appearance are inextricably linked to their self-esteem. Indeed, physical appearance is all-important, even in specific situations where one might expect other attributes—such as intelligence in a learning-disabled group—to be paramount. Cultural and media messages about the importance of good looks as a measure of self-worth appear to contribute strongly to our excessive valuation of physical appearance. People whose self-esteem depends on their appearance and who seek to reach standards of attractiveness (especially for women) that are virtually unattainable are vulnerable to low self-esteem, which in turn may contribute to the life-threatening eating disorders associated with slenderness, namely bulimia and anorexia nervosa.

Research has uncovered important individual differences in the links between self-esteem and assessments of attractiveness. Beginning at age four, some children's self-esteem depends on their view of how they look, while for others self-esteem is independent of appearance. The former orientation has been shown to be particularly pernicious for girls; as a group, they report more dissatisfaction with their appearance and more depressed mood than girls with the latter orientation. Greater knowledge about the factors underlying these different perspectives on the self should aid in encouraging young people to adopt standards for self-worth that are less superficial and less threatening to mental health.

Child-rearing practices. The behavior of parents and other caregivers also influences the early development of self-esteem. Recent studies reveal that children of depressed mothers in particular are at risk for low self-esteem; depressed mood; and lack of energy to engage in activities that foster physical, intellectual, and social development. However, more must be learned about which specific aspects of the parent–child relationship, in addition to genetic factors, contribute to these effects.

School environment. A new line of research indicates how changes in the school environment influence self-esteem and motivation for learning. As children move from elementary to middle, junior, and high school, the school environment becomes increasingly more competitive and impersonal. In addition, growing emphasis is placed on social comparisons and scholastic ability.

The negative impact of this environment is most serious as students enter junior high school. Just as children are becoming more self-conscious, the emphasis on social comparison escalates, leading many students with lesser abilities to notice their deficiencies and possibly become "turned off" to school. Similarly, just as adolescents are trying to develop greater autonomy from their parents—and therefore need other adults to support their self-esteem—attention from teachers becomes less abundant, less personal, and more focused on the students' academic performance. These findings suggest that broader intervention efforts in schools, communities, and institutions outside the family may encourage a more positive self-concept in children and adolescents.

The finding that many women have a diminished sense of self-esteem compared with men invites further study of the social and other factors that contribute to this important difference. For example, in one long-term study, researchers found that during the adolescent years, self-esteem tends to increase in boys and decrease in girls. In another study, conducted at an all-women's college that became coeducational, women's self-esteem levels decreased after men were admitted. Following the men's arrival, the women also participated less in class discussions and showed less interest in the academic subject matter of their classes.

Such findings call for more research on how environments, including coeducational and same-sex school settings, influence and alter self-esteem. Since not all students are negatively affected by entering junior high, researchers may be able to reliably identify those whose self-esteem decreases, determine what factors and circumstances contribute to that outcome, and discover how to prevent that loss.

Research Directions

Important directions for future research on vulnerability and resilience include the following:

- Research has revealed that low self-esteem plays a powerful role in depression and eating disorders. Future research should explore the developmental pathways leading to low self-esteem and its maintenance. These pathways include comparisons to others in scholastic, athletic, social, and physical appearance domains. Self-esteem is also affected by specific socialization processes transmitted by parents, peers, schools, and the media. This is a vital research priority given the fact that low self-esteem is associated with self-destructive actions and antisocial behaviors.

- Considerable research suggests that complex relations exist among coping strategies, ethnicity, and culture. More research is needed to clarify different cultural orientations and define those cultural strengths that maintain a solid sense of self among members of ethnic minority groups, collectively and individually.
- Personality assessment can be useful in determining possible antecedents of mental illness as well as the outcomes of interventions intended to improve mental health. Future research in personality evaluation should move beyond the use of self-report questionnaires to the more frequent inclusion of judgments by other informants and observations of behavior in natural settings and in laboratory settings that can provide concurrent psychophysiological recordings. Such research will have practical applications in the prediction and diagnosis of psychopathological behavior.
- More precise theories of personality and more sophisticated and broadly based assessment tools must be developed to follow for extended periods individuals with specific personality patterns. Such studies can reveal how, when, and under what circumstances these patterns lead to harmful life outcomes and develop into mental disorders.
- Severe early problems in the emotional attachment between infant and caregiver create increased risk for certain mental disorders, such as borderline personality disorder, as well as impaired peer relations. Future studies of attachment need to examine in more detail both stability and change in parent–child attachment relationships. In addition, because, as their social network expands, children form attachments to siblings, friends, grandparents, day care personnel, and teachers, the developmental impact of these understudied aspects of attachment also requires examination.
- Confirmed connections between parental depression and disordered parent–child attachment raise the possibility that a mentally disturbed caregiver influences many aspects of the child-rearing environment. Future research should explore the possible contributions of other major life stressors, such as parental divorce and severe medical illness, to emerging attachment security.

REFERENCES

Block, J. (1993). Studying personality the long way. In D. Funder, R. Parke, C. Tomlinson-Keasey, & K. Widaman (Eds.), *Studying lives through time: Personality and development*. Washington, DC: American Psychological Association.

Dunn, J. (1993). *Young children's close relationships: Beyond attachment*. Newbury Park, CA: Sage Publications.

Kagan, J. (1989). *Unstable ideas: Temperament, cognition, and self*. Cambridge, MA: Harvard University Press.

Loehlin, J. C. (1992). *Genes and environment in personality development*. Newbury Park, CA: Sage Publications.

Plomin, R. (1990). *Nature and nurture: An introduction to human behavioral genetics*. Pacific Grove, CA: Brooks/Cole.

Sampson, R. J., & Laub, J. H., II (1993). *Crime in the making: Pathways and turning points through life*. Cambridge, MA: Harvard University Press.

Werner, E. E., & Smith, R. S. (1992). *Overcoming the odds: High-risk children from birth to adulthood*. Ithaca, NY: Cornell University Press.

Insanity Pleas Fail a Lot of Defendants As Fear of Crime Rises

RICHARD B. SCHMITT

Staff Reporter of THE WALL STREET JOURNAL

Brian McMonagle, a Philadelphia criminal-defense lawyer, no longer has delusions about the insanity defense.

A few years ago, he thought he had a good shot at using it successfully in a murder case. His client had a history of schizophrenia, had been confined to a psychiatric hospital and considered his victim—an insurance executive on a lunch break—a neo-Nazi hit man.

But the jury returned a guilty verdict, and the client was sentenced to life in prison without the possibility of parole. "It was clear that mental illness was the reason he committed the crime," Mr. McMonagle says, adding, "I'm glad I don't make a living out of winning insanity cases."

In recent years, the insanity defense has veered far from the stereotype of guilty people literally getting away with murder, as legislators, prosecutors and juries have grown impatient with violent crime. Over the past decade or so, some states have rewritten their insanity laws to severely limit the availability of the defense, and a handful have abolished it outright.

Some Pending Cases

Today, the insanity defense is on trial again. Lawyers for John du Pont, the wealthy heir, indicate they will use it in connection with the shooting death of Olympic wrestler David Schultz—thus putting Pennsylvania's tough law to possibly its biggest test.

The insanity defense also is planned in the case of Mark Bechard, his attorney says. Mr. Bechard, a mental patient who has been hospitalized more than a dozen times, has been charged in the bludgeoning deaths of two nuns last month in Waterville, Maine. And in Dedham, Mass., the insanity defense has been raised in the trial of John Salvi, charged with the 1994 murder of two abortion-clinic workers.

To critics, such cases raise anew the prospect of clever—and rich or well-connected—defendants feigning illness to beat the rap for horrible crimes.

Unjust Convictions Feared

But some doctors and prisoner-rights advocates contend that because of the weakening of the insanity defense, some sick people are convicted unjustly. Fred Berlin, a Johns Hopkins University psychiatrist and prison consultant for the state of Maryland, notes cases of inmates whose illnesses were never raised at trial.

"We want to be careful not to allow someone to escape responsibility for their actions by mistakenly labeling them mentally ill," he says. "But nobody thinks to worry about people who may be impaired and who slip through the cracks and have their lives taken away from them."

Defense lawyers complain of a chipping away of a bedrock legal principle. "The whole moral authority of our criminal law is that we only punish people who are bad, who did something intentionally, and that is what is at the bottom of the insanity defense," says Harvey Silverglate, a Boston lawyer. "The idea of getting rid of it makes a lot of people uncomfortable."

Major Paradox

Paradoxically, many defense lawyers believe, the more insane the crime, the less likely that the defense will succeed, no matter what the defendant's mental problems. In the case of Jeffrey Dahmer, the jury never reached the issue of insanity because it believed he wasn't suffering from any mental disease, a conclusion that suggests the serial murderer was "just a normal guy misbehaving," says Dr. Berlin, who testified for the defense and finds the guilty verdict "troublesome." Mr. Dahmer, a necrophiliac who murdered and dismembered 17 men and boys, was himself murdered in prison.

But prosecutors and judges note the narrow scope of the insanity defense. "People can act for a crazy reason and still be legally sane" because they knew what they were doing was wrong and intended to kill, explains Ronald Tochterman, a Superior Court judge in Sacramento, Calif. Years ago, he successfully prosecuted a man known as the Vampire Killer, who drank his victims' blood. "There was no question he was severely mentally ill," Mr. Tochterman says. "It was truly an awful, shocking, grisly case. But I knew, under the legal test, he was sane."

The idea that certain mentally disturbed people shouldn't be held accountable for crimes has been debated for ages. A strict version of the insanity defense, an inability to distinguish right from wrong, originated in early Victorian England after a Scottish woodturner, Daniel M'Naghten, was acquitted in the killing of an aide to the prime minister. In the U.S., such concern coalesced with John Hinckley's 1982 acquittal on insanity grounds in the assassination attempt on President Reagan. Two years later, Congress responded with the "Insanity Defense Reform Act," and many states soon followed suit.

Because the legal test for insanity focuses on the defendant's mental state at the time of the alleged crime, seriously ill people whose delusions come and go are still likely to be convicted. And the threshold is even lower for people to be considered "competent" to stand trial; prosecutors need show only that defendants understand the charges and can assist their lawyers in their own defense.

But the new laws weaken the defense even more. For example, many states eliminated a part of it intended for people so mentally ill they can't control their impulses. In most places the test has boiled down to the old standard of whether a defendant can distinguish right from wrong.

"We were leaving to psychiatrists the ultimate question of criminal accountability," says Lynn Thomas, solicitor gen-

Reprinted with permission from the *Wall Street Journal*, February 29, 1996, pp. A1, A8. © 1996 by Dow Jones & Company, Inc. All rights reserved worldwide.

eral of Idaho, one of the states that abolished the defense. Idaho still allows limited evidence of mental illness in the sentencing phase of trials, but according to Mr. Thomas, "that is such a rare occurrence, it hardly even counts."

A study by Policy Research Associates, a Delmar, N.Y., think tank, shows that, nationwide, the insanity defense is raised in only about 1% of felony indictments and succeeds in only a small fraction of those, mostly where prosecutors have conceded the issue before trial. In Seattle, "There hasn't been a jury verdict of insanity in a murder case for at least 15 or 20 years," Lenell Nussbaum, a defense lawyer, says.

Some Questionable Cases

Even so, the defense still raises eyebrows. Just last year, a Massachusetts psychiatrist tried to convince a jury that a psychotic delusion was the reason he massively overbilled insurance plans, including Medicare. (The jury didn't buy it.) Even proponents of the defense say the acquittal by reason of insanity of Lorena Bobbitt, the Virginia woman who cut off her husband's penis, was going a bit far.

Defense lawyers still raise the insanity defense along with a jumble of other mental woes—syndromes relating to child and spousal abuse and even socioeconomic factors—in seeking reduced charges or lenient sentences. Joyce David, a Brooklyn lawyer, says she used the insanity defense to drum up sympathy for a man accused of stabbing the Rev. Al Sharpton. The man was convicted of assault and illegal weapons possession but was acquitted on charges of attempted murder. "I probably use the insanity defense more than any attorney I know," Ms. David says, even though juries often reject it.

Such cases are hit or miss. The defendant in a 1993 Washington state case—the first in the country that recognized child abuse as a possible defense to murder—eventually pleaded guilty to manslaughter. The Menendez brothers are being retried in Los Angeles after a 1994 mistrial in their murder case sparked national debate over the so-called abuse excuse.

The attention such cases get is misleading, says Richard Bonnie, an expert at the University of Virginia law school. "If anything, there is a hardening public attitude, not a forgiving one," he says.

The Legal Result

Today, the true legacy of the narrower laws, from procedural devices to newfangled verdicts that enhance the odds of conviction, is becoming clear.

Mr. McMonagle's client, for example, was convicted under a Pennsylvania law that allows juries to find defendants "guilty but mentally ill." Such verdicts give a judge the authority to order a defendant to get psychiatric treatment and then serve out the full sentence like any other prisoner. Mr. McMonagle's client is still hospitalized.

Proponents of such verdicts, which are allowed in about a dozen states, say they are compassionate because they increase the likelihood that a defendant will receive some care. Critics contend that they merely ensure hard time—or worse—for people who otherwise might be acquitted. An Indiana court saw no reason why persons found guilty but mentally ill couldn't still receive the death penalty.

Defendants are finding the tables turned against them in other ways. The federal rule changes now put the burden on the defense to prove insanity by clear and convincing evidence. Previously, the defense only had to raise the insanity issue, and the prosecution then had to prove otherwise beyond a reasonable doubt. The difficulty of that task was considered a crucial reason Mr. Hinckley was acquitted and sent to a psychiatric hospital.

Last year, the case of another would-be presidential assassin, Francisco Martin Duran, showed the difference the new rules make: He was sentenced to 40 years in prison for spraying the White House with bullets. The change in federal law "has cast into a net some people who really are not criminally responsible," asserts A. J. Kramer, the public defender who represented Mr. Duran, who allegedly suffered from hallucinations and voices inside his head and reported seeing an evil mist hanging over the White House before he emptied a 30-round clip.

Uninformed Jury

Juries' fear that acquittal would someday let murders and other violent offenders walk the streets has hardly been allayed by some recent court rulings. In 1994, the U.S. Supreme Court held that juries needn't be told that people acquitted by reason of insanity will probably be confined to psy-

chiatric hospitals for years. The case involved Terry Lee Shannon, who tried to commit suicide after being stopped by police and was charged with illegally carrying a handgun. His lawyer, T. R. Trout, says jurors might have viewed him more sympathetically if they had known that if he were found not guilty by reason of insanity, he probably would have been hospitalized until no longer considered a threat to himself or society. Instead, they sent him to prison for 15 years.

In the du Pont case, of course it is hard to tell what may happen. On the one hand, the accused man was a man who heard voices, called himself the Dalai Lama and barreled around his suburban-Philadelphia estate in a tank. On the other hand, the prosecution has hired Park Dietz, a Newport Beach, Calif., forensic psychiatrist who helped make the case against Mr. Dahmer as well as Joel Rifkin, the Long Island, N.Y., landscaper who a few years ago admitted killing 17 women and carrying them around in the trunk of his car.

Vincent Fuller, a Washington lawyer who represented Mr. Hinckley, thinks Mr. du Pont has "a very strong" insanity defense. "From what I can see, the man became detached from reality some time ago," Mr. Fuller says. He adds that although wealth doesn't guarantee anything, "the best insanity defenses are done by people with financial resources."

Already, Mr. du Pont's lawyers, including two former Philadelphia-area prosecutors, have hired two psychiatric experts and a team of University of Pennsylvania neurologists, prompting speculation that they are trying to corner the market for local experts.

But Pennsylvania's insanity law may be hard to crack. Despite the bizarre behavior that Mr. du Pont exhibited, all that matters, under the law, is what was going through his head while he shot Mr. Schultz. Possibly dooming Mr. du Pont's chances is the way he fled into his mansion after the shooting and holed up for two days; it suggests to some observers that he may have known his actions were wrong. Court-appointed doctors will examine him and determine whether he is competent to stand trial before he enters his plea at a hearing scheduled for March 21.

Mr. du Pont's lawyers say they haven't decided whether to try an insanity defense but acknowledge it would be a fight. Pennsylvania's insanity law, one of them, William Lamb, says, is "a tough rule."

Anxiety Disorders, Mood Disorders, and Suicide

Standing in front of a class of students preparing to deliver a required presentation, you begin your talk and become keenly aware that your mouth is dry, your voice is quivering, and your body is shaking. A few months later, you receive the distressing news that all of your applications to graduate school were rejected. You think there is a cloud hovering over you, and you find it almost impossible to drag yourself out of bed each day. Experiences like these suggest that many of us have had some of the symptoms of anxiety and mood disorders. These disorders account for a large percentage of individuals who are diagnosed with mental problems.

Large-scale epidemiological surveys provide needed information about the prevalence of mental disorders. One of the most distressing anxiety disorders is panic disorder; its victims often believe that they are having a heart attack. A recent survey has shown that an occasional panic attack is not uncommon. Moreover, we now know that a significant number of panic disorder cases occur without agoraphobia. The social and demographic characteristics of these disorders are helping investigators to understand and treat this debilitating and frightening disorder.

Post-traumatic stress disorder is one of the most terrifying of all disorders, and it usually begins after someone experiences an extremely terrifying event (as in war or a plane crash). The major feature of this disorder is reliving the experience, especially through intrusive and disturbing flashbacks and dreams. But why do the symptoms continue well after the frightening event has passed? Researchers are finding that post-traumatic stress disorder may result from changes in the brain, especially those associated with the stress hormones.

Depression has been called the common cold of mental disorders. The symptoms are familiar to many of us, but their severity may not be familiar. A mild to moderate form of depression often occurs along with other disorders and medical problems. Major depression is a seriously debilitating disorder; as a result, researchers have identified a number of possible causes and continue to evaluate an array of possible treatments.

Convincing evidence indicates that artists and writers have a higher rate of manic-depressive (bipolar) disorder than the general population. Although most artists and writers do not have mood disorders, the association between mood disorders and creativity is intriguing to researchers and therapists. The manic high may provide the energy, exuberance, and flow of ideas that lead to creative products. However, this creative productivity comes with a price. For example, one of the most serious consequences of mood disorders is suicide. A number of demographic, psychological, and social factors are related to suicide rates. For example, suicide rates increase with age. Most people who commit suicide have some type of mental or emotional disorder.

Looking Ahead: Challenge Questions

Anxiety and mood disorders are quite common in the general population. What symptoms do they share? Do we need separate categories for anxiety and mood disorders?

Why are some people prone to altered hormonal levels when faced with serious stressors, whereas other people are not affected?

How are some people with bipolar disorder able to channel their energy into creative productions?

How can depression be more effectively identified and treated?

What social changes might be instituted to reduce the rate of suicide?

UNIT 2

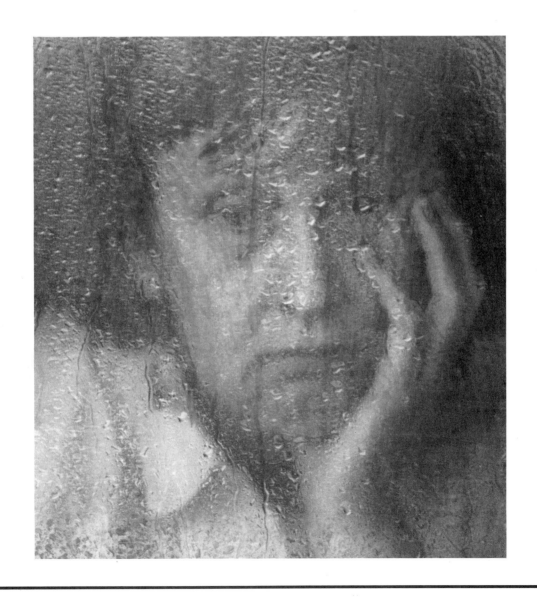

Panic and Panic Disorder in the United States

William W. Eaton, Ph.D., Ronald C. Kessler, Ph.D.,
Hans Ulrich Wittchen, Ph.D., and William J. Magee, M.S.

Objective: The goal of this study was to determine the prevalence of DSM-III-R panic disorder and to describe its correlates. Method: The study was part of the National Comorbidity Survey, the first psychiatric epidemiologic survey of the entire U.S. population and the first to use DSM-III-R criteria for diagnosis. The 8,098 survey respondents, aged 15–54 years, were given the Composite International Diagnostic Interview. For this report, the data on panic were analyzed, and from them the prevalence of panic disorder and related experiences in the U.S. population was estimated. Results: About 15% of the survey respondents reported the occurrence of a panic attack over their lifetimes, and 3% reported a panic attack in the preceding month. About 1% met the DSM-III-R criteria for panic disorder in the month preceding the interview. Panic attacks and panic disorder had a bimodal age distribution and were associated with female sex and lower educational achievement. Fifty percent of the survey respondents with panic disorder reported no symptoms of agoraphobia. The pattern of prevalence of correlated sociodemographic factors was similar for persons with panic attacks, panic disorder, and panic disorder with agoraphobia. Conclusions: There appears to be no obvious threshold for the diagnosis of panic disorder. Panic disorder and agoraphobia, although highly comorbid, also occur separately.

Epidemiologic research on panic has burgeoned in the last decade for two principal reasons. First, although the particular phenomenology of panic had been described before the turn of the century and was recognized by Freud (1), it was not until 1980, in DSM-III, that panic was codified as a stand-alone diagnosis. Second, more recent research on the biochemical stimulation of panic, its association with cardiovascular problems, possible neuroanatomical locations, and distinctive physiological concomitants has stimulated intense interest (2–4).

The first major epidemiologic study to incorporate the DSM-III criteria for panic disorder was the National Institute of Mental Health Epidemiologic Catchment Area (ECA) program (5). There have been publications from that study on the prevalence (6, 7) and

incidence (8, 9) of panic, as well as on the strong tendency of persons suffering panic attacks to use health services (10). The ECA study sample originated from the populations of five metropolitan areas in the United States. Panic is rare enough to require a large sample for estimation of prevalence, and there have been no studies in the United States similar to the ECA study since 1980. Wittchen and Essau (11) reviewed several studies since 1980 that were conducted outside the United States.

In this article we present epidemiologic data on panic and panic disorder from the National Comorbidity Survey, the first epidemiologic study to represent the population of the entire continental United States. The age range of the population targeted for the survey was 15–54 years, which is an advantage over the ECA study's range of 18 years or older, since it is suspected that persons aged 15–18 years have high rates of panic (12). The National Comorbidity Survey is also the first study to use the operational criteria of DSM-III-R, published in 1987.

METHOD

The method used in the National Comorbidity Survey has been described in detail in an initial paper by Kessler et al. (13). We discuss briefly here the details important for understanding the results presented in this article.

Received Jan. 14, 1993; revision received June 1, 1993; accepted July 14, 1993. From the National Comorbidity Survey, Institute for Social Research, University of Michigan, Ann Arbor. Address reprint requests to Dr. Eaton, The Johns Hopkins University School of Hygiene and Public Health, Department of Mental Hygiene, 624 North Broadway, Rm. 880, Baltimore, MD 21205.

This report was supported by NIMH grant MH-47447 to Dr. Eaton and NIMH grant MH-00507 to Dr. Kessler. The National Comorbidity Study was supported by grant MH-46376 from the Alcohol, Drug Abuse, and Mental Health Administration and by the W.T. Grant Foundation.

From *The American Journal of Psychiatry,* March 1994, pp. 413-420. © 1994 by the American Psychiatric Association. Reprinted by permission.

TABLE 1. Estimated Prevalence of DSM-III-R Panic Disorder and Related Experiences in the U.S. Population Based on Data From Respondents in the National Comorbidity Survey

| | Preceding Month | | | | | | Lifetime (N=8,098) | |
| | Men (N=3,847) | | Women (N=4,251) | | Total Sample (N=8,098) | | | |
Item	%	SE	%	SE	%	SE	%	SE
Fearful spell	2.2	0.3	5.3	0.4	3.8	0.3	15.6	0.7
Intense fearful spell	1.7	0.2	4.4	0.4	3.0	0.3	11.3	0.5
Panic attack	1.1	0.2	3.2	0.3	2.2	0.2	7.3	0.3
Recurrent panic attacks	0.9	0.2	2.5	0.3	1.7	0.2	4.2	0.3
Panic disorder	0.8	0.2	2.0	0.3	1.5	0.2	3.5	0.3
With criterion of four panic attacks in 1 month	0.8	0.2	1.7	0.2	1.3	0.2	2.3	0.2
With expanded criterion including 1 month of worry about panic attacks	0.0	0.0	0.3	0.2	0.2	0.1	1.2	0.2
Panic disorder with agoraphobia	0.4	0.2	1.0	0.3	0.7	0.1	1.5	0.2

The National Comorbidity Survey was a nationwide survey designed to produce data on the prevalence of psychiatric morbidity and comorbidity. It was based on a stratified, multistage, area probability sample of the noninstitutionalized civilian population in the 48 coterminous states. The 8,098 respondents who participated in the survey were selected with the use of probability methods from 1,205 block-level segments. The segments were created within a stratified sample of small areas in 172 counties in 34 states throughout the United States. The survey was administered by the staff of the Survey Research Center at the University of Michigan. The period of data collection in the field was between Sept. 14, 1990, and Feb. 6, 1992. The 8,098 respondents represent a response rate of 82.4%.

The National Comorbidity Survey included a supplemental sample of students living in campus group housing. This is an important design feature because there are approximately two million such students in the United States who would be unrepresented in a more conventional household survey that excludes persons living in institutional housing (14). Also, a survey was carried out in a group of 353 persons who did not respond initially to the main survey and who were offered a substantial financial incentive to complete a short form of the diagnostic interview. Significantly higher rates of both lifetime and current psychiatric disorders were found among these initial nonrespondents than among respondents in the main survey. This result is consistent with previous research showing that persons with histories of psychiatric disorders are underrepresented in cross-sectional surveys (15) as well as in reinterview surveys (16) of the general population. The survey data were weighted to compensate for the nonrespondents. The data were also weighted to adjust for variation in probabilities of selection across households and within households, and they were then stratified by means of an iterative procedure to approximate the national population distributions of the cross-classification of age, sex, race/ethnicity, marital status, education, living arrangement, locality, and region as defined by the 1989 U.S. National Health Interview Survey (17).

DSM-III-R diagnoses were based on a modified version of the Composite International Diagnostic Interview (18), a structured diagnostic interview developed in a collaborative project of the World Health Organization (WHO) and the U.S. Alcohol, Drug Abuse, and Mental Health Administration (19) to foster epidemiologic and cross-cultural comparative research by producing diagnoses according to the definitions and criteria of DSM-III-R and the diagnostic criteria for research of ICD-10. Diagnoses were generated with the use of the Composite International Diagnostic Interview diagnostic program (20).

The architecture of the Composite International Diagnostic Interview is based on the National Institute of Mental Health Diagnostic Interview Schedule (DIS) (21). The subsets of interview questions and probes used to make DSM-III-R diagnoses are very similar to those in the DIS. This means that the reliability and validity of the Composite International Diagnostic Interview sections that remained unchanged after the introduction of DSM-III-R might reasonably be assumed to be similar to those found in the validation of DIS version III (21–23).

More direct evidence for the reliability and validity of the Composite International Diagnostic Interview comes from a series of international studies that were in large part conducted as part of the WHO field trials of the instrument. The field trials documented good acceptance and cultural appropriateness of the interview (24, 25), excellent interrater reliability (26, 27), and good test-retest reliability (28, 29) for all diagnoses. The good validity of the Composite International Diagnostic Interview has been documented in relation to concordance with clinical diagnoses (30–33), and it compares well in procedural validity with the Present State Examination (30, 34, 35). The interrater reliability kappa for the instrument was 0.92 for panic disorder and 0.94 for panic attacks (26). The test-retest reliability kappa value was 0.86 for panic disorder (36) and 0.69 for panic attacks (30).

The National Comorbidity Survey was administered by the field staff of the Survey Research Center at the University of Michigan. The 158 interviewers working on the survey had an average of 5 years' prior interviewing experience with the Survey Research Center. The interviewers underwent a 7-day study-specific training program for the survey. During the phase of data collection, each regional supervisor was responsible for roughly 15 interviewers. Supervisors reviewed and edited all interviews and recontacted a subgroup of respondents throughout the study to verify responses and guarantee high-quality interviewer performance.

The data analyzed in this report were weighted to adjust for differential probabilities of selection and lack of response by using the total U.S. population in the target age range. Estimates of standard errors of proportions were obtained with the Taylor series linearization method (37). The PSRATIO program in OSIRIS (38) was used to make these calculations. Estimates of standard errors of logistic regression coefficients were obtained with the method of balanced repeated replication (39). The LOGISTIC program in SAS (40) was used to make individual calculations for each of 44 replicate subsamples.

RESULTS

Panic and Panic Disorder

Panic disorder relates to a range of fearful experiences. The threshold at which a disorder is considered to be present is operationally defined in DSM-III-R but is still a subject of interest to researchers and clinicians (41). Therefore, table 1 presents prevalence rates at several thresholds. The thresholds are operationally defined in the interview situation by positive answers to successive questions that are increasingly specific. Over 15% of the respondents reported a sudden experience of unexplained fear, or a *fearful spell*, over their lifetimes, and 3.8% reported this occurrence in the month before the interview. The concept of fearful spell used here corresponds to the concept of "simple panic attack" in the ECA analyses. The 15.6% lifetime prevalence we report is higher than the ECA report of 9.7% (7) and higher than that of the equivalent "limited symptom attack" in the work of Katerndahl and Realini (41), who found a lifetime prevalence of 11.6% in a household-residing sample in San Antonio, Texas.

Following a positive response to an initial question in the diagnostic interview about a spell of unexplained fear are questions about 13 specific psychophysiological symptoms. A large majority of the persons reporting a sudden, unexplained fearful spell also reported experiencing four or more accompanying psychophysiological symptoms. The combination of a fearful spell with four or more symptoms is labeled an *intense fearful spell* in table 1; it occurred in more than 11% of the respondents over their lifetimes and in 3% during the month preceding the interview. The estimated lifetime prevalence is higher than the ECA study prevalence of 5.9% for the equivalent "intense panic attack" (7). The study in San Antonio reported a lifetime prevalence for "panic attack," the closest equivalent to our intense fearful spell, of 9.4% (41).

Panic attacks are defined here as unexplained fearful spells, with accompanying psychophysiological symptoms, that are limited to only a few minutes' duration—sometimes called the "crescendo" quality. About half of the respondents with fearful spells had one or more panic attacks, for an estimated lifetime prevalence of over 7% and a prevalence in the preceding month of 2.2% (table 1). The crescendo quality was added to the criteria for panic disorder in DSM-III-R. The question operationalizing this additional criterion was not asked in the ECA surveys, and there are therefore no data on panic attacks that are strictly comparable. This is an important addition from the epidemiologic point of view, in that it excludes about one-third of respondents with intense fearful spells from the possibility of receiving a diagnosis of panic disorder (i.e., the prevalence for the preceding month in table 1 drops from 3.0% to 2.2%).

To qualify for a diagnosis of panic disorder, an individual must experience *recurrent panic attacks,* that is, have four or more attacks within 1 month or have a period of 1 month during which he or she is constantly worried about the possibility of an attack. More than half of the respondents who experienced a panic attack met this criterion of recurrence (estimated lifetime prevalence=4.2%, prevalence in preceding month=1.7%) (table 1). Panic attacks are unpleasant but perhaps tolerable if isolated; the recurrence criterion brings the phenomenon to the level of clinical importance.

As in the earlier ECA data (9), most individuals with recurrent panic attacks had at least one spontaneous attack (that is, an attack in the absence of an identifiable phobic object or situation). These individuals met the criteria for *panic disorder.* The estimated lifetime prevalence of 3.5% is more than double the ECA study prevalence of 1.6% (7) but close to the San Antonio study lifetime prevalence of 3.8% (41); the point prevalence of 1.5% is three times as high as the ECA study prevalence of 0.5%.

A major addition to the criteria for panic disorder in DSM-III-R was the expansion of the recurrence criterion to include a month of worry about panic, even if there are fewer than four panic attacks during the month. To examine the possibility that this expansion may have unduly enlarged the estimated prevalence of panic disorder in this study, table 1 shows the prevalence of panic disorder when the expanded criterion is omitted and in the next row shows the effect of adding this operational definition of recurrence. The two rows add up to the prevalence of DSM-III-R panic disorder. For prevalence in the preceding month, the effect is trivial for men and very small (less than 20% increase in rate) for women. For lifetime prevalence, the effect is to increase the rate by about 50%.

A subcategory of panic disorder is *panic disorder with agoraphobia,* for persons meeting the criteria for panic disorder who also have agoraphobia. This is a particularly severe form of the disorder, with lower prevalence. Over their lifetimes, an estimated 1.5% of the population meet the criteria for panic disorder with agoraphobia, and 0.7% have this disorder within the preceding month. Respondents with panic disorder were divided into those with and those without agoraphobia, with no residual or undefined category. Thus, the reader can estimate the prevalence of panic disorder without agoraphobia by subtraction of the percentages in table 1 (e.g., for women, the one-month prevalence of panic disorder without agoraphobia is 2.0% – 1.0%, or 1.0%). In terms of cases, there were 274 respondents who met the criteria for panic disorder, of whom 106 (less than 40%) also met the criteria for agoraphobia. Of the 168 persons with panic disorder without agoraphobia, 30 responded positively to the initial questions on agoraphobic fears but were not sufficiently embarrassed or incapacitated to meet the criteria for the diagnosis of agoraphobia. Thus, 138 (50%) of the 274 persons with panic disorder reported no evidence of agoraphobia.

The panic disorder diagnosis requires the occurrence of at least one panic attack outside a situation of phobic stimulus, but the diagnosis of phobia requires avoidance above a threshold of severity. There was a small group of respondents who had intense and recurrent panic attacks, always in a phobic situation, but who did not meet diagnostic criteria of avoidance. These individuals are diagnostic anomalies, because they present with many symptoms but meet criteria for no disorder. They are excluded from the diagnosis of panic disorder by the situational nature of their attacks and excluded from the diagnosis of phobic disorder by not meeting avoidance criteria. This group was not included in the analyses presented here, and the issue will be dealt with in a later report.

Age and Sex

The estimated prevalence of panic and related experiences is very different in men and women, as shown

TABLE 2. Estimated Prevalence of Panic Attacks and Panic Disorder in the U.S. Population, by Age Groups, in the Preceding Month Based on Data From Respondents in the National Comorbidity Survey

Diagnosis/Age Group	Men (N=3,847)		Women (N=4,251)		Total Sample (N=8,098)	
	%	SE	%	SE	%	SE
Panic attacks						
15–24 years	1.7	0.6	3.5	0.8	2.6	0.5
25–34 years	0.9	0.4	2.9	0.6	2.0	0.3
35–44 years	1.1	0.3	3.6	0.9	2.3	0.4
45–54 years	0.9	0.4	3.0	1.1	1.9	0.6
Total group	1.1	0.2	3.2	0.3	2.2	0.2
Panic disorder						
15–24 years	1.3	0.6	2.5	0.7	1.9	0.5
25–34 years	0.7	0.4	1.6	0.5	1.2	0.3
35–44 years	0.6	0.2	2.1	0.8	1.3	0.4
45–54 years	0.7	0.4	2.2	1.0	1.4	0.6
Total group	0.8	0.2	2.0	0.2	1.5	0.2

in the left-hand columns of table 1. In every category of increasing severity, the prevalence is slightly more than twice as great among women as among men, as in the ECA results (6). There appears to be no particular threshold where male-female differences are especially stronger or weaker.

The total estimated prevalence of panic attacks and panic disorder is greatest in persons aged 15–24 years, as shown in table 2, but the association with age seems to differ by sex. For men, the highest rates for both panic attacks and panic disorder are in the lowest age group, but for women, the peak is in the age range of 35–44 for attacks. The pattern for both men and women suggests a bimodality revealed in fine-grained analyses of the ECA data on age at onset (42). The pattern in table 2 suggests that the early mode for panic disorder is in the same age range of 15–24 for both men and women and that the later mode occurs in the age range of 45–54 for both men and women.

Tests of the significance of the overall relation of sex and age to panic attacks and panic disorder were conducted using the log-linear model and the likelihood ratio chi-square. The effects of sex were strong and significant ($\chi^2=26.65$, df=1, p<0.005, and $\chi^2=12.47$, df=1, p<0.005, for panic attacks and panic disorder, respectively). However, the relation of age to panic attacks or panic disorder and the Age by Sex interaction were not significant. Thus, the pattern of bimodality of age of panic attacks and disorder, while intriguing, is not statistically significant in these data.

The relation of age to panic disorder may differ by race/ethnicity, although the data (not shown) are quite sparse. Tests of the overall relation of age, sex, and race/ethnicity to panic attacks and panic disorder were conducted with the likelihood ratio chi-square test. The main effect for race/ethnicity was not significant. For panic disorder and panic disorder with agoraphobia (but not for panic attacks), the Age by Race/Ethnicity interactions were large and significant. The data revealed that for each of the three nonwhite racial/ethnic

categories (black, Hispanic, other), there were no cases in the age range 45–54, leading to prevalence estimates of zero. For the Hispanic and "other" category, there were no cases in the age range 35–44 as well. Thus, for young adults, differences between racial/ethnic groups are trivial; racial/ethnic differences are concentrated in the older age groups.

Correlates of Panic and Panic Disorder

The patterns of association of panic attacks and panic disorder with age, sex, and other sociodemographic variables are shown in table 3. The method of logistic regression was used to produce odds ratios. Each variable in table 3 has a reference group for which the odds ratio is 1.00, and the other numbers in the table show the odds that an individual has had a panic attack or has met the criteria for panic disorder in the preceding month as compared to the reference group. Thus, males are the reference group for the variable "sex," with an odds ratio of 1.00, and in comparison with them, females have 2.89 times the odds for a panic attack and 2.48 times the odds for meeting criteria for panic disorder. In the 95% confidence intervals for odds ratios, when the interval does not include the value of 1.00, as is the case for sex differences in panic attacks and panic disorder, one might describe the relationship as significant at the 0.05 level. The number of cases of panic disorder with agoraphobia was so small (31 cases among 8,098 respondents) that the 95% confidence interval includes 1.00 for almost all predictors.

Table 3 presents crude, not adjusted, odds ratios, even though the technique of logistic regression permits multiple covariates. Adjusted odds ratios are not presented because the adjustment procedure had only trivial effects on the odds ratios.

The odds ratios for age reveal the suggestion of bimodality for panic attacks and panic disorder, as we have discussed. For panic disorder with agoraphobia, the pattern is unimodal, with a peak in the age range of 35–44. The crude odds ratios for race/ethnicity were not significant, as we have said.

Number of years of education produced strong and significant differences in odds for panic attacks, panic disorder, and panic disorder with agoraphobia. Persons with fewer than 12 years of education were more than four times as likely to have a panic attack, more than 10 times as likely to have panic disorder, and more than seven times as likely to have panic disorder with agoraphobia as the reference group with a college education (16 or more years). The pattern is not linear, in that those with some college education have odds similar to the odds of those who finish college, and those who do not complete high school have odds similar to the odds of those who complete high school but obtain no further education.

The strength of the finding for education contrasts markedly with the other variable related to general socioeconomic standing, income. Large differences in income—e.g., less than $20,000 per year versus $70,000

TABLE 3. Population Estimates of Sociodemographic Variables Associated With Panic Attacks, Panic Disorder, and Panic Disorder With Agoraphobia During the Preceding Month Based on Data From 8,098 Respondents in the National Comorbidity Survey

Variable	Panic Attacks (N=136)[a]		Panic Disorder (N=77)[a]		Panic Disorder With Agoraphobia (N=31)[a]	
	Odds Ratio[b]	95% Confidence Interval	Odds Ratio[b]	95% Confidence Interval	Odds Ratio[b]	95% Confidence Interval
Sex						
Female	2.89	1.83–4.54	2.48	1.40–4.39	2.64	0.82–8.49
Male	1.00		1.00		1.00	
Age (years)						
15–24	1.35	0.62–2.92	1.32	0.45–3.90	3.08	0.50–18.94
25–34	1.04	0.45–2.43	0.82	0.24–2.79	3.25	0.59–17.88
35–44	1.21	0.59–2.50	0.93	0.34–2.34	5.11	1.12–23.24
45–54	1.00		1.00		1.00	
Race/ethnicity						
White	0.75	0.34–1.67	1.30	0.21–8.20	0.78	0.05–12.61
Black	0.58	0.19–1.81	0.85	0.08–9.14	0.95	0.02–42.00
Other	0.92	0.16–5.22	1.84	0.12–27.01	1.16	0.04–31.68
Hispanic	1.00		1.00		1.00	
Education (years)						
<12	4.93	2.46–9.86	10.38	2.78–38.69	7.62	1.39–41.72
12	4.73	2.37–9.44	8.55	2.16–33.80	5.76	1.29–25.59
13–15	3.51	1.91–6.46	4.82	1.38–16.87	1.00	
≥16	1.00		1.00		1.00	
Annual income (dollars)						
≥70,000	0.72	0.34–1.54	0.69	0.22–2.17	0.58	0.06–6.06
35,000–69,000	0.60	0.30–1.20	0.51	0.18–1.42	0.54	0.13–2.15
20,000–34,000	0.77	0.39–1.50	0.82	0.32–2.12	0.97	0.17–5.41
<20,000	1.00		1.00		1.00	
Employment						
Student	1.99	1.12–3.55	2.48	1.19–5.16	2.22	0.41–11.93
Housekeeping	3.21	1.05–9.77	2.78	0.51–15.01	0.55	0.17–1.75
Other	1.97	0.94–4.16	1.54	0.63–3.77	1.43	0.40–5.07
Working outside the home	1.00		1.00		1.00	
Marital status						
Married	0.66	0.32–1.36	0.50	0.19–1.31	0.37	0.09–1.44
Never married	0.66	0.32–1.37	0.65	0.26–1.62	0.31	0.05–2.04
Widowed/divorced	1.00		1.00		1.00	
Living arrangement						
With spouse	0.71	0.43–1.16	0.59	0.26–1.34	0.89	0.29–2.69
With parents	0.87	0.39–1.93	0.79	0.31–2.03	0.88	0.16–4.90
Other	0.70	0.34–1.43	0.85	0.26–2.77	1.60	0.22–11.73
Alone	1.00		1.00		1.00	
Religion						
Protestant	0.74	0.43–1.27	0.83	0.44–1.55	2.65	0.88–7.92
Other	0.61	0.29–1.31	0.44	0.15–1.27	1.00	
No preference	0.55	0.26–1.61	0.47	0.10–2.29	1.00	
Catholic	1.00		1.00		2.71	0.91–8.04
Locality						
Metropolitan	1.77	0.94–3.34	1.44	0.66–3.14	1.20	0.38–3.78
Urban	1.52	0.82–2.84	1.33	0.51–3.43	1.21	0.43–3.40
Rural	1.00		1.00		1.00	
Region						
Northeast	1.62	0.92–2.86	1.73	0.74–4.06	1.21	0.14–10.60
Midwest	1.22	0.72–2.08	1.17	0.60–2.29	0.94	0.32–2.78
West	1.32	0.79–2.18	1.06	0.38–2.98	0.48	0.09–2.60
South	1.00		1.00		1.00	

[a]N=number of cases in the group of respondents.
[b]Based on the reference group for each variable with the odds ratio of 1.00.

per year—were associated with trivial and nonsignificant differences in odds ratios.

For other sociodemographic variables, the patterns of association are neither strong nor significant and might have been predicted from the general literature on distress (43). Working people, married persons, and those living with others have a generally lower estimated prevalence of panic than their counterparts. Crude categories of religion have little influence on the prevalence of panic. Persons living in cities appear to have a somewhat greater prevalence of panic, but the result is not stable statistically.

Respondents living in the northeast had a higher prevalence of panic attacks, panic disorder, and panic disorder with agoraphobia than those living in other regions. In a multivariate logistic model including all the variables in table 3 (not shown), the adjusted odds ratio for the northeast was 6.11, with a 95% confidence interval of 1.11–33.56. (This was the only group for which the adjusted odds were importantly different from the crude odds.)

DISCUSSION

This is the first presentation of data on panic attacks and panic disorder in a large sample that is representative of the population of the United States. The prevalence rates based on data from this study are higher than the rates based on the only other comparable data, those from the ECA program. Differences in the samples and the diagnostic conventions preclude close comparison of the two studies, but there are several possible explanations for the higher rates we report from the National Comorbidity Survey: age distribution, order of questions, intensity of probing, and response bias.

The age ranges of the ECA and National Comorbidity Survey samples are different: the National Comorbidity Survey had a lower minimum (15 years, compared to the ECA minimum of 18 years) and no one over the age of 54 (compared to about one-third of the ECA sample who were over the age of 54). Since the prevalence of panic is higher in younger people, the National Comorbidity Survey sample would be expected to have a higher rate. Therefore, we examined the rates of panic disorder in the ECA study within age categories constructed to be as similar as possible to those reported in table 2. In every age category that could be identically constructed, the National Comorbidity Survey prevalence rate was substantially larger than the ECA study rate (e.g., the ECA prevalence of DSM-III panic disorder in the preceding month was 0.68%, 0.73%, and 0.84% in the age ranges 25–34, 35–44, and 45–54 years, respectively). The greatest discrepancy was in the youngest age category, which we could not match exactly (i.e., prevalence of 0.38% for the 18–24 age group in the ECA study, compared with 1.9% in our study). This discrepancy is consistent with other reports of a high prevalence of panic in adolescents (12). The ECA rate for persons over the age of 55 was also much smaller (0.23%) than for younger persons.

Other methodologic differences between the National Comorbidity Survey and the ECA study concern the order of questions, probing, and lack of response. The Composite International Diagnostic Interview was revised for the National Comorbidity Survey to place all stem questions (including the question on the lifetime occurrence of panic attacks) at the beginning of the interview instead of at the beginning of the relevant sections. This placement was based on the judgment that respondents learn, over the course of the interview, that positive responses generate probes that are time-consuming; as a result, respondents increasingly avoid positive responses as the interview progresses. The strategy is to capture the positive response prior to the learned avoidance later in the interview by placing the stem questions at the beginning. A probing strategy developed by Cannell et al. (44, 45) was used in the National Comorbidity Survey, but not the ECA study, to increase the intensity of memory search. Finally, in the

National Comorbidity Survey, a survey of nonrespondents was conducted, and this showed that nonrespondents had higher rates of panic. This response bias was corrected by a weighting procedure. These methodologic differences contributed to the higher rates found in the National Comorbidity Survey as compared with the ECA study. Although the overall prevalence of panic was higher in the National Comorbidity Survey, the patterns of relation to age, sex, and education are roughly similar to those found in the ECA data.

The relation of sociodemographic variables to categories of panic defined by a variety of thresholds reveals no obvious point at which pathology, deviance, or disorder should be considered to be present. The crucial threshold appears to be the occurrence of a simple panic attack, as suggested in earlier analyses of this issue (6).

Less than one-half of the respondents with panic disorder also met criteria for agoraphobia. These results support continuing research on the distinction between the two disorders.

The strong results of the analysis of the data on education are intriguing. In studies of variables related to social class, such as education and income, many overlapping but not well-measured factors come into play. The various social class indicators are not always equally associated with psychopathology, as shown in analyses of schizophrenia (46), distress (47), and, now, panic. The occurrence of panic might well be related to stressful situations in which the individual is at a disadvantage relative to others, such as might be experienced by poor people. On the other hand, panic might also be strongly mediated by cognitive factors involving the appraisal of risk. These cognitive factors are probably more closely measured by level of education than by income. These issues can be fruitfully explored in future research. Since education had a much stronger association with panic than did income, these analyses suggest that appraisal of cognitive factors may be a more fruitful line of research than investigation of the effects of social disadvantage.

ACKNOWLEDGMENTS

The National Comorbidity Survey (Ronald C. Kessler, Principal Investigator) was conducted with the participation of the following collaborating sites and investigators: Addiction Research Foundation (Robin Room); Duke University Medical Center (Dan Blazer, Marvin Swartz); Johns Hopkins University (James Anthony, William Eaton, Philip Leaf); Max Planck Institute of Psychiatry (Hans Ulrich Wittchen); Medical College of Virginia (Kenneth Kendler); University of Michigan (Lloyd Johnston, Ronald C. Kessler); National Institute of Mental Health (Darrel Kirsch, Darrel Regier); New York University (Patrick Shrout); State University of New York at Stony Brook (Evelyn Bromet); University of Toronto (R. Jay Turner); and Washington University School of Medicine (Linda Cottler).

REFERENCES

1. Breier A, Charney DS, Heninger GR: The diagnostic validity of anxiety disorders and their relationship to depressive illness. Am J Psychiatry 1985; 142:787–797
2. Ballenger JC: Biological aspects of panic disorder (editorial). Am J Psychiatry 1986; 143:516–518
3. Woods SW, Charney DS, McPherson CA, Gradman AH, Heninger GR: Situational panic attacks: behavioral, physiologic, and biochemical characterization. Arch Gen Psychiatry 1987; 44: 365–375

4. Gelder MG: Panic disorder: fact or fiction? (editorial). Psychol Med 1989; 19:277–283

5. Eaton WW, Regier DA, Locke BZ, Taube CA: The Epidemiologic Catchment Area Program of the NIMH. Public Health Rep 1981; 96:319–325

6. Von Korff MR, Eaton WW, Keyl PM: The epidemiology of panic attacks and panic disorder: results of three community surveys. Am J Epidemiol 1985; 122:970–981

7. Eaton WW, Dryman A, Weissman MM: Panic and phobia, in Psychiatric Disorders in America: The Epidemiologic Catchment Area Study. Edited by Robins LN, Regier DA. New York, Free Press, 1991

8. Eaton WW, Kramer M, Anthony JC, Dryman A, Shapiro S, Locke BZ: The incidence of specific DIS/DSM-III mental disorders: data from the NIMH Epidemiologic Catchment Area program. Acta Psychiatr Scand 1989; 79:163–178

9. Keyl P, Eaton WW: Risk factors for the onset of panic attacks and panic disorder. Am J Epidemiol 1990; 131:301–311

10. Boyd JH: Use of mental health services for the treatment of panic disorder. Am J Psychiatry 1986; 143:1569–1574

11. Wittchen HU, Essau CA: Epidemiology of anxiety disorders, in Psychiatry 1993. Edited by Michels R. Philadelphia, JB Lippincott (in press)

12. Hayward C, Killen JD, Taylor CB: Panic attacks in young adolescents. Am J Psychiatry 1989; 146:1061–1062

13. Kessler RC, McGonagle KA, Zhao S, Nelson CB, Hughes M, Eshleman S, Wittchen HU, Kendler KS: Lifetime and 12-month prevalence of DSM-III-R psychiatric disorders in the United States: results from the National Comorbidity Survey. Arch Gen Psychiatry (in press)

14. US Bureau of the Census: Statistical Abstract of the United States 1991: The National Data Book. Washington, DC, US Government Printing Office, 1991

15. Allgulander C: Psychoactive drug use in a general population sample, Sweden: correlates with perceived health, psychiatric diagnoses, and mortality in an automated record-linkage study. Am J Public Health 1989; 79:1006–1010

16. Eaton WW, Anthony JC, Tepper S, Dryman A: Psychopathology and attrition in the Epidemiologic Catchment Area study. Am J Epidemiol 1992; 135:1051–1059

17. US Department of Health and Human Services: National Health Interview Survey, 1989 (computer file). Hyattsville, Md, National Center for Health Statistics, 1992

18. World Health Organization: Composite International Diagnostic Interview (CIDI), version 1.0. Geneva, WHO, 1990

19. Robins LN, Wing J, Wittchen HU, Helzer JE, Babor TF, Burke J, Farmer A, Jablenski A, Pickens R, Regier DA, Sartorius N, Towle LH: The Composite International Diagnostic Interview: an epidemiologic instrument suitable for use in conjunction with different diagnostic systems and in different cultures. Arch Gen Psychiatry 1988; 45:1069–1077

20. World Health Organization: Composite International Diagnostic Interview Computer Programs, version 1.1. Geneva, WHO, 1990

21. Robins LN, Helzer JE, Croughan J, Ratcliff KS: The National Institute of Mental Health Diagnostic Interview Schedule: its history, characteristics, and validity. Arch Gen Psychiatry 1981; 38:381–389

22. Robins LN, Helzer JE, Ratcliff KS, Seyfried W: Validity of the Diagnostic Interview Schedule, version II: DSM-III diagnoses. Psychol Med 1982; 12:855–870

23. Anthony JC, Folstein M, Romanoski AJ, Von Korff MR, Nestadt GR, Chahal R, Merchant A, Brown CH, Shapiro S, Kramer M, Gruenberg EM: Comparison of the lay Diagnostic Interview Schedule and a standardized psychiatric diagnosis: experience in eastern Baltimore. Arch Gen Psychiatry 1985; 42:667–675

24. Wittchen HU, Robins LN, Cottler L, participants in the Multicentre WHO/ADAMHA Field Trials: Interrater reliability of the Composite International Diagnostic Interview (CIDI): results from the multicenter WHO/ADAMHA Field Trials (wave I), in Psychiatry: A World Perspective, vol 1: Proceedings of the VIII World Congress of Psychiatry. Edited by Stefanis CN, Rabavilas AD, Soldatos CR. Amsterdam, Elsevier, 1990

25. Cottler LB, Robins LN, Helzer JE: The reliability of the CIDI-SAM: a comprehensive substance abuse interview. Br J Addict 1989; 84:801–814

26. Wittchen HU, Robins LN, Cottler LB, Sartorius N, Burke JD, Regier D, and participants in the Multicentre WHO/ADAMHA Field Trials: Cross-cultural feasibility, reliability and sources of variance of the Composite International Diagnostic Interview (CIDI). Br J Psychiatry 1991; 159:645–653

27. Cottler LB, Robins LN, Grant BF, Blaine J, Towle LH, Wittchen HU, Sartorius N, and participants in the Multicentre WHO/ADAMHA Field Trials: The CIDI-core substance abuse and dependence questions: cross-cultural and nosological issues. Br J Psychiatry 1991; 159:653–658

28. Semler G, Von Cranach M, Wittchen HU (eds): Comparison Between the Composite International Diagnostic Interview and the Present State Examination: Report to the WHO/ADAMHA Task Force on Instrument Development. Rockville, Md, Alcohol, Drug Abuse, and Mental Health Administration, 1987

29. Wacker HR, Battegay R, Mullejans R, Schlosser C: Using the CIDI-C in the general population, in Psychiatry: A World Perspective, vol 1: Proceedings of the VIII World Congress of Psychiatry. Edited by Stefanis CN, Rabavilas AD, Soldatos CR. Amsterdam, Elsevier, 1990

30. Semler G (ed): Reliabilitat und Validitat des Composite International Diagnostic Interview. Inauguraldissertation zur Erlangung des akademischen Grades eines Doktors der Philosophie. Mannheim, Germany, Universitat Mannheim, 1989

31. Spengler P, Wittchen HU: Procedural validity of standardized symptom questions for the assessment of psychotic symptoms: a comparison of the CIDI with two clinical methods. Compr Psychiatry 1989; 29:309–322

32. Janca A, Robins LN, Cottler LB, Early TS: Clinical observation of CIDI assessments: an analysis of the CIDI field trials—wave II at the St Louis site. Br J Psychol 1992; 160:815–818

33. Leitmeyer P (ed): Zur Symptomerfassung mit dem standarisierten Interview CIDI-C in der Allgemeinpraxis. Inauguraldissertation zur Erlangung des medizinischen Doktorgrades fur Klinische Medizin. Mannheim, Germany, Universitat Mannheim, 1990

34. Farmer AE, Katz R, McGuffin P, Bebbington P: A comparison between the Present State Examination and the Composite International Diagnostic Interview. Arch Gen Psychiatry 1987; 44:1064–1068

35. Farmer AE, Jenkins PL, Katz R, Ryder L: Comparison of CATEGO-derived ICD-8 and DSM-III classifications using the Composite International Diagnostic Interview in severely ill subjects. Br J Psychiatry 1991; 158:177–182

36. Semler G, Wittchen HU, Joschke K, Zaudig M, von Geiso T, Kaiser S, von Cranach M, Pfister H: Test-retest reliability of a standardized psychiatric interview (DSI/CIDI). Eur Arch Psychiatry Neurol Sci 1987; 236:214–222

37. Woodruff RS, Causey BD: Computerized method for approximating the variance of a complicated estimate. J Am Statistical Assoc 1976; 71:315–321

38. University of Michigan: OSIRIS VII. Ann Arbor, University of Michigan, Institute for Social Research, 1981

39. Kish L, Frankel MR: Balanced repeated replications for standard errors. J Am Statistical Assoc 1970; 65:1071–1094

40. SAS Introductory Guide, release 6.03. Cary, NC, SAS Institute, 1988

41. Katerndahl DA, Realini JP: Lifetime prevalence of panic states. Am J Psychiatry 1993; 150:246–249

42. Anthony JC, Aboraya A: The epidemiology of selected mental disorders in later life, in Handbook of Mental Health and Aging, 2nd ed. Edited by Birren JE, Sloane RB, Cohen GD. San Diego, Academic Press, 1992

43. Mirowsky J, Ross CE: Social Causes of Psychological Distress. New York, Aldine de Gruyter, 1989

44. Cannell CF, Oksenberg L, Converse JM: Experiments in Interviewing Techniques. Ann Arbor, University of Michigan, Survey Research Center, 1979

45. Cannell CF, Miller PV, Oksenberg L: Research on interviewing techniques, in Sociological Methodology. Edited by Leinhardt S. San Francisco, Jossey-Bass, 1981

46. Eaton WW: Residence, social class, and schizophrenia. J Health Soc Behav 1974; 15:289–299

47. Kessler RC: A disaggregation of the relationship between socioeconomic status and psychological distress. Am Sociological Rev 1982; 47:752–764

MAKING SENSE of Mania & Depression

We all feel moments of gloom or exhilaration on occasion. But few of us truly understand how far off-key the melodies of mood can drift. Here, a leading psychiatrist eloquently recounts two real-life tales of mania and depression—and shows how these disorders are indeed moods apart from our everyday experience.

By Peter C. Whybrow, M.D.

TRY FOR A MOMENT TO IMAGINE a personal world drained of emotion, a world where perspective disappears. Where strangers, friends, and lovers are all held in similar affection, where the events of the day have no obvious priority. There is no guide to deciding which task is most important, which dress to wear, what food to eat. Life is without meaning or motivation.

This colorless state of being is exactly what happens to some victims of melancholic depression, one of the most severe mood disorders. Depression—and its polar opposite, mania—are more than illnesses in the everyday sense of the term. They cannot be understood merely as an aberrant biology that has invaded the brain; for by disturbing the brain the illnesses enter and disturb the *person*—the feelings, behaviors, and beliefs that uniquely identify the individual self. These afflictions invade and change the very core of our being. And the chances are overwhelming that most of us, during our lifetime, will come face to face with mania or depression, seeing them in ourselves or in somebody close to us. It's estimated that in the United States 12 to 15 percent of women and eight to 10 percent of men will struggle with a serious mood disorder during their lifetime.

While in everyday speech the words *mood* and *emotion* are often used interchangeably; it is important to distinguish them. Emotions are usually transient—they con-

stantly respond to our thoughts, activities, and social situations throughout the day. Moods, in contrast, are consistent extensions of emotion over time, sometimes lasting for hours, days, or even months in the case of some forms of depression. Our moods color our experiences and powerfully influence the way we interact. But moods can go wrong. And when they do, they significantly alter our normal behavior, changing the way we relate to the world and even our perception of who we are.

CLAIRE'S STORY. Claire Dubois was such a victim. It was the 1970s, when I was professor of psychiatry at Dartmouth Medical School. Elliot Parker, Claire's husband, had telephoned the hospital desperately worried about his wife, who he suspected had tried to kill herself with an overdose of sleeping pills. The family lived in Montreal, but were in Maine for the Christmas holidays. I agreed to see them that afternoon.

Before me was a handsome woman approaching 50 years of age. She sat mute, eyes cast down, holding her husband's hand without apparent anxiety or even interest in what was going on. In response to my questioning she said very quietly that it was not her intention to kill herself but merely to sleep. She could not cope with daily existence. There was nothing to look forward to and she felt of no value to her family. And she could no longer

From *Psychology Today*, May/June 1997, pp. 34-38, 71-72. Adapted from *A Mood Apart* by Peter C. Whybrow. © 1997 by Peter C. Whybrow. Reprinted by permission of BasicBooks, a division of HarperCollins Publishers, Inc.

concentrate sufficiently to read, which had been her greatest passion.

Claire was describing what psychiatrists call anhedonia. The word literally means "the absence of pleasure," but in its most severe form anhedonia becomes an absence of *feeling*, a blunting of emotion so profound that life itself loses meaning. This lack of feeling is most frequently present in melancholia, which lies on a continuum with depression, extending the illness to its most disabling and frightening form. It is a depression that has taken root and grown independent, distorting and choking the feeling of being alive.

SLIP SLIDING AWAY.

In Claire's mind and in Elliot's, the whole thing began after an automobile accident the winter before. On a snowy evening, while on her way to pick up her children from choir practice, Claire's car had slid off the road and down an embankment. The injuries she sustained were miraculously few but included a concussion from her head hitting the windshield. Despite this good fortune, she began to experience headaches in the weeks following the accident. Her sleep became fragmented, and with this insomnia came increasing fatigue. Eating held little attraction. She was irritable and inattentive, even to her children. By the spring, Claire was complaining of dizzy spells. She was seen by the best specialists in Montreal, but no explanation could be found. In the words of the family doctor, Claire was "a diagnostic puzzle."

The summer months, when she was alone in Maine with her children, brought minor improvement, but with the onset of winter the disabling fatigue and insomnia returned. Claire withdrew to the world of books, turning to Virginia Woolf's novel *The Wave*, for which she had a particular affection. But as the shroud of melancholy fell upon her, she found sustaining her attention increasingly difficult, and a critical moment arrived when Woolf's woven prose could no longer occupy Claire's befuddled mind. Deprived of her last refuge, Claire had only one thought, drawn possibly from her identification with Woolf's own suicide: that the next chapter in Claire's life should be to fall asleep forever. This stream of thought, almost incomprehensible to those who have never experienced the dark vortex of melancholy, is what preoccupied Claire in the hours before she took the sleeping pills that brought her to my attention.

Why should sliding off an icy road have precipitated Claire into this black void of despair? Many things can trigger depression. In a sense it is the common cold of emotional life. In fact, depression can literally follow in the wake of the flu. Just about any trauma or debilitating illness, especially if it lasts a long time and limits physical activity and social interaction, increases our vulnerability to depression. But the roots of serious depression grow slowly over many years and are usually shaped by numerous separate events, which combine in a way unique to the individual. In some, a predisposing shyness is amplified and shaped by adverse circumstance, such as childhood neglect, trauma, or physical illness. In those who experience manic depression, there are also genetic factors that determine the shape and course of the mood disturbance. But even there the environment plays a major role in determining the timing and frequency of illness. So the only way to understand what kindles depression is to know the life story behind it.

THE TRIP THAT WASN'T.

Claire Dubois was born in Paris. Her father was much older than her mother and died of a heart attack shortly after Claire's birth. Her mother remarried when Claire was eight, but drank heavily and was in and out of hospital with various ailments until she died in her late forties. By necessity a solitary child, Claire discovered literature at an early age. Books offered a fairy-tale adaptation to the reality of daily life. Indeed, one of her fondest memories of adolescence was of lying on the floor of her stepfather's study, sipping wine and reading *Madame Bovary*. The other good thing about adolescence was Paris. Within walking distance were all the bookstores and cafes an aspiring young woman of letters could desire. These few blocks of the city became Claire's personal world.

Just before the second World War, Claire left Paris to attend McGill University in Montreal. There, she spent the war years consuming every book she could lay her hands on, and after college she became a freelance editor. When the war ended, she returned to Paris at the invitation of a young man she had met in Canada. He proposed marriage, and Claire accepted. Her new husband offered her a sophisticated life among the city's intellectual elite, but after only 10 months he declared that he wanted a separation. Claire never fathomed the reason for his decision; she assumed he had discovered some deep flaw in her that he would not reveal. After months of turmoil she agreed to a divorce and returned to Montreal to live with her stepsister.

Much saddened by her experience and considering herself a failure, she entered psychoanalysis and her life stabilized. Then, at age 33, Claire married Elliot Parker, a wealthy business associate of her brother-in-law's, and soon the couple had two daughters.

Claire initially valued the marriage. The sadness of her earlier years did not return, although at times she drank rather heavily. With her daughters now growing rapidly, Claire proposed that the family live in Paris for a year. She eagerly planned the year in every detail. "The children were signed up for school. I had rented houses and cars; we had paid deposits," she recalled. "Then, one month before it was to begin, Elliot came home to say that money was tight and it couldn't be done.

"I remember crying for three days. I felt angry but totally impotent. I had no allowance, no money of my own, and absolutely no flexibility." Four months later, Claire slid off the road and into the snowbank.

As Claire and Elliot and I explored her life story together, it was clear to all that the event that kindled her melancholia was not her automobile accident but the devastating disappointment of the canceled return to France. That was where her energy and emotional investment had been placed. She was grieving the loss of the dream of introducing her adolescent daughters to what she herself had loved as an adolescent: the streets and bookshops of Paris, where she had crafted a life for herself out of her lonely childhood.

Elliot Parker loved his wife, but he had not truly understood the emotional trauma of canceling the year in Paris. And it was not Claire's nature to explain how important it was to her or to request an explanation of Elliot's decision. After all, she had never received one from her first husband when he left her. The accident itself further obscured the true nature of her disability: Her restlessness and fatigue were taken as the residue of a nasty physical encounter.

THE LONG ROAD TO RECOVERY.

Those bleak midwinter days marked the nadir of Claire's melancholia. Recovery required a hospital stay, which Claire welcomed, and she soon missed her daughters—a reassuring sign that the anhedonia was cracking. What she found difficult was our insistence that she follow a routine—getting out of bed, showering, eating breakfast with others. These simple things we do everyday were for Claire giant steps, comparable to walking on the moon. But a regular routine and social interaction are essential emotional exercises in any recovery program—calisthenics for the emotional brain. Toward the third week of her hospital stay, as the combination of behavioral treatment and antidepressant drugs took hold, Claire's emotional self showed signs of reawakening.

It was not difficult to imagine how her mother's whirlwind social life and repeated illnesses, plus the early death of her father, had made Claire's young life a chaotic experience, depriving her of the stable attachments from which most of us securely explore the world. She longed for intimacy and considered her isolation a mark of her unworthiness. Such patterns of thinking, common in those who suffer depression, can be shed through psychotherapy, an essential part of the recovery from any depression. Claire and I worked on reorganizing her thinking while she was still in the hospital, and we continued after she returned to Montreal. She was committed to change; each week she employed her commuting time to review the tape of our therapy session. All together, Claire and I worked intensively together for almost two years. It was not all smooth sailing. On more than one occasion, in the face of uncertainty, hopelessness returned, and sometimes Claire succumbed to the anesthetic beckoning of too much wine. But slowly she was able to put aside old patterns of behavior. While it is not the case for all, for Claire Dubois the experience of depression was ultimately one of renewal.

One reason that we do not diagnose depression earlier is that—as in Claire's case—the right questions are not asked. Unfortunately, this state of ignorance is often present as well in the lives of those who experience mania, the colorful and deadly cousin of melancholia.

STEPHAN'S TALE. "In the early stages of mania I feel good—about the world and everybody in it. There's a sense that my life will be full and exciting." Stephan Szabo, elbows on the bar, leaned closer as voices rose from the crush of people around us. We had met years earlier in medical school, and on one of my visits to London he agreed to a few beers at the Lamb and Flag, an old pub in the Covent Garden district. Despite the jostle of the evening crowd, Stephan seemed unperturbed. He was warming to his topic, one he knew well: his experience with manic depression.

"It's a very infectious thing. We all appreciate somebody who's positive and upbeat. Others respond to the energy. People I don't know very well—even people I don't know at all—seem happy around me.

"But the most extraordinary thing is how my thinking changes. Usually I think about what I'm doing with the future in mind; I'm almost a worrier. But in the early manic periods everything focuses upon the present. Suddenly I have the confidence that I can do what I had set out to do. People give me compliments about my insight, my vision. I fit the stereotype of the successful, intelligent male. It's a feeling that can last for days, sometimes weeks, and it's wonderful."

A TERRIBLE TORNADO. I felt fortunate Stephan was willing to talk openly about his experience. A Hungarian refugee, Stephan had begun his medical studies in Budapest before the Russian occupation of 1956, and in London we had studied anatomy together. He was a wry political commentator, an extraordinary chess player, an avowed optimist, and a good friend to all. Everything Stephan did was energetic and purposeful.

Then two years after graduation came his first episode of mania, and during the depression that followed he tried to hang himself. In recovery, Stephan had been quick to blame two unfortunate circumstances: He had been denied entry to the Oxford University graduate program and, worse, his father had committed suicide. Insisting that he was not ill, Stephan refused any long-term treatment and over the next decade suffered several further bouts of illness. When it came to describing mania from the inside, Stephan knew what he was talking about.

He lowered his voice. "As time rolls on, my head speeds up; ideas move so fast they stumble over each other. I begin to think of myself as having special insight, understanding things that others do not. I recognize now that these are warning signs. But typically, at this stage people still seem to enjoy listening to me, as if I have some special wisdom.

"Then at some point I start to believe that because I feel special, maybe I am special. I have never actually thought I was God, but a prophet, yes, that has occurred to me. Later—probably as I cross into psychosis—I sense that I am losing my own will, that others are trying to control me. It's at this stage that I first feel twinges of fear. I become suspicious; there's a vague feeling that I am the victim of some outside force. After that everything becomes a terrifying, confusing slide that is impossible to describe. It's a crescendo—a terrible tornado—that I wish never to experience again."

I asked at what point in the process he considered himself ill.

Stephan smiled. "It's a tough question to answer. I think the 'illness' is there, in muted form, in some of the most successful among us—those leaders and captains of industry who sleep only four hours a night. My father was like that, and so was I in medical school. It's a feeling that you have the ability to live life fully in the present. What's different about mania is that it goes higher until it blows away your judgment. So it is not simple to determine when I go from being normal to being abnormal. Indeed, I'm not sure I know what a 'normal' mood is."

EXHILARATION AND DANGER

I believe there is much truth in Stephan's musing. The experience of hypomania—of early mania—is described by many as comparable to the exhilaration of falling in love. When the extraordinary energy and self-confidence of the condition are harnessed with a natural talent—for leadership or the arts—such states can become the engine of achievement. Cromwell, Napoleon, Lincoln, and Churchill, to name a few, appear to have experienced periods of hypomania and discovered the ability to lead in times when lesser mortals failed. And many artists—Poe, Byron, Van Gogh, Schumann—had periods of hypomania in which they were extraordinarily productive. Handel, for example, is said to have written *The Messiah* in just three weeks, during an episode of exhilaration and inspiration.

But where early mania may be exciting, mania in full flower is confusing and dangerous, seeding violence and even self-destruction. In the United States, a suicide occurs every 20 minutes—some 30,000 people a year. Probably two-thirds are depressed at the time, and of those half will have suffered manic-depression. Indeed, it's been estimated that of every 100 people who suffer manic-depressive illness, at least 15 will eventually take their own lives—a sobering reminder that mood disorders are comparable to many other serious diseases in shortening the life span.

The crush of revelers in the Lamb and Flag had diminished. Stephan had changed little with the years. True, he had less hair, but there before me was the same nodding head, the long neck and square shoulders, the dissecting intellect. Stephan had been lucky. Over the past decade, since he had decided to accept his manic depression as an illness—something he had to control lest it control him—he had done well. Lithium carbonate, a mood stabilizer, had smoothed his path, reducing the malignant manias to manageable form. The rest he had achieved for himself.

While we may aspire to the vivacity of early mania, at the other end of the continuum depression is still commonly considered evidence of failure and a lack of moral fiber. This will not change until we can speak openly about these illnesses and recognize them for what they are: human suffering driven by dysregulation of the emotional brain.

I reflected this to Stephan. He readily agreed. "Look at it this way," he said as we got up from the bar, "things are improving. Twenty years ago neither of us would have dreamed about meeting in a public place to discuss these things. People are interested now because they rec-

> **Emotion is an instrument of self correction—when we are happy or sad, it has meaning. Seeking ways to blot out variation in mood is equivalent to an airline pilot ignoring his navigational devices.**

ognize that mood swings, in one form or another, touch everybody every day. Times really are changing."

I smiled to myself. Here was the Stephan I remembered. He was still in the saddle, still playing chess, and still optimistic. It was a good feeling.

THE MEANING OF MOODS

During a recent interview, I was asked what hope I could give those who suffer the "blues." "In the future," my interviewer asked, "will antidepressants eliminate sadness, just as fluoride has eradicated cavities in our teeth?" The answer is no—antidepressants are not mood elevators in those without depression—but the question is provocative for its cultural framing. In many countries, the pursuit of pleasure has become the socially accepted norm.

Behavioral evolutionists would argue that our increasing intolerance of negative moods perverts the function of emotion. Transient episodes of anxiety, sadness, or elation are part of normal experience, barometers of experience that have been essential to our successful evolution. Emotion is an instrument of social self-correction—when we are happy or sad, it has meaning. Seeking ways to blot out variation in mood is equivalent to the airline pilot ignoring his navigational devices.

Perhaps mania and melancholia endure because they have had survival value. The generative energy of hypomania, it can be argued, is good for the individual and social groups. And perhaps depression is the built-in braking system required to return the behavioral pendulum to its set point after a period of acceleration. Evolutionists have also suggested that depression helps maintain a stable social hierarchy. After the fight for dominance is over, the vanquished withdraws, no longer challenging the leader's authority. Such withdrawal provides a respite for recovery and an opportunity to consider alternatives to further bruising battles.

Thus the swings that mark mania and melancholia are musical variations that play easily but with a tendency to become progressively off-key. For a vulnerable few the adaptive behaviors of social engagement and withdrawal unravel under stress into mania and melancholic depression. These disorders are maladaptive for the individuals who suffer them, but their roots draw upon the same genetic reservoir that has enabled us to be successful social animals.

Several research groups are now searching for genes that increase vulnerability to manic depression or recurrent depression. Will neuroscience and genetics bring wisdom to our understanding of the disorders of mood and spur new treatments for those who suffer these painful afflictions? Or will some members of our society harness genetic insights to sharpen discrimination and drain compassion to deprive and stigmatize? We must remain vigilant, but I am confident that humanity will prevail, for all of us have been touched by these disorders of the emotional self. Mania and melancholia are illnesses with a uniquely human face.

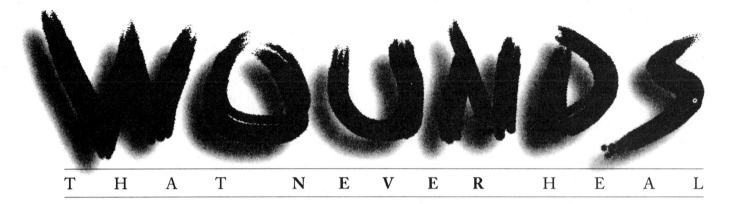

HOW TRAUMA CHANGES YOUR BRAIN

Daniel Goleman

Daniel Goleman is a psychologist who covers behavioral sciences for the New York Times.

"I see a fleeting shadow out of my field of vision. I hear the crunch of leaves or a car whizzing by. And it starts again," says Deb Mulligan, a 38-year-old advertising executive who was brutally raped on the sidewalk in front of her rural Ohio home one moonless fall night eight years ago. "Twigs snapping around me are enough to send me into a sweat. The wind will whip up, and suddenly I can feel the knife cutting into my throat, my blouse being ripped from body. I almost think, just for a moment, that there is blood running down my neck."

Robert Morris was thankful when US-Air flight #5050 pulled away from the LaGuardia airport gate on time. A traveling salesman, Morris closed his eyes in hopes of refreshing himself for the next day's sales presentation. When next he opened them, the wing of his DC-10 was slamming into the East River break wall.

"The fuselage had broken into three pieces, and I was sinking fast," recalls Morris. Handicapped with prostheses below both knees, it took incredible strength for Morris to pull himself to the surface for air. Then the debris hit his body. "I stayed underwater as long

as I could to avoid the smoke. As I came up, a woman grabbed onto my already weighted body and screamed 'don't let me die.' " I hung on to her, and we treaded water together until the helicopters pulled us out."

More than two years later, Morris still gets terrified in situations he can't control. And swimming is out of the question.

Twenty years after he watched a Jeep hit a land mine in Vietnam and explode, Jerry still sees that moment as if he were there. Although he can conjure the image from memory all too easily, it usually comes unbidden. He can be watching a television comedy when suddenly he sees and feels the smoke and thump of the explosion, the Jeep flying into the air, his buddies sprawling—mangled and dead. Every time Jerry relives that scene, he repeats the same, all-too-familiar thoughts: "It shouldn't have happened. We were in a convoy. The road had been checked. I had been on the team that cleared it."

The traumatic scene always brings back the same flood of intense fear, guilt, and sadness—feelings that break through the numbness blanketing Jerry's emotions since that day.

THE SCENE RETURNED AGAIN for him in 1988 as he sat in a room at the West Haven VA Medical Center, just outside New Haven, Connecticut. Jerry, along with 14 other Vietnam veterans, was given a dose of the drug yohimbine—an extract from the bark of a tropical African tree—as part of an experiment to explore the links between traumatic events and changes in brain chemistry.

Jerry, like all the other veterans in the study, was suffering from posttraumatic stress disorder, or PTSD. Common symptoms include flashbacks, jumpiness and irritability, insomnia and nightmares, guilt, and intense panic—often in response to something only vaguely reminiscent of the original trauma. PTSD is not confined to combat veterans; its symptoms can afflict victims of violent crimes, airplane crashes, earthquakes, or other natural disasters—and the number of Americans who experience such trauma in a given year could be in the millions.

Nine of the 15 veterans in the study, including Jerry, experienced a panic attack when the yohimbine became active in their

   Reprinted with permission from *Psychology Today,* January/February 1992, pp. 62-66, 88. © 1992 by Sussex Publishers, Inc.

brain; the six others experienced flashbacks. These particular symptoms occurred along with other PTSD symptoms.

Yohimbine is used clinically to boost the heart rate and blood pressure in patients whose systems are failing. The drug energizes the sympathetic nervous system, causing it to act as though it were confronting an emergency: The heart races, pupils dilate, and blood rushes to the muscles in the "fight or flight" response.

In most people the changes do not induce panic or even discomfort. But Jerry and eight other Vietnam veterans in the study reacted so severely that they felt they were reliving the dangers of the battlefield.

That a drug should trigger most of the posttraumatic stress symptoms in many of those who suffer from the emotional aftermath of trauma is but one of several pieces of evidence pointing to a new and surprising scientific consensus: Traumatic events—even a single episode like Jerry's—can alter the brain's chemistry.

ever there's been a major disaster or war, you see a wave of descriptions of the same problem," says John Krystal, M.D., who directs the West Haven VA Medical Center's Laboratory of Clinical Psychopharmacology.

That consistency in descriptions was one of the early clues that suggested there might be underlying neurological changes resulting from trauma.

"The persistence of these symptoms over several decades was evidence that they were long-lasting changes," Dr. Krystal says.

By the 1980s, evidence from studies with laboratory animals was pointing to a specific site of those brain changes: the noradrenaline system, which rouses the body for emergencies. Trauma seems to reset the brain's noradrenaline system, making people prone to adrenaline surges even decades later. Such surges can be triggered by anything resembling

These changes may also occur in the locus coeruleus, which coordinates the secretion of the hormones adrenaline and noradrenaline, which course through the body to prepare it for an emergency. About 90 percent of the cells for the brain's noradrenaline-controlling system are in the locus coeruleus or connect directly to it. One major trunk of these connections runs to the limbic system, the system that modulates emotions; another runs to the frontal cortex, which involves planning and rational decision-making.

In other words, researchers found a series of neurobiological changes that left PTSD sufferers with an altered brain metabolism—vulnerable to surges of noradrenaline—thus prompting the alarm states.

Millions of Americans endure intense trauma each year, and many of them may be suffering the symptoms of PTSD. A 1989 study of 1,007 men and women ages 21 to 30 who are members of a large health plan in Detroit found 39 percent had at sometime in their lives endured the type of trauma that can lead to PTSD. Of those, one in four developed symptoms of posttraumatic stress, according to Naomi Breslau, Ph.D., a sociologist specializing in psychiatric epidemiology at the Henry Ford Hospital in Detroit.

If Dr. Breslau's findings are confirmed by other studies, as many as one in 10 young Americans is likely to suffer from the symptoms of PTSD at some point in his or her life. Yet only a small number of PTSD victims recognize the source of their trouble, let alone seek help for their symptoms.

Scientists have yet to determine what type of person is most susceptible to PTSD, but one clue may come from dozens of studies with animals that show that suffering severe trauma in early life increases susceptibility to the impact of other trauma later on. One implication is that people who were victims of abuse as children may be among the most vulnerable to PTSD as adults. "Once you're exposed to early kinds of stresses, you're more reactive to later ones," says the VA's Dr. Krystal.

As researchers have focused on trauma and the brain, they have found two other major shifts in addition to the noradrenaline system's increased vulnerability to adrenaline rushes: One of the main changes is in the brain circuit linking the hypothalamus and the pituitary gland. During stress, this circuit triggers the

MORE THAN 20 YEARS AFTER HE WATCHED A JEEP HIT A LAND MINE IN VIETNAM AND EXPLODE, JERRY STILL SEES THAT MOMENT AS IF HE WERE THERE.

"Our hypothesis is that people who have been through intense trauma may never be the same biologically," says Dennis Charney, M.D., chief of clinical neuroscience at the National Center for PTSD, in West Haven, Connecticut, and one of the investigators in the yohimbine study.

Dr. Charney is linked through the center to a network of other researchers who are trying to pierce the mystery of PTSD—with an eye toward developing more effective treatment. A six-year-old project of the Department of Veterans Affairs (formerly known as the Veterans Administration), this network is a unique research-and-treatment consortium located at four VA medical centers. The Clinical Neuroscience Division, in West Haven, is devoted to studying the biology and psychopharmacology of the aftermath of trauma.

Posttraumatic stress disorder is a new name for an old phenomenon. "Whenever

the original trauma—or they can come out of the blue.

One site of changes in the brain has been pinpointed: Yohimbine blocks the action of the alpha-2 receptor located on the noradrenaline neuron. This allows more noradrenaline to be released for a longer time in the brain, which mobilizes the body for an emergency that exists only in the mind.

OTHER STUDIES AT THE WEST Haven research center show that a trauma could sensitize people to adrenaline. In one, John Mason, M.D., found that PTSD sufferers had abnormally high levels of adrenaline and noradrenaline in their bodies. In another, led by Bruce Perry, M.D. (now at the University of Chicago), PTSD patients were found to have 40 percent fewer alpha-2 receptors on their blood platelets.

release of CRF, an important stress hormone. Trauma seems to leave this brain system prone to oversecreting CRF, thereby reacting to emergencies that do not exist in reality.

In a study similar to the yohimbine experiment, PTSD patients at Duke University Medical School were injected with CRF, which typically causes people to secrete large amounts of ACTH, a chemical that then triggers the stress reaction. But the PTSD victims had an unusual response: They secreted far less ACTH. That apparent paradox is actually a sign that the PTSD victims had been secreting ACTH far more than usual before their injection.

"That implies that these patients have been chronically hypersecreting CRF," says Charles Nemeroff, M.D., the psychiatrist at Duke University who did the study. "The reason is that if you continually oversecrete CRF, the brain compensates by decreasing the number of receptors for CRF."

But the decrease in receptors is not steep enough to mute the effects of too much CRF. The CRF oversecretion may explain many of the symptoms of PTSD, compounding the effects of adrenaline surges. "Too much CRF makes you exaggerate the danger of things, so you overreact," says Dr. Nemeroff. "If you have PTSD from battle in the Gulf War and you hear a car backfire in the shopping-mall parking lot, too much CRF floods you with the same feelings you had in combat: You're scared; you start sweating or begin to get the chills."

DR. SHELLEY NEIDERBACH had sped out of Lincoln Center and was still humming Carmen McRae as she crossed the Brooklyn Bridge. She was already thinking about her head hitting the pillow. A longtime resident of New York's friendly Brooklyn Heights, she didn't think much of the two teenagers on the sidewalk near her car as she waited for the light to turn. She wasn't the slightest bit concerned until she found herself staring at a revolver.

"One guy stood in front of the car; another pointed the gun at my head through the window. I only fully comprehended what was going on when he tapped on the window and said, 'Move over or I'll blow your head off.'"

Neiderbach slid over as one of the men took the wheel and the other climbed in behind her, wrapped his left arm around her neck, and held the gun to the back of her head. Then he began repeatedly smashing her skull with the butt of his gun. She thought briefly about giving in to unconsciousness until she noticed that both of her captor's hands were wrapped around the gun, not her. She reached for the door latch and hit the pavement at 30 mph.

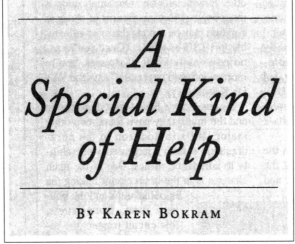

A Special Kind of Help

By Karen Bokram

The legal aspect of her trauma ended rather quickly. A psychotherapist who had spent her first few years treating "garden-variety neurotics," Neiderbach suddenly found herself in the role of victim—and patient. After she wore out the sympathy of friends by telling of the experience again and again (as many victims must), Neiderbach began to deteriorate. There followed a hospitalization for "severe depression and other behaviors" and a search for help that exhausted five therapists.

A full year and a half after the assault, Dr. Pauline Swede told Neiderbach she wasn't sure what Neiderbach had—it was four years before PTSD was named or defined—but she thought she could help her. "I wish I could say something magical about the treatment," says Neiderbach, "but the key was that she understood what I was feeling. She let me sort out my feelings and let me go over it again and again until it was okay."

Neiderbach was on the road to recovery when, one day in 1980, she and a friend surprised a pair of burglars in her house. Neiderbach offered her ring, cash, and watch. Suddenly, one of the thieves put a knife to her throat. "I don't know where I got the calm voice," she says, "but I just looked him in the eye and said, 'Look, you've got enough.' He grabbed the other guy and ran."

She had no trouble picking the burglars from the mug shots. But when she learned that the chances of the thieves—juveniles—getting anything more than probation were slim, she opted not to prosecute. "The thought of some guy being able to get his revenge on me was too much to bear."

The next day Neiderbach had her "first and only vision in life"—the entire organization chart for what would become Crime Victims' Counseling Services. "There were no organizations where people could go and get the kind of support that they needed. All the services were geared to the legal system—you need a coherent witness, after all—but nothing to help victims deal with the trauma. And what we needed was a place where victims could talk to other victims, realize they are not crazy, and go over the incident again and again, if need be, until they reached a level of acceptance and developed a rationale enabling them to resume normal, day-to-day functioning."

A few years later, Neiderbach observed a disturbing trend. "People were being traumatized again by therapists, who simply didn't know how to treat PTSD." Thus Neiderbach launched the International Association of Trauma Counselors last September, to train and accredit those who can help trauma victims.

As for her own recovery, "there is always a little piece hanging around," she says. "I just recently became able to tolerate the New York street-corner window washers. I was driving down the West Side Highway one day, and it was pouring. I looked and saw only a solitary figure in the road. The paranoia started again, but as I drew closer, I noticed a sign in his hands. It said, 'Due to inclement conditions, window washing has been canceled today.' I laughed myself silly. Sometimes that's all it takes."

The third brain area that shows a change in PTSD is the opioid system, which serves to blunt the sensations of pain during an injury. The best-known class of opioids are the endorphins—brain chemicals that, like the other opioids, act at the same site in the brain as opium and, like that drug, dull pain while evoking a pleasant, detached dreaminess.

The changes in the opioid system might account for what are called the "negative" symptoms of PTSD: emotional numbness, apathy, and lack of zest or interest in life. These negative symptoms often alternate with more flamboyant ones such as nightmares or nervousness, or mix with them in a confusing welter of ups and downs.

In a study by the Harvard Medical School and the VA Medical Center in Manchester, New Hampshire, men with PTSD were shown a harrowing ambush scene from the movie *Platoon*—twice. The first time, they were given a placebo; the second time, they got naloxone, a drug which acts to block the opioid system.

"We found that veterans with PTSD who watched the movie after having taken the placebo showed a strong drop in their sensitivity to pain while watching," says Roger Pitman, M.D., an associate professor of psychiatry at Harvard Medical School.

Researchers consider such a drop in pain sensitivity to be a direct clue to the workings of the veterans' opioid systems.

Their drop in pain sensitivity, says Dr. Pitman, was blocked by the naloxone. This suggests that the combat stimulus did activate the opioid system to release endorphins, which blunt pain. That may explain the perplexing accounts of mortally wounded soldiers who have continued to fight on, oblivious to the severity of their wounds: Under extreme duress, the body secretes substances that dull the very sensation of pain.

In PTSD, that response seems to continue, sensitizing the nerve pathways regulating endorphins so that they continue to blunt pain—even in reaction to mere images of battle.

This research is all directed toward one ultimate goal: developing new, more effective treatments for PTSD. The preliminary findings have prompted leading pharmaceutical firms to seek medications that will restore a balance to the brain systems that have been altered by trauma. For instance, medication that would block the action of CRF could compensate for that compound's oversecretion. No such drug currently exists.

While there is no medication yet that is specifically effective for all of the brain changes underlying PTSD, some offer partial relief. One is clonidine; another propranolol. Both have been useful for other disorders where there is an excess of adrenaline. But no drugs relieve all of the PTSD symptoms. And no one sees medication as the sole answer.

"Drugs are an adjunct to psychotherapy," says Matthew Friedman, M.D., executive director of the National Center for PTSD and a professor of psychiatry and pharmacology at Dartmouth.

But, he adds, "many PTSD patients are so anxious they can't even participate in therapy. Drugs that tone down their symptoms can make them able. People feel less driven and anxious and can sleep better with fewer nightmares," Dr. Friedman says. "But there are other problems such as alienation, emotional numbness, guilt, and moral pain that only psychotherapy can help solve."

It's no news that stress can make you sick. But recent research says the solution isn't working less or playing more. It's having someone to confide in.

DON'T FACE STRESS ALONE

By Benedict Carey

THE CURE FOR EXCESSIVE STRESS SHOULD be excessive cash. A fat pile of Microsoft common that provides for limo service and trips to the Seychelles and nannies and someone to vacuum those tumbleweed pet hairs that breed in every corner of the house. Better still, a house that cleans itself. That way we'd have time to read Emerson, learn to play some baroque stringed instrument, and sample Eastern gurus like finger food, accumulating vast reserves of inner peace and healing energy. . . .

We're fooling ourselves. Even stinking rich, most of us would often feel rushed, harassed, afraid that the maid's boyfriend had designs on our Swedish stereo components. We'd lose sleep, lose our tempers, and continue to wonder whether stress was killing us. Not because money doesn't buy

From *Health*, April 1997, pp. 74-76, 78. © 1997 by Time Publishing Ventures, Inc. Reprinted by permission.

Almost half of Americans say they'd rather be alone when they're stressed. Only 18 percent would call a friend.

tranquility; it buys plenty. But because what we call stress is more than the sum of our chores and responsibilities and financial troubles. It's also a state of mind, a way of interpreting the world, a pattern of behavior.

Think of the people you know. There are those who are so consumed with work that they practically sleep with their cell phones, who go wild when they just have to wait in line at the checkout. And then there are those who breeze through the day as pleased as park rangers—despite having deadlines and kids and a broken-down car and charity work and scowling Aunt Agnes living in the spare bedroom. Back in the 1960s cardiologists Ray Rosenman and Meyer Friedman labeled these polar opposites Type A and Type B. They described Type As as "joyless strivers," people who go through life feeling harried, hostile, and combative. Type Bs, by contrast, are unhurried, even tempered, emotionally secure. In person Type As may be twitchy, prone to interrupt, resentful of conversational diversions. Type Bs are as placid as giraffes, well mannered, affectionately patient. In a landmark 1971 study Rosenman and Friedman found that Type As were about twice as likely to develop coronary artery disease as Type Bs. This was the first evidence of a phenomenon that we now take for granted: People consumed by stress often live short lives.

Often. But not always. Some Type As live long and prosper. Some Type Bs succumb to heart attacks before they turn 50. Rosenman and Friedman's theory represented a giant step in tracing a link between disease and personality. But it only partly explained why stress sometimes damages the heart. So the search has been under way to discover a more specific connection between personality and illness. In the past decade findings in fields as seemingly unrelated as sociology and immunology have begun to converge on a surprising answer. Of course it matters if your life is a high-wire act of clamoring demands and pressing deadlines. And yes, it does make a difference whether you're angry or retiring, effusive or shy, belligerent or thoughtful. But what really matters appears to be something much simpler: whether you have someone in your life who's emotionally on call, who's willing to sit up late and hear your complaints.

HUMAN EMOTIONS ARE a messy affair, fleeting, contradictory, and as hard to define as human beings themselves. So it's no wonder researchers have found themselves groping around the dim and convoluted catacombs of personality, trying to locate the core of the trouble with Type As. Some suspect the real villain may be a specific trait such as hostility, cynicism, or self-centeredness. And indeed, all of these characteristics are prevalent in many people who develop coronary disease. But none has proved terribly useful for predicting who will get sick. The search has been a little like being fitted for glasses: Lens two looks clearer than lens one at first, but then you're not so sure. Still, something's there, all right, and several studies conducted in the late eighties and early nineties have finally brought its ghostly shape into focus.

"If you look across all of these studies for a pattern," says psychologist Margaret Chesney, who has spent the past 20 years doing precisely that, "you see that the hostility questionnaires and the Type A interview and all the other measures—they're all picking up the same thing. It's this person who's often suspicious; who sees people as being in their way; who, when they meet someone new, asks, 'What do you do? Where did you go to school?'—not to make a connection but to assess the competition."

More details emerged in 1989 when psychologists Jerry Suls and Choi Wan of the State University of New York at Albany reviewed the Type A research to look for a common thread. They concentrated on stud-

and fear associated with the garden-variety neurotic. These are the sort of people who need counseling but consider therapists overpriced palm-readers. "The picture we're getting is of someone who has deep problems but doesn't admit them," says Suls. "So there are a couple of possibilities here. Either they're in denial. Or they really don't have rich inner lives. They never really think about these things."

They aren't Oprah Winfrey fans, in short. They're happy enough talking about work, fashion, sports—anything but the mushy personal stuff. "If you confront them with that," says Suls, "they get angry. They blow up." As one researcher puts it, "They never let their guard down. If you come close, they wonder, What is this person after?" Spare me the advice, Sigmund, can't you see I'm busy?

This evidence, admittedly raw, is still the subject of much debate, but it has even the most authoritative, skeptical, hard-line figures in the field talking like late-night radio shrinks. Just listen to founding father Rosenman, who has guarded the Type A franchise like a hawk, staring down dozens of psychologists whose work he deemed soft or flawed. "After 40 years of observing and treating thousands of patients, and doing all of the studies, I believe that what's underneath the inappropriate competitiveness of Type As is a deep-seated insecurity. I never would have said that before, but I keep coming back to it. It's different from anxiety in the usual sense, because Type As are not people who retreat. They constantly compete because it helps them suppress the insecurity they're afraid others will sense.

"If I felt this way, how would I cover it up? I'd distract myself, go faster and faster, and win over everybody else. I'd look at everyone as a threat, because they might expose me."

Avoiding exposure inevitably means avoiding close relationships. The person

The people most vulnerable to stress are those who are emotionally isolated. They might have the biggest Rolodex, but they're alone.

ies whose authors had performed general psychological profiles as well as Type A assessments. As a rule, general psych profiles ask directly about fears, insecurities, childhood traumas, and so on, while the Type A diagnosis focuses on how pressured a person feels and how pleasantly he or she answers aggressive questions.

Suls and Wan had suspected that Type A behavior would be associated with emotional distress. But they found something strange. The Type As did show strains of insecurity and emotional isolation—but none of the anxiety

Rosenman is describing has friends, sure, but no genuine confidants, no one who's allowed so much as a whiff of frailty. That's why many researchers now believe that the symptom most common among those vulnerable to stress is emotional isolation. As Chesney puts it, "These people might have the biggest Rolodex, but they're alone. They're busy looking for more connections, charming more people. When they feel isolated they get busy. It's a defense mechanism."

According to Jonathan Schedler, a research psychologist affiliated with Harvard

They Touched a Nation

THANKS TO PUBLIC FIGURES who spoke out about their illnesses, we have all grown more comfortable in the past decade confronting health problems that were long shrouded in lonely silence.
—*Rita Rubin*

MUHAMMAD ALI

It was the most arresting moment of the 1996 Olympics in Atlanta: the former boxer, arm trembling, face frozen, raising the torch to the light the ceremonial flame. Calls flooded the National Parkinson's Foundation, which adopted a torch as its symbol.

ANNETTE FUNICELLO

In 1992, when the onetime Mickey Mouse Club girl publicly revealed her diagnosis, we all suddenly knew at least one person with MS: Annette. "She is everyone's extended family member," says Arney Rosenblat of the National Multiple Sclerosis Society.

LINDA ELLERBEE

Months after the journalist underwent a double mastectomy, she produced an emotionally charged special on breast cancer. "I can be fair and honest," she says of the disease. "But objective I cannot be."

RONALD REAGAN

Ever-folksy, the former president announced he had Alzheimer's disease in a handwritten letter addressed to "my fellow Americans" in 1994. He called his gesture "an opening of our hearts."

WILLIAM STYRON

The novelist told of his depression in the New York Times and later in *Darkness Visible: A Memoir of Madness*. "The overwhelming reaction made me feel that inadvertently I had helped unlock a closet from which many souls were eager to come out."

CHRISTOPHER REEVE

"You only have two choices," says the actor whose 1995 fall from a horse left him permanently paralyzed and who has raised millions for spinal injury research. "Either you vegetate and look out the window or activate and try to effect change."

GREG LOUGANIS

Mortified that he'd hid his HIV-positive status when his head wound bloodied the Olympic pool in 1988, the diver finally told his story during an interview with Barbara Walters in 1995.

ball: from "slow down, spend more time with your family, and don't sweat the little things" to "control your anger, read more poetry, and verbalize affection." Hardly the sort of wisdom that transforms lives.

If these interventions have anything in common, though, it is the presence of other people. This makes sense if you think of stress the way most doctors do, as a hormonal response to pressure. The body perceives a threat, mental or physical, and releases hormones that hike blood pressure and suppress immune response. According to the theory, some of us (the hostile, the troubled, the Type As) have a higher risk of heart disease or cancer because we secrete more of these hormones more frequently than the average joe. This stress response isn't easy to moderate, but one of the few things that seems to help is contact with a supportive person. In several lab experiments, for instance, psychologists have shown that having a friend in the room calms the cardiovascular response to distressing tasks such as public speaking. It's the secret of group therapy: We relax around our own. The simple grace of company can keep us healthy.

Humans are, after all, social by nature. So perhaps it makes sense that the healthiest among us might be the ones who find solace in companionship, who can defuse building pressure by opening up our hearts to someone else. As the late biologist and writer Lewis Thomas observed, human beings have survived by being useful to one another. We are as indispensable to each other as hummingbirds are to hibiscus.

And by finding ways to help each other out, the latest research hints, we forge the emotional connections that could very well sustain us. Thomas understood this. In a *New York Times* interview in 1993, just two weeks before his death, the reporter asked him, "Is there an art to dying?"

"There's an art to living," Thomas replied. "One of the very important things that has to be learned around the time dying becomes a real prospect is to recognize those occasions when we have been useful in the world. With the same sharp insight that we all have for acknowledging our failures, we ought to recognize when we have been useful, and sometimes uniquely useful. All of us have had such times in our lives, but we don't pay much attention to them. Yet the thing we're really good at as a species is usefulness. If we paid more attention to this biological attribute, we'd get a satisfaction that cannot be attained from goods or knowledge."

Benedict Carey has been a staff writer at the magazine since 1988.

University, the tests researchers use to identify hostile personalities essentially measure something he calls interpersonal warmth. "It has to do with whether you see the people in your life as benevolent or malevolent, whether they offer nourishment or frustration," he says. "The fact is, humans are emotionally frail. We need real support from other people, and those who don't acknowledge it are going to feel besieged."

These notions could easily collapse into sentimentality. Yet scientific evidence for the physical benefits of social support is coming in from all sides. At Ohio State University, for example, immunologist Ron Glaser and psychologist Janice Kiecolt-Glaser have found that the biggest slump in immunity during exam periods occurs in medical students who report being lonely. Analyzing data from the Tecumseh Community Health Study, sociologist James House calculated

that social isolation was as big a risk factor for illness and death as smoking was. And these were just the warm-up acts. In 1989 David Spiegel of Stanford Medical School measured the effect of weekly group therapy on women being treated for breast cancer. As expected, those who met in groups experienced less pain than those who didn't. But that wasn't all. The women in counseling survived an average of 37 months—nearly twice as long as those without the group support. Other researchers, including Friedman, have also lengthened some heart patients' lives through group therapy.

The reason remains anyone's guess. Perhaps, as Spiegel has suggested, being in a group makes patients more likely to take their medications, perform prescribed exercise, and so on. Patients may also benefit from advice offered in therapy, which can range from the commonsensical to the corn-

Dysthymic Disorder: The Chronic Depression

RANDY A. SANSONE, M.D., and LORI A. SANSONE, M.D.
University of Oklahoma College of Medicine, Tulsa, Oklahoma

Dysthymic disorder is defined as chronic depression of a mild to moderate degree for at least two years' duration. The disorder tends to be underdiagnosed despite a prevalence of 5 to 15 percent in primary care settings. Both the diagnosis and treatment of dysthymic disorder may be complicated by a variety of comorbid psychiatric and medical conditions as well as chronic stressors. Treatment may be determined by the accompanying comorbid condition. Antidepressant drugs are moderately efficacious in the treatment of dysthymia, with selective serotonin reuptake inhibitors preferred over tricyclic antidepressants. However, patients may report oversensitivity to antidepressants, experience only partial remission with treatment and suffer relapses. Adjunctive support or psychodynamic psychotherapy should also be considered.

Dysthymic disorder, also known as dysthymia, is a depressive disorder characterized by mild to moderate symptoms with a duration of two or more years.[1] In contrast, major depression is a relatively discrete disorder with moderate to severe symptoms (*Table 1*).

Dysthymia has an insidious onset and a waxing and waning course. Individuals with the disorder may have brief periods of normal mood, but these periods seldom last longer than two months. This smoldering mood disturbance, which intensifies and remits throughout its course, has an average duration of 16 years.[2] Dysthymic disorder may be as debilitating as major depression.

The disorder can have an early or late onset (i.e., before or after the age of 21 years). Criteria for the diagnosis of dysthymic disorder, as outlined in the *Diagnostic and Statistical Manual of Mental Disorders* (*DSM-IV*), are listed in *Table 2*.[1]

Etiology

As with many psychiatric disorders, the etiology of dysthymic disorder is unknown. Several investigators suspect serotonergic dysfunction,[3,4] but the validity of this theory requires further investigation. In addition to possible neurotransmitter abnormalities, there appear to be several clinical disorders in which dysthymic disorder is more common, including personality disorder, other affective disorders and/or chronic life stressors.[5,6]

Because of the multiple possible determinants, it is feasible to conceptualize dysthymia as a "final common pathway" disorder, or one in which multiple etiologic factors independently cause the same symptom complex (*Figure 1*). The relation-

---

TABLE 1

Major Depression and Dysthymic Disorder

Parameter	Major depression	Dysthymic disorder
Minimum duration of symptoms	Two weeks	Two years
Minimum number of depressive symptoms*	Five symptoms	Two symptoms
Neurovegetative features	Typically present	May be present
Intensity of symptoms	Moderate to severe	Mild to moderate
Onset of symptoms	Fairly defined	Insidious
Persistence of symptoms	Sustained and continuous	Waxing and waning quality with periods of normal mood lasting up to two months in duration

—Depressive symptoms according to the Diagnostic and Statistical Manual of Mental Disorders (DSM-IV).

From *American Family Physician*, June 1996, pp. 2588-2594. © 1996 by the American Academy of Family Physicians. Reprinted by permission.

TABLE 2

**Diagnostic Criteria
for Dysthymic Disorder**

1. Depressed mood for most of the day for at least two years (one year for children)

2. Two or more of the following symptoms while depressed:
   a. Poor appetite or overeating
   b. Insomnia or hypersomnia
   c. Low energy or fatigue
   d. Low self-esteem
   e. Poor concentration or difficulty making decisions
   f. Feelings of hopelessness

3. During the two-year period, no symptom-free period for more than two months at a time

4. No major depressive episode during the first two years (one year for children)

5. No prior history of a manic or hypomanic episode or a cyclothymic disorder

6. Symptoms do not exclusively occur during a chronic psychotic disorder

7. Symptoms are not due to the direct physiologic effects of a substance or a general medical condition

8. Symptoms cause clinically significant distress or impairment in social, occupational or other important areas of functioning

Adapted with permission from American Psychiatric Association. Diagnostic and statistical manual of mental disorders. 4th ed. Washington, D.C.: American Psychiatric Association, 1994:349. Copyright 1994.

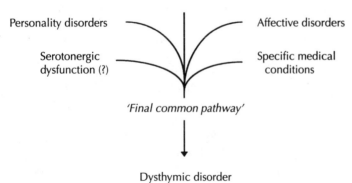

FIGURE 1. Dysthymic disorder as a "final common pathway" from a variety of different substrates.

ship, if any, among these etiologic variables is unknown.

Prevalence

Dysthymic disorder is relatively common, regardless of the population studied. According to the Epidemiological Catchment Area study,[7] the prevalence of dysthymia in the general population is around 3 percent. Other studies of community samples have shown similar prevalence rates for the disorder.[8] As expected, the prevalence of dysthymia in mental health settings is much higher, ranging from 22 to 36 percent.[5,9] In primary care settings, the prevalence of dysthymic disorder is between 5 and 15 percent.[6,10] In community samples, the disorder has been found to be twice as common in women as in men.[11]

Comorbidity

Investigators have consistently noted a strong association of dysthymic disorder with other psychiatric and medical conditions.[5,6] Indeed, dysthymia without any associated comorbidity appears to be rare.[2] Comorbid conditions include several psychiatric disorders, as well as a variety of medical conditions. In addition, there appears to be a relationship between psychosocial stressors and dysthymic disorder, with this relationship being more common in older adults than in persons in other age groups.

PSYCHIATRIC COMORBIDITY

The most common comorbid psychiatric condition is major depression, which occurs in up to 70 percent of individuals with dysthymia.[5] When both major depression and dysthymia coexist, the clinical phenomenon is described as "double depression." The clinical significance of these comorbid depressions is twofold. First, double depression is more difficult to treat than major depression alone. Second, because of the potential coexistence of the two disorders, it is reasonable to screen all patients who present with major depression for comorbid dysthymic disorder.

A second possible psychiatric comorbidity is a personality disorder. Several personality disorders have been associated with dysthymia, including avoidant, self-defeating, dependent and borderline personalities.[5,12] In an outpatient psychiatric setting, we found the prevalence of borderline personality traits or borderline personality disorder in patients with major depression, major depression with dysthymia or dysthymia to be 21 percent, 47 percent, and 50 percent, respectively (unpublished data). The existence of a relationship between dysthymic disorder and borderline personality in some individuals is not surprising. According to the Kolb and Gunderson criteria,[13] one of the five diagnostic features of borderline personality is long-standing dysphoria. The *DSM-IV* also incorporates several criteria that relate to longstanding affective disturbance, such as an enduring pattern of affective instability due to a marked reactivity of mood, chronic feelings of emptiness or inappropriate and intense anger.[1]

Some investigators believe that the likelihood of a comorbid personality disorder is greater with early-onset dysthymia than with late-onset dysthymic disorder.[14,15] This impression is based on the belief that the foundation of an individual's personality is established at a fairly early age and that some of the personality disorders are characterized by enduring patterns of inner experience and behavior that appear to reflect a mood disturbance. Although investigators have compared various aspects of early-onset and late-onset dysthymia,[16,17] between-group differences in the prevalence of personality disorders are undetermined at the present time.

The third area of psychiatric comorbidity is social phobia. Investigators report that up to 15 percent of dysthymic individuals have comorbid social phobia.[6] This observation may be related to dysthymic individuals with comorbid avoidant personality traits or avoidant personality disorder.

MEDICAL COMORBIDITY

A variety of medical conditions have been associated with dysthymia.[6] These include several neurologic disorders (e.g., cerebrovascular accident, multiple sclerosis), acquired immunodeficiency syndrome, premenstrual dysphoric disorder, postcardiac transplantation, hypothyroidism and several psychophysiologic disorders (e.g., fibromyalgia, chronic fatigue syndrome).

Despite the intuitive sense of a predictable association between chronic med-

ical conditions and dysthymia, there appears to be a low prevalence of dysthymic disorder in patients with cancer.[6] Therefore, the relationship between medical conditions and chronic depression is not simply due to the imposition of the medical condition and its resulting effect on mood.

Various theories have been advanced to explain the relationship between dysthymia and medical conditions. First, the medical condition may alter the status of neurotransmitters, thereby precipitating a psychiatric illness (e.g., the effect of Parkinson's disease on serotonin). Second, dysthymia may be a risk factor for medical morbidity. Third, pharmacologic treatment (e.g., corticosteroids, beta blockers) of medical conditions may precipitate psychiatric illness. Finally, it may be that dysthymia and medical conditions coexist in a complicated reinforcing cycle. At present, the interrelationship and validity of these theories remain speculative.

OTHER COMORBIDITY

A subgroup of patients with late-onset dysthymia report severe psychosocial stressors and do not appear to have comorbid psychiatric disorders.[18,19] These psychosocial stressors represent losses, which may include the death of a spouse, changes in income or housing and/or abandonment by adult children. We have noted a relationship between dysthymia and psychosocial stressors more frequently in older individuals in primary care settings than in mental health settings.

DIFFERENCES IN COMORBIDITY
ACCORDING TO CLINICAL SETTING

No studies to date have explored the relationship between clinical setting (i.e., primary care versus mental health settings) and comorbidity in dysthymia. However, dysthymic individuals may preselect their treatment setting so that those with significant psychiatric comorbidity (e.g., severe personality disorder, superimposed major depression) may be more likely to present for treatment to mental health professionals. In comparison, those with psychosocial stressors and somatic manifestations of stress may be more likely to present to primary care physicians.

Clinical Assessment

It is important to distinguish between dysthymic disorder and major depression. Because of its dramatic symptomatology, major depression is often easier to detect. The smoldering nature and low-grade intensity of dysthymia probably contribute to its underdiagnosis.[20]

Differentiation of the two disorders can be accomplished by determining the duration and quality of the depressive episode. For example, the symptoms of major depression are more intense and sustained than those of dysthymic disorder. However, major depression and dysthymia may coexist.

When dysthymia is diagnosed, the age of onset (i.e., before or after 21 years of age) should be determined. This is important because individuals with early-onset dysthymic disorder appear more likely to have a comorbid personality disorder.

Once the diagnosis of dysthymic disorder has been confirmed, the patient should be assessed for comorbid conditions, including associated psychiatric conditions (e.g., major depression, a personality disorder such as borderline personality or social phobia), medical conditions and psychosocial stressors. In primary care settings, the rapid and accurate assessment for multiple psychiatric diagnoses may be facilitated by the use of instruments such as the Primary Care Evaluation of Mental Disorders (PRIME-MD)[10] and the Symptom-Driven Diagnostic System for Primary Care (SDDS-PC).[21]

Treatment

OVERVIEW OF PHARMACOLOGIC INTERVENTION

General guidelines for antidepressant therapy in dysthymia are summarized in *Table 3*. Antidepressants are the foundation for the treatment of dysthymic disorder. Selective serotonin reuptake inhibitors (SSRIs), including sertraline (Zoloft), fluoxetine (Prozac) and paroxetine (Paxil), are preferred because they are well tolerated and have fewer side effects than other antidepressant drugs. Their primary limitation is sexual dysfunction. Tricyclic antidepressants may be poorly tolerated because of their anticholinergic and cardiovascular effects.

Antidepressant therapy should be initiated in a low dose. This does not preclude titrating to higher doses. However, drug sensitivity, particularly among those individuals with personality disorder[22] and medical conditions,[6] may deter the standard psychiatric doses of antidepressants in many primary care patients with dysthymic disorder.

The physician's expectations concerning drug response need to be conservative, particularly in patients with comorbid personality disorders. While several investigators have reported significant antidepressant responses in dysthymic subjects,[23,24] others have found a lower response rate in subjects with dysthymic disorder than in those with major depression alone.[25] When improvement occurs, it is often mild to moderate at best.[26,27] Furthermore, relapses occur. We have found that in patients with dysthymia and a comorbid personality disorder, a 25 to 30 percent reduction in overall symptoms appears to be a realistic expectation following intervention with antidepressant medication.

In patients with dysthymic disorder, the treatment response to antidepressant med-

---

TABLE 3

General Guidelines for Antidepressant Therapy in Dysthymic Disorder

---

1. Selective serotonin reuptake inhibitors are recommended.

2. Initiate antidepressant treatment with a low daily dosage, such as 25 mg of sertraline (Zoloft), 10 mg of fluoxetine (Prozac) or 10 mg of paroxetine (Paxil).

3. Titrate the dose upward until side effects preclude higher titration or the recommended dose is attained: 50 to 150 mg per day of sertraline, 20 to 40 mg per day of fluoxetine and 20 to 40 mg per day of paroxetine.

4. If the recommended daily dosage cannot be attained, continue treatment at the lower dosage if the patient is responding to the drug.

5. Contract with the patient for a three-month drug evaluation trial.

6. Educate the patient with comorbid personality disorder to expect only a moderate response to antidepressant drug therapy (i.e., an overall reduction in symptoms of perhaps 25 to 30 percent).

7. In a patient who is also receiving other medications, be alert to potential drug interactions with serotonin reuptake inhibitors.

8. If one drug trial is unsuccessful, attempt a second or third drug trial, particularly in a patient with comorbid major depression.

9. If the patient continues to be unresponsive after several drug trials, consider adjunctive medications, such as buspirone (BuSpar) or lithium, or consultation with a psychiatrist.

10. For the patient who responds to drug therapy, continue the antidepressant for two to three years, or for life.

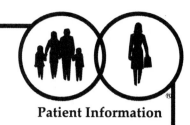

Dysthymic Disorder: When Depression Lingers

What is dysthymic disorder?

Dysthymic disorder, or dysthymia, is a type of depression that lasts for at least two years. Some people suffer from dysthymia for years. The depression is usually mild or moderate, rather than severe. Most people with dysthymia cannot tell for sure when they first became depressed.

Symptoms of dysthymic disorder include a poor appetite or overeating, difficulty sleeping or sleeping too much, low energy, fatigue and feelings of hopelessness. But people with dysthymic disorder may have periods of normal mood that last up to two months. Family members and friends may not even know that their loved one is depressed. Even though this type of depression is mild, it may make it difficult for a person to function at home and at school or work.

When does dysthymic disorder begin?

Dysthymia can begin in childhood or in adulthood. Like most types of depression, it appears to be more common in women. No one knows why depression is more common in women.

How common is dysthymic disorder?

Dysthymic disorder is a fairly common type of depression. Up to 3 percent of people have dysthymia. From 5 to 15 percent of patients in a family doctor's office have dysthymia.

What causes dysthymic disorder?

No one knows for sure what causes dysthymia. There may be some changes in the brain that involve a chemical called serotonin. Personality problems, medical problems and chronic life stresses may also play a role.

How is dysthymic disorder diagnosed?

If you think you have dysthymia, discuss your concerns with your doctor. Your doctor will ask you questions to find out if you have depression and to identify the type of depression you have. Your doctor may ask you questions about your health and your symptoms, such as how well you're sleeping, if you feel tired all of the time, if you

This handout is provided to you by your family doctor and the American Academy of Family Physicians.

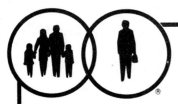

Patient Information

have trouble concentrating. Your doctor will also consider medical reasons that may cause you to feel depressed, such as problems with your thyroid or a medicine you may be taking.

What is the treatment for dysthymic disorder?

Dysthymic disorder can be treated with an antidepressant medicine. This type of drug relieves depression. Antidepressants are commonly prescribed, and they are safe. They do not create an artificial "high," and they are not addicting.

If you are given an antidepressant, it may take a number of weeks or even several months before you and your doctor know whether the drug is helping you. It is important for you to take the medicine as it is prescribed. If the antidepressant drug helps you feel better, you may need to take this medicine for several years. In other words, continue to take the antidepressant drug even though you begin to feel better. If you stop taking the medicine, you may get depressed again.

Will I have to see a psychiatrist?

You will probably not have to see a psychiatrist unless the medication is not working or you have problems taking the drugs that are usually prescribed for depression. Sometimes, in addition to taking an antidepressant medicine, patients are referred for psychotherapy to help them deal with specific problems. This type of therapy can be very helpful for some people. In general, the treatment of dysthymic disorder is adjusted to the person.

Is there anything else I can do to help me feel better?

Talking to your doctor about how you're feeling and getting treatment for the dysthymic disorder are the first steps to feeling better.

Getting involved in activities that make you feel good or make you feel like you've accomplished something may help you. For example, going to a movie, taking a drive on a pleasant day, going to a ball game, working in the garden are a few activities that may help you feel better.

Eat well-balanced, healthy meals. Don't use drugs or alcohol. Both can make depression worse.

Exercise may help lift your mood. Do it as much as you can. Exercising three times a week for 30 minutes to one hour is a good goal.

This information provides a general overview on dysthymic disorder and may not apply to everyone. Talk to your family doctor to find out if this information applies to you and to get more information on this subject.

ication may occur later than the four to six weeks reported for patients with major depression.[28] Therefore, it is prudent to consider longer drug evaluation trials (perhaps up to three months). This may be particularly important in patients whose chaotic lives may mask a positive response to medication during a brief drug evaluation period.

If a patient has a reasonable treatment response to antidepressant therapy (i.e., a 25 to 30 percent or more reduction in symptoms), therapy should be continued for at least two to three years, if not for life, depending on the initial severity of the symptoms and the extent of the patient's response.

DYSTHYMIC DISORDER
AND MAJOR DEPRESSION

In cases of double depression, titration of antidepressant medication to standard psychiatric doses should be attempted. If this is unsuccessful, a second or even a third antidepressant may be tried. In addition, consideration should be given to adjunctive medications, such as buspirone (BuSpar) or lithium, which may be initiated in consultation with a psychiatrist. Lithium augmentation should be done using a low dose, with serum levels ranging from 0.6 to 0.8 mEq per L (0.6 to 0.8 mmol per L). For patients who fail to respond to several drug trials, consultation with a psychiatrist is recommended to evaluate for other comorbidity, such as personality disorder, and/or to initiate more complex treatment, if indicated, such as psychodynamic psychotherapy or anticonvulsant drugs.

DYSTHYMIC DISORDER
AND PERSONALITY DISORDER

As an adjunct to antidepressant therapy, psychodynamic psychotherapy may be useful in higher functioning patients with dysthymia and a personality disorder. This type of intervention typically continues for several years, with sessions occurring about once a week.

For lower functioning patients (e.g., low educational and occupational achievement, poor social and marital adjustment), supportive interventions may be indicated. These interventions may include supportive psychotherapy, 12-step programs when appropriate, vocational rehabilitation, training in life management skills, and/or enhancement of environmental structure through schedules and activities.

DYSTHYMIC DISORDER
AND MEDICAL COMORBIDITY

Treatment with an SSRI is recommended for patients with dysthymic disorder and a concomitant medical condition. Drug therapy should be initiated in a low dosage and titrated upward as tolerated. Potential drug interactions should be monitored, as should medication sensitivity and synergistic effects with other medications. In addition, the medical condition should be stabilized to the extent possible.

In many cases, patients with medical conditions may also benefit from psychotherapy. The focus of psychotherapy may vary, from resolving anger at the limitations imposed by the medical condition to facing loss due to impending death. Whether psychodynamic or supportive psychotherapy is indicated depends on the particular clinical circumstance.

DYSTHYMIC DISORDER
AND CHRONIC STRESSORS

Patients with dysthymia and chronic psychosocial stressors should be treated with SSRIs, and the nature of the stressors should also be explored. Time-limited stressors are usually alleviated by strengthening immediate social supports and helping patients recognize and deal with their own limitations.

Ongoing stressors (e.g., a physically abusive spouse, a parent with Alzheimer's disease) require more detailed assessment to determine the best form of intervention, which is often specific to the situation. These types of psychosocial stressors may require consultation with other professionals, such as a psychiatrist, a lawyer and/or a financial advisor, to formulate a plan for intervention. Ongoing stressors typically require a long time to resolve. Again, antidepressants may significantly alleviate some of the associated depression and stress.

Final Comment

Dysthymic disorder is commonly encountered in both primary care and psychiatric settings. Medical and/or psychiatric morbidity is common in patients with this disorder. While antidepressants help to alleviate depression, treatment may be complicated by medication sensitivity, partial response to drug therapy (particularly in those with personality disorder) and possible delayed onset of response to medication. Consequently, the management of dysthymic disorder can be challenging.

The Authors

RANDY A. SANSONE, M.D.
is associate professor in the Department of Psychiatry at the University of Oklahoma College of Medicine, Tulsa, where he is also medical director of the psychiatric outpatient clinic. He received his medical degree from Ohio State University College of Medicine, Columbus, and completed a residency in psychiatry at the same institution.

LORI A. SANSONE, M.D.
is clinical assistant professor in the Department of Family Medicine at the University of Oklahoma College of Medicine, Tulsa, and is also a staff physician at Medical Care Associates of Tulsa. After graduating from Ohio State University College of Medicine, she completed a residency in family practice at Miami Valley Hospital, Dayton, Ohio.

REFERENCES

1. American Psychiatric Association. Diagnostic and statistical manual of mental disorders. 4th ed. Washington, D.C.: American Psychiatric Association, 1994:345-9.
2. Klein DN, Riso LP, Anderson RL. DSM-III-R dysthymia: antecedents and underlying assumptions. Prog Exp Pers Psychopathol Res 1993;16:222-53.
3. Ravindran AV, Chudzik J, Bialik RJ, Lapierre YD, Hrdina PD. Platelet serotonin measures in primary dysthymia. Am J Psychiatry 1994;151:1369-71.
4. Bersani G, Pozzi F, Marini S, Grispini A, Pasini A. Ciani N. 5-HT2 receptor antagonism in dysthymic disorder: a double-blind placebo-controlled study with ritanserin. Acta Psychiatr Scand 1991;83:244-8.
5. Markowitz JC, Moran ME, Kocsis JH, Frances AJ. Prevalence and comorbidity of dysthymic disorder among psychiatric outpatients. J Affect Disord 1992;24:63-71.
6. Howland RH. General health, health care utilization, and medical comorbidity in dysthymia. Int J Psychiatry Med 1993;23:211-38.
7. Weissman MM, Leaf PJ, Bruce ML, Florio L. The epidemiology of dysthymia in five communities: rates, risks, comorbidity, and treatment. Am J Psychiatry 1988;145:815-9.
8. Robins LN, Helzer JE, Weissman MM, Orvaschel H, Gruenberg E, Burke JD Jr, et al. Lifetime prevalence of specific psychiatric disorders in three sites. Arch Gen Psychiatry 1984;41:949-58.
9. Klein DN, Dickstein S, Taylor EB, Harding K. Identifying chronic affective disorders in outpatients: validation of the General Behavior Inventory. J Consult Clin Psychol 1989;57:106-11.
10. Spitzer RL, Williams JB, Kroenke K, Linzer M, de Gruy FV 3d, Hahn SR, et al. Utility of a new procedure for diagnosing mental disorders in primary care. The PRIME-MD 1000 study. JAMA 1994; 272:1749-56.
11. Kessler RC, McGonagle KA, Zhao S, Nelson CB, Hughes M, Eshleman S, et al. Lifetime and 12-month prevalence of DSM-III-R psychiatric disorders in the United States. Results from the National Comorbidity Survey. Arch Gen Psychiatry 1994; 51:8-19.
12. Sanderson WC, Wetzler S, Beck AT, Betz F. Prevalence of personality disorders in patients with major depression and dysthymia. Psychiatry Res 1992;42:93-9.
13. Kolb JE, Gunderson JG. Diagnosing borderline patients with a semistructured interview. Arch Gen Psychiatry 1980;37:37-41.
14. Schrader G. Chronic depression: state or trait? J Nerv Ment Dis 1994;182:552-5.
15. Hirschfeld R. Personality and dysthymia. In: Burton SW, Akiskal HS, eds. Dysthymic disorder. London: Gaskell, 1990:69-77.
16. Kovacs M, Akiskal HS, Gatsonis C, Parrone PL. Childhood-onset dysthymic disorder. Clinical features and prospective naturalistic outcome. Arch Gen Psychiatry 1994;51:365-74.
17. McCullough JP, Braith JA, Chapman RC, Kasnetz MD, Carr KF, Cones JH, et al. Comparison of early and late onset dysthymia. J Nerv Ment Dis 1990; 178:577-81.
18. Devanand DP, Nobler MS, Singer T, Kiersky JE, Turret N, Roose SP, et al. Is dysthymia a different disorder in the elderly? Am J Psychiatry 1994;151: 1592-9.
19. Pahkala K, Kivela SL, Laippala P. Social and environmental factors and dysthymic disorder in old age. J Clin Epidemiol 1992;45:775-83.
20. Keller MB. Dysthymia in clinical practice: course, outcome and impact on the community. Acta Psychiatr Scand Suppl 1994;383:24-34.
21. Broadhead WE, Leon AC, Weissman MM, Barrett JE, Blacklow RS, Gilbert TT, et al. Development and validation of the SDDS-PC screen for multiple mental disorders in primary care. Arch Fam Med 1995;4:211-9.
22. Sansone RA, Johnson CL. Treating the eating disorder patient with borderline personality: theory and technique. In: Barber JP, Crits-Christoph P, eds. Dynamic therapies for psychiatric disorders (axis I). New York: Basic Books, 1995:230-66.
23. Marin DB, Kocsis JH, Frances AJ, Parides M. Desipramine for the treatment of "pure" dysthymia versus "double" depression. Am J Psychiatry 1994;151:1079-80.
24. Bakish D, Ravindran A, Hooper C, Lapierre Y. Psychopharmacological treatment response of patients with a DSM-III diagnosis of dysthymic disorder. Psychopharmacol Bull 1994;30:53-9.
25. Howland RH. Pharmacotherapy of dysthymia: a review. J Clin Psychopharmacol 1991;11:83-92.
26. Fawcett J. Antidepressants: partial response in chronic depression. Br J Psychiatry Suppl 1994; 165:37-41.
27. Ormel J, Oldehinkel T, Brilman E, vanden Brink W. Outcome of depression and anxiety in primary care. A three-wave 3 1/2-year study of psychopathology and disability. Arch Gen Psychiatry 1993;50:759-66.
28. Keller MB, Russell CW. Refining the concept of dysthymia. Hosp Community Psychiatry 1991; 42:892-3,896.

UPDATE ON MAJOR DEPRESSION

John Zajecka, M.D.*

Major depression is a serious medical illness that afflicts nearly 9.5 million people in the U.S. in any six-month period. The potential consequences of untreated depression can be devastating for the depressed individual as well as for family members, significant others, and society in general. A medical-outcome study published in 1989 showed greater physical impairment associated with major depression than with other chronic medical illnesses such as chronic lung disease, diabetes, arthritis, and hypertension. Untreated depression may be accountable for as much as $44.7 billion spent per year as a result of its consequences, usually days away from work and unnecessary use of physical health services.

Studies suggest that 15 percent of people with major depression die by suicide, which remains one of the leading causes of death in younger individuals. Ironically, major depressive disorder is among the most treatable illnesses encountered in medicine, which means that the potential personal and social tragedies associated with the illness can be prevented when the disorder is recognized and appropriate intervention occurs. Despite the availability of effective treatments for major depression, studies suggest that only one-third of those with this often devastating brain disorder ever seek treatment. Unfortunately, numerous barriers contribute to its under-recognition and undertreatment. A significant amount of work needs to be done to educate the public, the medical professions, the work industry, and government agencies about the recognition and availabilities of effective treatments for depression.

*About the author: John Zajecka, M.D., an assistant professor of psychiatry at Rush Medical College, is the clinical director of the Woman's Board Depression Treatment and Research Center, Rush Institute for Mental Well-Being, Rush-Presbyterian-St. Luke's Medical Center, Chicago. He is also the president of the Midwestern Division of the American Suicide Foundation, a scientific advisory board member of the Obsessive-Compulsive Foundation of Metropolitan Chicago, and a psychiatric consultant on the depression task force of the Joint Commission on Accreditation of Health Care Organizations. Dr. Zajecka has authored or co-authored more than 30 publications for scientific journals and has been an investigator in more than 50 studies on mood and anxiety disorders.

Major depression is a medical illness defined as a syndrome with a core cluster of symptoms. It is specifically identified when five or more of the following symptoms are present for two or more weeks: diminished interest or pleasure in activities; depressed mood and feelings of sadness; weight gain or loss; increased or decreased appetite; sleep disturbances (difficulty falling asleep, restless sleep, early morning awakening, or sleeping too much); fatigue or lack of energy; difficulty concentrating and/or making decisions; agitation or anxiety; a slowdown in thoughts and/or physical activity; feelings of hopelessness and/or helplessness; and recurrent thoughts of death or suicide. Other physical symptoms that commonly occur with depression include headaches, gastrointestinal problems, and musculoskeletal pain. Clinical depression is not always accompanied by feeling "depressed" or sad, so the absence of this feeling should not exclude the existence of the disorder, particularly in the presence of other symptoms.

There is no "good reason to be depressed." Major depression is a treatable medical illness that is often written off or rationalized as attributable to other problems such as concomitant medical illnesses and/or significant psychosocial stress—both of which, however, can precipitate or exacerbate depression in susceptible individuals. Up to 25 percent of individuals with certain medical conditions—diabetes, myocardial infarction, stroke, or cancer, for example—will develop major depression during the course of their medical illness. The management of the medical condition may be more complex and the prognosis less favorable if depression is present and not recognized and treated. Drug and/or alcohol abuse or dependence may also contribute to the onset or exacerbation of depressive illness. And episodes may follow significant psychosocial stressors that can play a significant role in the precipitation of early depressive episodes, but may play a lesser role in later episodes, which can occur spontaneously without any precipitating events.

The lifetime risk for major depression in community samples ranges from 10 percent to 25 percent for women and five percent to 12 percent for men. Prevalence rates

From *The Decade of the Brain,* Summer 1996, pp. 1-3. © 1996 by the National Alliance for the Mentally Ill. Reprinted by permission.

appear unrelated to ethnicity, education, income, or marital status. The average age of onset is the mid-twenties, but episodes can begin as early as prepuberty or in the later decades of life.

The course of major depression is variable. Recurrent depression can be characterized by isolated episodes that are separated by years without any symptoms or by increasing frequency of episodes over time. The number of previous episodes predicts the likelihood of developing future episodes: approximately 50 percent to 60 percent of first episodes will be followed by a second episode, 70 percent of second episodes will be followed by a third, and there is a 90 percent chance of developing a fourth episode after three episodes.

Major depression can be accompanied by psychotic symptoms, often mood-congruent (depressive themes) in nature. Individuals may hear voices telling them that they are bad or to kill themselves, or they may have delusions that they have a terminal illness or are responsible for some disaster. Appropriate treatment should result in improvement of both depressive and psychotic symptoms.

Major depression can also exist as part of a bipolar disorder. When it does, the depressive episodes are interspersed with mania, hypomania, or mixed episodes of depression and mania, in which case treatment must include management and prevention of different cycles of the illness.

Major depression is 1.5 to 3 times more common among first-degree biological relatives of persons with the illness than it is in the general population. There is increased risk of alcohol-dependence in adult first-degree biological relatives, and there may be increased incidence of attention deficit disorder in children of adults with the illness.

Etiology

Depression was accurately described as far back as the days of Hippocrates when it was referred to as "melancholia." Hippocrates himself described the illness as a cluster of symptoms that was suspected to have a physiological origin, mainly "black bile." Throughout the centuries, the pathophysiological basis of depression has evolved from "black bile" to theories involving genetic vulnerability and an intricate dysregulation of brain neurotransmitter and hormone systems. Current theories implicate at least three neurotransmitter systems: norepinephrine, serotonin, and dopamine. Early hypotheses speculated that depression is the result of a depletion of one or more of these neurotransmitters in areas of the brain that then exhibit a dysregulation of normal brain functions associated with depression such as sleep, appetite, energy, and pleasure. These hypotheses have been central to understanding the causes of the illness and finding effective treatments. Currently available treatments for depression appear to increase the levels of these neurotransmitters in varying degrees to restore the central nervous system to a functional state.

From an etiological standpoint, depression may be a heterogeneous illness, meaning that different physiological and/or anatomical abnormalities may exist. Such abnormalities may account for: 1) different clinical presentations of the subtypes of depression; 2) the variability of biological "markers" found in depression; and 3) the varying responses to treatment among depressed individuals. While there is no single "biological test" for depression, there are a number of findings in subpopulations of depressed individuals that are present only when depressive symptoms are present, but not present following successful treatment or remission of the illness. Examples of such findings include electroencephalograph-recorded changes in sleep architecture; decreased brain activity of specific brain areas seen with brain-imaging studies; dysregulation of the hypothalamic-pituitary-adrenal axis hormones (i.e., cortisol); and changes in the levels of the metabolites of norepinephrine, serotonin, and dopamine when measured in blood, urine, or spinal fluid of depressed persons.

Compared to many other medical disorders, there has been an enormous amount of information that has emerged over the last decade about the proposed etiologies of depression. The result has been the development and refinement of effective treatments.

Treatment

Depression is among the most treatable illnesses in medicine. Once depression is diagnosed, appropriate management of the illness with the numerous effective available treatments can prevent the unnecessary toll the illness can take on individuals and society. As with any other medical condition, the consumer and any significant others should be informed that symptoms are caused by a disorder that is readily treatable. Clinicians must address misperceptions about depression, including the stigma often attached to it and wrong assumptions that it is a "normal" reaction or a "weakness of character."

Pharmacotherapy with antidepressants is often the treatment of choice for major depression. The clinician may need to educate those who believe that antidepressants are "happy pills," tranquilizers, addicting, "a crutch," or responsible for inadvertently changing one's personality.

Approximately 20 different antidepressants are currently available in the United States, and several others are being evaluated in clinical trials with the hope for public availability within the next two years. Currently available antidepressants include tricyclic/heterocyclic antidepressants (i.e., amitriptyline [Elavil] and nortriptyline [Pamelor]); monoamine oxidase inhibitors (MAOIs) (i.e., phenelzine [Nardil]); selective serotonin reuptake inhibitors (SSRIs) (i.e., fluoxetine [Prozac]), bupropion (Wellbutrin), venlafaxine (Effexor), and nefazodone (Serzone). All of the currently available antidepressants are equally effective, although certain individuals may respond to some but not others. They primarily differ in their mechanism of action (i.e., varying effects on increasing norepinephrine, serotonin, and/or dopamine) and potential side-effect profile. The older compounds—the tricyclic/heterocyclic antidepressants and the MAOIs—tend to have side effects or dietary restrictions that are less easily tolerated than those of the newer antidepressants. This difference is significant because quality of life is appropriately becoming more important in the treatment of many disorders, and side effects of treatment are an issue.

Electroconvulsive therapy (ECT) is a safe and effective treatment for depression, particularly when a fast antidepressant response is crucial. Results can take weeks with the use of antidepressants. ECT can be particularly useful for postpartum depression, depression with psychotic symptoms, treatment-refractory depression, or for the seriously suicidal patient whose life may be endangered by waiting for an antidepressant medication to become efficacious.

Time-limited psychotherapies such as cognitive therapy or interpersonal therapy can be useful for mild depressions and as an adjunct to pharmacotherapy for optimal treatment outcomes of more serious depressive illness. Studies suggest that these psychotherapies may not only optimize short-term treatment outcomes, but may also reduce future relapses.

Phototherapy—using specific light intensities for specified amounts of time on a daily basis—has been shown to improve depressive symptoms when used alone or in combination with antidepressants in some individuals who suffer from seasonal affective disorder.

While not formally approved by the FDA for the treatment of depression, some antidepressant combinations and antidepressant potentiation strategies have been reported to be useful for individuals who otherwise achieve only a partial response to monotherapy with an antidepressant. Some antidepressant combinations that have had success in such situations include SSRI's combined with low doses of tricyclic/heterocyclic antidepressants and SSRI's combined with low doses of bupropion. Potentiating antidepressants with one of the following pharmacotherapies has also been at times useful for the treatment of partial responders to monotherapy antidepressant treatment: lithium; thyroid hormone (T_3); stimulants (ie. methylphenidate[Ritalin]; buspirone; pindolol; bromocriptine); and estrogen replacement in postmenopausal women. Such pharmacotherapy strategies should be managed by clinicians who are familiar with such treatment modalities.

Given the breadth of effective interventions available for depression, there are few, if any, reasons why a person with this disorder in the 1990s should be allowed to suffer the potential consequences of nontreatment. Unfortunately, barriers to recognition and treatment still exist. For some consumers and families, there is a lack of available resources from which to obtain effective treatments. And, among others, government agencies, employee assistant programs, and managers of health care utilization must understand why resources must be available to prevent personal suffering, tragedies, and economic burdens. The message that depression is a medical illness for which treatment works has to reach the future opinion leaders in this country.

Manic-Depressive Illness and Creativity

Does some fine madness plague great artists?
Several studies now show that creativity
and mood disorders are linked

Kay Redfield Jamison

KAY REDFIELD JAMISON is professor of psychiatry at the Johns Hopkins University School of Medicine. She wrote *Touched with Fire: Manic-Depressive Illness and the Artistic Temperament* and co-authored the medical text *Manic-Depressive Illness.* Jamison is a member of the National Advisory Council for Human Genome Research and clinical director of the Dana Consortium on the Genetic Basis of Manic-Depressive Illness. She has also written and produced a series of public television specials about manic-depressive illness and the arts.

"Men have called me mad," wrote Edgar Allan Poe, "but the question is not yet settled, whether madness is or is not the loftiest intelligence—whether much that is glorious—whether all that is profound—does not spring from disease of thought—from moods of mind exalted at the expense of the general intellect."

Many people have long shared Poe's suspicion that genius and insanity are entwined. Indeed, history holds countless examples of "that fine madness." Scores of influential 18th- and 19th-century poets, notably William Blake, Lord Byron and Alfred, Lord Tennyson, wrote about the extreme mood swings they endured. Modern American poets John Berryman, Randall Jarrell, Robert Lowell, Sylvia Plath, Theodore Roethke, Delmore Schwartz and Anne Sexton were all hospitalized for either mania or depression during their lives. And many painters and composers, among them Vincent van Gogh, Georgia O'Keeffe, Charles Mingus and Robert Schumann, have been similarly afflicted.

Judging by current diagnostic criteria, it seems that most of these artists—and many others besides—suffered from one of the major mood disorders, namely, manic-depressive illness or major depression. Both are fairly common, very treatable and yet frequently lethal diseases. Major depression induces intense melancholic spells, whereas manic-depression, a strongly genetic disease, pitches patients repeatedly from depressed to hyperactive and euphoric, or intensely irritable, states. In its milder form, termed cyclothymia, manic-depression causes pronounced but not totally debilitating changes in mood, behavior, sleep, thought patterns and energy levels. Advanced cases are marked by dramatic, cyclic shifts.

Could such disruptive diseases convey certain creative advantages? Many people find that proposition counterintuitive. Most manic-depressives do not possess extraordinary imagination, and most accomplished artists do not suffer from recurring mood swings. To assume, then, that such diseases usually promote artistic talent wrongly reinforces simplistic notions of the "mad genius." Worse yet, such a generalization trivializes a very serious medical condition and, to some degree, discredits individuality in the arts as well. It would be wrong to label anyone who is unusually accomplished, energetic, intense, moody or eccentric as manic-depressive.

All the same, recent studies indicate that a high number of established artists—far more than could be expected by chance—meet the diagnostic criteria for manic-depression or major depression given in the fourth edition of the *Diagnostic and Statistical Manual of Mental Disorders* (*DSM-IV*). In fact, it seems that these diseases can sometimes enhance or otherwise contribute to creativity in some people.

Diagnosing Mood Disorders

By virtue of their prevalence alone, it is clear that mood disorders do not necessarily breed genius. Indeed, 1 percent of the general population suffer from manic-depression, also called bipolar disorder, and 5 percent from a major depression, or unipolar disorder, during their lifetime. Depression affects twice as many women as men and most often, but not always, strikes later in life. Bipolar disorder afflicts equal numbers of women and men, and more than a third of all cases surface before age 20. Some 60 to 80 percent of all adolescents and adults who commit suicide have a history of bipolar or unipolar illness. Before the late 1970s, when the drug lithium first became widely available, one person in five with manic-depression committed suicide.

Major depression in both unipolar and bipolar disorders manifests itself through apathy, lethargy, hopelessness, sleep disturbances, slowed physical movements and thinking, impaired memory and concentration, and a loss of pleasure in typically enjoyable events. The diagnostic criteria also include suicidal thinking, self-blame and inappropriate guilt. To distinguish clinical depression from normal periods of unhappiness, the common guidelines further require that these symptoms persist for a minimum of two to four weeks and also that they significantly interfere

Reprinted with permission from *Scientific American*, February 1995, pp. 62-67. © 1995 by Scientific American, Inc. All rights reserved.

The Tainted Blood of the Tennysons

Alfred, Lord Tennyson, who experienced recurrent, debilitating depressions and probable hypomanic spells, often expressed fear that he might inherit the madness, or "taint of blood," in his family. His father, grandfather, two of his great-grandfathers as well as five of his seven brothers suffered from insanity, melancholia, uncontrollable rage or what is today known as manic-depressive illness. His brother Edward was confined to an asylum for nearly 60 years before he died from manic exhaustion. Lionel Tennyson, one of Alfred's two sons, displayed a mercurial temperament, as did one of his three grandsons.

Modern medicine has confirmed that manic-depression and creativity tend to run in certain families. Studies of twins provide strong evidence for the heritability of manic-depressive illness. If an identical twin has manic-depressive illness, the other twin has a 70 to 100 percent chance of also having the disease; if the other twin is fraternal, the chances are considerably lower (approximately 20 percent). A review of identical twins reared apart from birth—in which at least one of the twins had been diagnosed as manic-depressive—found that two thirds or more of the sets were concordant for the illness.

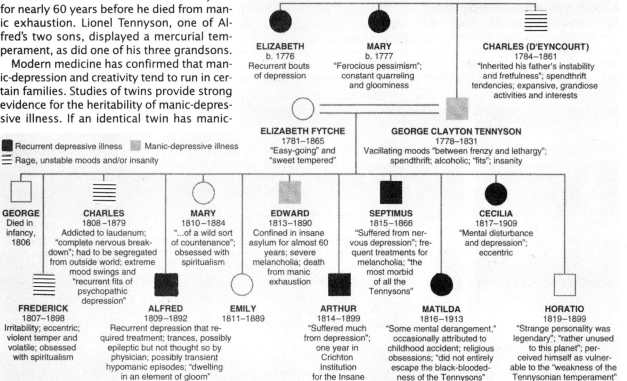

■ Recurrent depressive illness   ▨ Manic-depressive illness
☰ Rage, unstable moods and/or insanity

SOURCE: Adapted from Touched with Fire: Manic-Depressive Illness and the Artistic Temperament; *based on biographies, autobiographical writings and letters.*

with a person's everyday functioning.

During episodes of mania or hypomania (mild mania), bipolar patients experience symptoms that are in many ways the opposite of those associated with depression. Their mood and self-esteem are elevated. They sleep less and have abundant energy; their productivity increases. Manics frequently become paranoid and irritable. Moreover, their speech is often rapid, excitable and intrusive, and their thoughts move quickly and fluidly from one topic to another. They usually hold tremendous conviction about the correctness and importance of their own ideas as well. This grandiosity can contribute to poor judgment and impulsive behavior.

Hypomanics and manics generally have chaotic personal and professional relationships. They may spend large sums of money, drive recklessly or pursue questionable business ventures or sexual liaisons. In some cases, manics suffer from violent agitation and delu-sional thoughts as well as visual and auditory hallucinations.

Rates of Mood Disorders

For years, scientists have documented some kind of connection between mania, depression and creative output. In the late 19th and early 20th centuries, researchers turned to accounts of mood disorders written by prominent artists, their physicians and friends. Although largely anecdotal, this work strongly suggested that renowned writers, artists and composers—and their first-degree relatives—were far more likely to experience mood disorders and to commit suicide than was the general population. During the past 20 years, more systematic studies of artistic populations have confirmed these findings [*see illustration on next page*]. Diagnostic and psychological analyses of living writers and artists can give quite mean-ingful estimates of the rates and types of psychopathology they experience.

In the 1970s Nancy C. Andreasen of the University of Iowa completed the first of these rigorous studies, which made use of structured interviews, matched control groups and strict diagnostic criteria. She examined 30 creative writers and found an extraordinarily high occurrence of mood disorders and alcoholism among them. Eighty percent had experienced at least one episode of major depression, hypomania or mania; 43 percent reported a history of hypomania or mania. Also, the relatives of these writers, compared with the relatives of the control subjects, generally performed more creative work and more often had a mood disorder.

A few years later, while on sabbatical in England from the University of California at Los Angeles, I began a study of 47 distinguished British writers and visual artists. To select the group as best I could for creativity, I purposefully

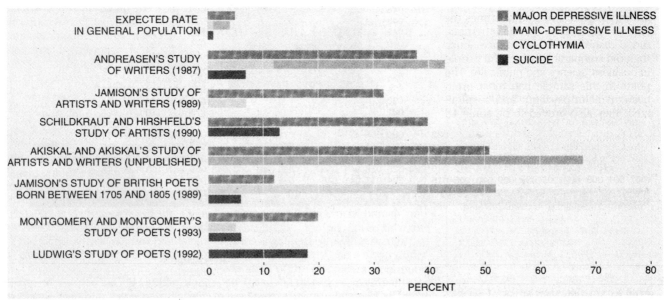

INCREASED RATES of suicide, depression and manic-depression among artists have been established by many separate studies. These investigations show that artists experience up to 18 times the rate of suicide seen in the general population, eight to 10 times the rate of depression and 10 to 20 times the rate of manic-depression and cyclothymia.

chose painters and sculptors who were Royal Academicians or Associates of the Royal Academy. All the playwrights had won the New York Drama Critics Award or the Evening Standard Drama (London Critics) Award, or both. Half of the poets were already represented in the *Oxford Book of Twentieth Century English Verse.* I found that 38 percent of these artists and writers had in fact been previously treated for a mood disorder; three fourths of those treated had required medication or hospitalization, or both. And half of the poets—the largest fraction from any one group—had needed such extensive care.

Hagop S. Akiskal of the University of California at San Diego, also affiliated with the University of Tennessee at Memphis, and his wife, Kareen Akiskal, subsequently interviewed 20 award-winning European writers, poets, painters and sculptors. Some two thirds of their subjects exhibited recurrent cyclothymic or hypomanic tendencies, and half had at one time suffered from a major depression. In collaboration with David H. Evans of the University of Memphis, the Akiskals noted the same trends among living blues musicians. More recently Stuart A. Montgomery and his wife, Deirdre B. Montgomery, of St. Mary's Hospital in London examined 50 modern British poets. One fourth met current diagnostic criteria for depression or manic-depression; suicide was six times more frequent in this community than in the general population.

Ruth L. Richards and her colleagues at Harvard University set up a system for assessing the degree of original think-ing required to perform certain creative tasks. Then, rather than screening for mood disorders among those already deemed highly inventive, they attempted to rate creativity in a sample of manic-depressive patients. Based on their scale, they found that compared with individuals having no personal or family history of psychiatric disorders, manic-depressive and cyclothymic patients (as well as their unaffected relatives) showed greater creativity.

Biographical studies of earlier generations of artists and writers also show consistently high rates of suicide, depression and manic-depression—up to 18 times the rate of suicide seen in the general population, eight to 10 times that of depression and 10 to 20 times that of manic-depressive illness and its milder variants. Joseph J. Schildkraut and his co-workers at Harvard concluded that approximately half of the 15 20th-century abstract-expressionist artists they studied suffered from depressive or manic-depressive illness; the suicide rate in this group was at least 13 times the current U.S. national rate.

In 1992 Arnold M. Ludwig of the University of Kentucky published an extensive biographical survey of 1,005 famous 20th-century artists, writers and other professionals, some of whom had been in treatment for a mood disorder. He discovered that the artists and writers experienced two to three times the rate of psychosis, suicide attempts, mood disorders and substance abuse than did comparably successful people in business, science and public life. The poets in this sample had most often been manic or psychotic and hospitalized; they also proved to be some 18 times more likely to commit suicide than is the general public. In a comprehensive biographical study of 36 major British poets born between 1705 and 1805, I found similarly elevated rates of psychosis and severe psychopathology. These poets were 30 times more likely to have had manic-depressive illness than were their contemporaries, at least 20 times more likely to have been committed to an asylum and some five times more likely to have taken their own life.

Cycles of Creative Accomplishment

These corroborative studies have confirmed that highly creative individuals experience major mood disorders more often than do other groups in the general population. But what does this mean for their work? How does a psychiatric illness actually contribute to creative achievement? First, the common features of hypomania seem highly conducive to original thinking; the diagnostic criteria for this phase of the disorder include "sharpened and unusually creative thinking and increased productivity." And accumulating evidence suggests that the cognitive styles associated with hypomania (namely, expansive thought and grandiose moods) can lead to increased fluency and frequency of thoughts.

Studying the speech of hypomanic patients has revealed that they tend to rhyme and use other sound associations, such as alliteration, far more often than do unaffected individuals. They

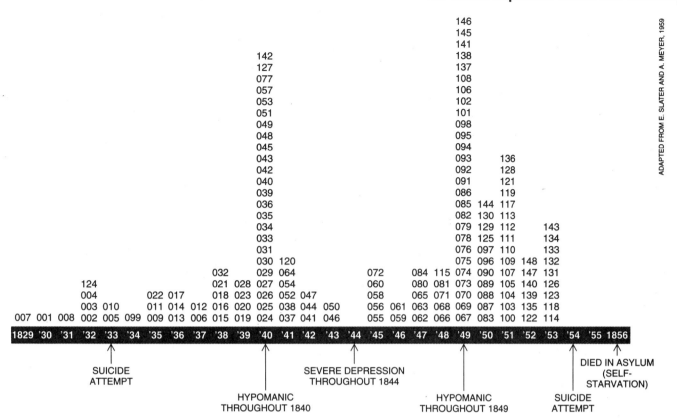

ADAPTED FROM E. SLATER AND A. MEYER, 1959

ROBERT SCHUMANN'S MUSICAL WORKS, charted by year and opus number (*above*), show a striking relation between his mood states and his productivity. He composed the most when hypomanic and the least when depressed. Both of Schumann's parents were clinically depressed, and two other first-degree relatives committed suicide. Schumann himself attempted suicide twice and died in an insane asylum. One of his sons spent more than 30 years in a mental institution.

also use idiosyncratic words nearly three times as often as do control subjects. Moreover, in specific drills, they can list synonyms or form other word associations much more rapidly than is considered normal. It seems, then, that both the quantity and quality of thoughts build during hypomania. This speed increase may range from a very mild quickening to complete psychotic incoherence. It is not yet clear what causes this qualitative change in mental processing. Nevertheless, this altered cognitive state may well facilitate the formation of unique ideas and associations.

Manic-depressive illness and creative accomplishment share certain noncognitive features: the ability to function well on a few hours of sleep, the focus needed to work intensively, bold and restless attitudes, and an ability to experience a profound depth and variety of emotions. The less dramatic daily aspects of manic-depression might also provide creative advantage to some individuals. The manic-depressive temperament is, in a biological sense, an alert, sensitive system that reacts strongly and swiftly. It responds to the world with a wide range of emotional, perceptual, intellectual, behavioral and energy

changes. In a sense, depression is a view of the world through a dark glass, and mania is that seen through a kaleidoscope—often brilliant but fractured.

Where depression questions, ruminates and hesitates, mania answers with vigor and certainty. The constant transitions in and out of constricted and then expansive thoughts, subdued and then violent responses, grim and then ebullient moods, withdrawn and then outgoing stances, cold and then fiery states—and the rapidity and fluidity of moves through such contrasting experiences—can be painful and confusing. Ideally, though, such chaos in those able to transcend it or shape it to their will can provide a familiarity with transitions that is probably useful in artistic endeavors. This vantage readily accepts ambiguities and the counteracting forces in nature.

Extreme changes in mood exaggerate the normal tendency to have conflicting selves; the undulating, rhythmic and transitional moods and cognitive changes so characteristic of manic-depressive illness can blend or harness seemingly contradictory moods, observations and perceptions. Ultimately, these fluxes and yokings may reflect truth in hu-

manity and nature more accurately than could a more fixed viewpoint. The "consistent attitude toward life," may not, as Byron scholar Jerome J. McGann of the University of Virginia points out, be as insightful as an ability to live with, and portray, constant change.

The ethical and societal implications of the association between mood disorders and creativity are important but poorly understood. Some treatment strategies pay insufficient heed to the benefits manic-depressive illness can bestow on some individuals. Certainly most manic-depressives seek relief from the disease, and lithium and anticonvulsant drugs are very effective therapies for manias and depressions. Nevertheless, these drugs can dampen a person's general intellect and limit his or her emotional and perceptual range. For this reason, many manic-depressive patients stop taking these medications.

Left untreated, however, manic-depressive illness often worsens over time—and no one is creative when severely depressed, psychotic or dead. The attacks of both mania and depression tend to grow more frequent and more severe. Without regular treatment the disease eventually becomes less re-

The Case of Vincent van Gogh

Many clinicians have reviewed the medical and psychiatric problems of the painter Vincent van Gogh posthumously, diagnosing him with a range of disorders, including epilepsy, schizophrenia, digitalis and absinthe poisoning, manic-depressive psychosis, acute intermittent porphyria and Ménière's disease. Richard Jed Wyatt of the National Institute of Mental Health and the author have argued in detail that van Gogh's symptoms, the natural course of his illness and his family psychiatric history strongly indicate manic-depressive illness. The extent of the artist's purported absinthe use and convulsive behavior remains unclear; in any event, his psychiatric symptoms long predate any possible history of seizures. It is possible that he suffered from both epilepsy and manic-depressive illness.

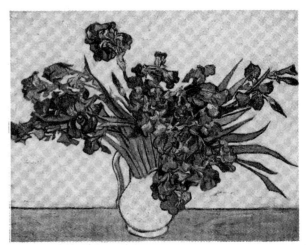

Irises, *1889*

METROPOLITAN MUSEUM OF ART, GIFT OF ADELE R. LEVY, 1958

sponsive to medication. In addition, bipolar and unipolar patients frequently abuse mood-altering substances, such as alcohol and illicit drugs, both of which can cause secondary medical and emotional burdens for manic-depressive and depressed patients.

The Goal of Treatment

The real task of imaginative, compassionate and effective treatment, therefore, is to give patients more meaningful choices than they are now afforded. Useful intervention must control the extremes of depression and psychosis without sacrificing crucial human emotions and experiences. Given time and increasingly sophisticated research, psychiatrists will likely gain a better understanding of the complex biological basis for mood disorders. Eventually, the development of new drugs should make it possible to treat manic-depressive in-

dividuals so that those aspects of temperament and cognition that are essential to the creative process remain intact.

The development of more specific and less problematic therapies should be swift once scientists find the gene, or genes, responsible for the disease. Prenatal tests and other diagnostic measures may then become available; these possibilities raise a host of complicated ethical issues. It would be irresponsible to romanticize such a painful, destructive and all too often deadly disease. Hence, 3 to 5 percent of the Human Genome Project's total budget (which is conservatively estimated at $3 billion) has been set aside for studies of the social, ethical and legal implications of genetic research. It is hoped that these investigations will examine the troubling issues surrounding manic-depression and major depression at length. To help those who have manic-depressive

illness, or who are at risk for it, must be a major public health priority.

FURTHER READING

TENNYSON: THE UNQUIET HEART. R. B. Martin. Oxford University Press, 1980.

CREATIVITY AND MENTAL ILLNESS: PREVALENCE RATES IN WRITERS AND THEIR FIRST-DEGREE RELATIVES. Nancy C. Andreasen in *American Journal of Psychiatry*, Vol. 144, No. 10, pages 1288-1292; October 1987.

MANIC DEPRESSIVE ILLNESS. Frederick K. Goodwin and Kay R. Jamison. Oxford University Press, 1990.

CREATIVE ACHIEVEMENT AND PSYCHOPATHOLOGY: COMPARISON AMONG PROFESSIONS. Arnold M. Ludwig in *American Journal of Psychotherapy*, Vol. 46, No. 3, pages 330–356; July 1992.

TOUCHED WITH FIRE: MANIC-DEPRESSIVE ILLNESS AND THE ARTISTIC TEMPERAMENT. Kay R. Jamison. Free Press/Macmillan, 1993.

Suicide — Part I

Suicide has been a topic of philosophical meditation, a legal and moral dilemma, and the climax of many great works of drama and fiction. It has been exalted as an honorable sacrifice and condemned as a mortal sin. Choosing to kill oneself has been contemplated as the ultimate human decision. Lawyers and ethical philosophers have discussed when suicide may be justified or desirable and when it must be condemned or prevented. In practice, however, the mental health system is the institution usually called on to cope with suicidal thoughts, threats, and behavior and the emotional consequences of suicide. From this point of view, suicide is not a moral or metaphysical issue but the most common serious psychiatric emergency, one of the most difficult problems in the treatment of mental illness and emotional disorders.

Suicide is almost impossible to predict. There is no test both sensitive enough to identify most people who will go on to kill themselves and so accurate that it will not falsely predict suicide for many others. Statistics can be compiled from death certificates, at least in advanced industrial countries, but they are not always reliable, since deaths are subject to highly varying degrees of official investigation. Family members and other survivors may have many reasons, emotional, legal, and financial, for denying that a death is suicide, and the authorities are often concerned more about ruling out homicide than about distinguishing suicide from accidents. When the cause is a fall, automobile accident, or drug or alcohol overdose, it may be difficult to tell. More reliable information can be obtained from a psychological autopsy, in which researchers examine medical and psychiatric records and interview relatives, doctors, employers, and others to judge the circumstances and intentions of the person who died. But this procedure is time-consuming and has not yet been used widely enough to judge when official records are inadequate.

The statistics of suicide

According to official figures, there were more than 32,000 suicides in the United States in 1994, about 11 per 100,000 persons. The actual number is undoubtedly higher, but no one knows by how much. Many more people die by suicide than by homicide. Officially, it is now the eighth leading cause of death in the United States, accounting for a little more than 1% of all deaths. More years of life are lost to suicide than to any other single cause except heart disease and cancer.

From *Harvard Mental Health Letter,* November 1996, pp. 1-5. © 1996 by the President and Fellows of Harvard College. Reprinted by permission.

Suicide rates are highest in old age: 20% of the population and 40% of suicides are over 60. After age 75, the rate is three times higher than average, and among white men over 80, it is six times higher than average. The suicide rate among the elderly declined from 1950 to 1980 but has been rising since then. A fear of chronic disabling illness and the growing social acceptability of ending a painful life may be contributing to this change.

Suicide patterns have also been changing among younger people. The age group 15–24, which once accounted for 5% of all suicides, now accounts for nearly 20% of male and 14% of female suicides. The rate at ages 15–19 quadrupled between 1950 (2.7 per 100,000) and 1988 (11.3 per 100,000). In a 1990 survey, 8% of American high school students said they had attempted suicide in the previous year, and 27% said they had thought about it seriously. Suicide attempts are among the most common causes of admission to hospital emergency rooms among people under 35.

The risk of suicide is also affected by nationality, race, religion, marital status, and place of residence. People who have never been married are twice as likely to take their own lives as currently married people; the highest rates of all occur among the divorced and widowed. The recorded suicide rate is usually lower in rural areas than in cities, although this difference may result from inadequate reporting. Steady churchgoers and people with strong religious convictions have a lower recorded suicide rate than average. Doctors have a higher than average rate, and psychiatrists have a higher rate than other medical specialists. Contrary to common opinion, Vietnam veterans do not commit suicide significantly more often than other men the same age.

National and ethnic factors

If official statistics can be believed, there are startling national differences in suicide rates. The frequency is highest in German-speaking countries, Switzerland, Scandinavia, Eastern Europe, and Japan. For many years Hungary has had the highest official suicide rate in the world — more than 40 per 100,000 per year, four times the American rate. Suicide is relatively uncommon (4–8 per 100,000) in Greece, Italy, and Spain. The American rate is about average for an industrial country. It is highest in the western states and lowest in the Northeast (in Nevada, 25 per 100,000; in New Jersey, 7 per 100,000. African-Americans commit suicide only half as often as whites, and the black suicide rate does not rise in old age. Native Americans have a higher suicide rate than whites at all ages. Suicide is thought to be less common in

underdeveloped than in industrially advanced countries, but their poor records make it difficult to tell.

Some of the regional, national, and ethnic differences in suicide rates may be a result of the political and religious pressures that affect coroners and other officials. But recording bias is probably not the full explanation, since national rankings for suicide plus accidents and undetected causes of death generally parallel rankings for suicide alone. The national differences have persisted steadily through changing political regimes and economic circumstances. The suicide rate in each European country is also highly correlated with the suicide rate among American descendants of emigrants from that country.

Cultures presumably influence the likelihood of suicide by the way they shape personality through upbringing or by the stresses they impose at different stages of life and in personal crises. The most influential sociological study of this subject was published in 1897 by Émile Durkheim, who claimed that the suicide rate varies with the strength of social control mechanisms he called integration and regulation. A type of suicide he named *egoistic* was associated with an absence of close social bonds or a lack of integration. This was said to explain the high suicide rates among unmarried people in modern industrial cities. Durkheim explained another type of suicide, the *anomic*, as resulting from emotional disorientation because of a disrupted social relationship — a loss of regulation. Such a suicide might be provoked, for example, by a death in the family or a sudden change in social status. Durkheim thought that both egoistic and anomic suicides were more common in modern industrial societies than in better integrated and regulated rural communities. He pointed out that the suicide rate declines during wars, when national solidarity provides integration, and rises in times of high unemployment, when anomie presumably becomes more pervasive. His ideas have been inconclusively challenged and defended for nearly a hundred years.

A person who commits suicide must have access to the means and be willing to tolerate the manner of death. In the United States today firearms account for proportionately twice as many suicides (50%–60%) as they did in 1900, although the suicide rate is no higher. Some European countries with strict gun control laws have high suicide rates; there most suicides use other means. But in this country suicide occurs more often where guns are easily available. A 1992 study found that after correction for arrests, drug and alcohol abuse, the use of prescription drugs, and limited education, the presence of a gun in the home increased the risk of suicide nearly five times. In a three-year study of two counties, one in Tennessee and one in Washington, 70% of suicides occurred in the home and 58% involved a firearm. In a study comparing Seattle and Vancouver, researchers found higher suicide rates among young adults and adolescents (but not older people) in the American city, where handguns were more freely available.

Conditions leading to suicide

Whatever the cultural background and manner of death, it is clear that the great majority of suicides have a mental or emotional disorder. The most common is depression: 30% to 70% of suicide victims suffer from major depression or bipolar (manic-depressive) disorder. More than two-thirds of moderately to severely depressed patients have suicidal thoughts, and suicide accounts for about 15% of deaths among people with major mood disorders. Anxiety disorders occur at a high rate in severely depressed people and may contribute independently to the risk of suicide.

Substance abuse is another great instigator of suicide; it may be involved in half of all cases. About 20% of suicides are alcohol abusers, and the lifetime rate of suicide among alcoholics is at least three or four times the average. Alcoholics who kill themselves are likely to be men over 30 who began addictive drinking early in life. The danger is greatest when alcohol abuse leads to a crisis such as arrest, divorce, or sudden unemployment. One study found that a quarter of all suicide victims had ended a love affair or marriage during the year before their deaths. About half of them were alcoholics; only 15% were depressed.

A drinking binge may lead to suicidal behavior even in nonalcoholics, since heavy drinkers sometimes become anxious and depressed while losing their inhibitions against impulsive action. One study of 50 people who had attempted suicide found blood levels of alcohol indicating drunkenness in 14 of them. In a study of completed suicides, a third had high blood alcohol levels. Suicidal depressions associated with heavy drinking usually clear within days of abstinence.

Illicit drug abusers also have a high rate of suicide. One study of narcotic addicts found a rate five times the average; the actual numbers are probably much higher, since addicts often die from overdoses and other questionable accidents or from homicide they may have provoked with suicidal intent. Tobacco smokers also have higher than average rates of both depression and suicide. When a depressed drug abuser or alcoholic commits suicide, it can be difficult to tell whether the depression caused the drug abuse (or vice versa) or whether the same depression that caused the drug abuse also led to suicide.

A third or more of schizophrenic patients attempt suicide and 5%–10% eventually succeed. Those most likely to kill themselves are young, unemployed men without families who have a severe illness with relapses that require repeated hospitalization. They are often isolated and abusing alcohol or other drugs. They may act either under the influence of hallucinations and delusions or at times when psychotic symptoms have faded and they can contemplate their lives despairingly. The apparent emotionlessness (blunted affect) of schizophrenia makes the moods and intentions of these patients difficult to discern. Some otherwise puzzling adolescent suicides may occur because of incipient schizophrenic symptoms.

It is almost impossible to tell whether homosexuality is associated with a higher rate of suicide than average. The only published survey considering sexual orientation found that 13 of 283 (5%) of consecutive male suicides were gay. This result is difficult to evaluate, since the proportion of homosexual men in the general population is not known. The suicide rate might be higher mainly among men who are concealing their sexuality. Some authors have claimed that homosexual adolescents are more likely than others both to attempt and to complete suicide, but again the evidence is weak, and concealment is an especially serious obstacle to judgment.

Rates of suicide are high in people with a record of bad temper, verbal abuse, fighting, wife-beating, sexual violence, or antisocial behavior (habitual lying, stealing, general irresponsibility). Murderers often kill themselves. The suicide rate among white murderers in the United States, for example, is almost 700 times the average. In a study of the 37 suicides that occurred during 25 years in a Detroit jail, researchers found that 14 of them were charged with homicide, although homicide offenders constituted only a tiny proportion of the jail population. Men who kill women are especially likely to be suicidal. The often-romanticized lovers' suicide pact is usually something closer to murder and suicide. Reports from survivors suggest that the man almost always subtly or crudely coerces the woman, insisting that she prove her love by dying with him.

Among elderly suicide victims, half or more suffer from a chronic physical illness. Any illness that may cause depression also heightens the risk of suicide. One study of 80 suicides found that 56 had an active illness, and in 40 cases it might have contributed to the suicide. (The illnesses included cancer, kidney disease, heart disease, respiratory disease, peptic ulcers, and arthritis.) Men who committed suicide, especially those over 60, were much more likely to be physically ill than women. Men who are unaccustomed to revealing their feelings or seeking help may take their own lives because they cannot tolerate the loss of mastery and self-sufficiency that results from illness. Among elderly men who kill themselves, only 25% have ever seen a mental health professional, but 70% have visited a doctor in the last month of life.

Genetic influences

Suicide and attempted suicide run in families, probably in part for genetic reasons. The risk of suicide is about four times higher than average in close relatives of a person who commits suicide and six times higher than average in the adopted-away children of a biological parent who commits suicide. The concordance (matching) rate for suicide among identical twins is at least five times as high as it is among fraternal twins. In one study, 10 of 26 identical twins and none of 9 fraternal twins of a suicide had themselves attempted suicide. Most of this family resemblance probably represents an inherited vulnerability to depression, alcoholism, and other psychiatric disorders, but there may also be an independent genetic factor involving the capacity to control impulses under stress. For example, among the Amish of Pennsylvania, 16% of all the family lines account for 73% of the suicides. Almost all Amish suicides are suffering from mood disorders, but not all Amish families with a high rate of these disorders also have a high rate of suicide.

If a genetically influenced tendency to impulsive violence exists, it may be associated with activity of the neurotransmitter serotonin (5-hydroxy tryptamine). Depressed patients with low serotonin levels apparently have stronger suicidal tendencies than those with normal levels. Among people hospitalized for violent suicide attempts, those with low levels of 5-HIAA (the metabolic product of serotonin) in their spinal fluid are ten times more likely to kill themselves within a year. Low serotonin levels are also found in nonsuicidal people with a tendency to impulsive violence. In postmortem studies of the brains of suicide victims, researchers have discovered an excess of nerve receptors for serotonin, which might be the brain's effort to compensate for a deficiency of the neurotransmitter. A combination of impulsive aggressiveness and feelings of hopelessness, associated with serotonin deficiency, is more common in men than in women and may partly explain why men kill themselves much more often even though women have a higher rate of depression.

Motives for suicide

It is easier to describe the psychiatric and physical conditions associated with suicide than to say what motivates people (consciously or unconsciously) to try to kill themselves. Karl Menninger defined it as a wish to kill, a wish to be killed, and a wish to die. Freud originally explained suicide as the result of anger at a loved person that is turned against the self. According to this theory, people kill themselves as a way of symbolically murdering someone (ultimately a parent) whose image they have incorporated. Other psychoanalysts have spoken of a desire to exert an infantile magical omnipotence by annihilating the world or a compulsion to masochistic surrender along with a secret hope of rescue.

More consciously, suicide may express a wish to be reunited with a lost person or convey a reproach to someone living. Sometimes a suicide attempt is a way to communicate misery and attract attention that reduces isolation. An unsuccessful or incomplete suicide attempt may create an opportunity for more direct and rational communication or lead to a needed change in a person's circumstances.

Among the immediate motives for suicide, almost by definition, despair is the most common. In one long-term study, hopelessness alone accounted for most of the association between depression and suicide, and a high level of hopelessness was the clearest sign that a person who had attempted suicide would try again. Intense guilt, psychotic delusions, and the severity of the depression in other respects were not nearly as significant. This despair may be longstanding or it may be temporary, brought on, for example, by illness, humiliation, the loss of a job, the collapse of a marriage, or a death in the family.

Adolescent suicide

Adolescent suicide presents special problems. Because they lack experience, adolescents may overreact to trivial frustrations — failure on a test means failure in life, a disappointing date means permanent loneliness. On the other hand, many suicidal adolescents, like suicidal adults, are deeply depressed, but the signs may be hard to recognize because their sadness and hopelessness are disguised as boredom, apathy, hyperactivity, or physical complaints. High school students who attempt suicide are often reckless and delinquent and abuse alcohol and other drugs. Sometimes they have been exposed to the suicidal thoughts and suicide attempts of family members or friends. When an unusually high number of suicides occurs in a small area in a brief time, it is almost always among adolescents and young adults. This contagion is sometimes blamed on television or newspaper stories, but it is much more likely to come from family, neighbors, schoolmates, and friends.

The disturbing rise in adolescent suicide over the last 30 years may be the result of alcoholism, drug abuse, and family and social disorganization. Separation, divorce, unemployment, imprisonment, and death are common in the families of adolescents who attempt suicide. These boys and girls are often alienated from indifferent or hostile parents, and some have suffered from child abuse and neglect. A recent study found that even after correction for depression, drug abuse, alcoholism, panic attacks, and other risk factors, the odds for attempting suicide were three to four times higher than average among women who report a sexual assault before age 16.

Part 2 can be found in the December 1996 issue of *The Harvard Mental Health Letter*.

FOR FURTHER READING

A. Alvarez. The Savage God: A Study of Suicide. *New York: Random House, 1972.*

Susan J. Blumenthal and David J. Kupfer, eds. Suicide over the Life Cycle: Risk Factors, Assessment, and Treatment of Suicidal Patients. *Washington, D.C.: American Psychiatric Press, 1990.*

John H. Chiles and Kirk Strohsall. The Suicidal Patient: Principles of Assessment, Treatment, and Case Management. *Washington, D.C.: American Psychiatric Press, 1995.*

Herbert Hendin. Assisted suicide, euthanasia, and suicide prevention: The implications of the Dutch experience. *Suicide and Life-threatening Behavior 25:1:193–204 (Spring 1995).*

Douglas Jacobs and Herbert N. Brown, eds. Suicide: Understanding and Responding. *Madison, Conn: International Universities Press, 1989.*

Schizophrenia

The central element of the psychotic disorders is a break with reality that frequently leads to hospitalization at some point. The most devastating of these disorders, schizophrenia, affects approximately one percent of the population. With only minor variations, the symptoms of schizophrenia are observed in patients throughout the world. The personal, social, and economic price of this disorder is very high. Schizophrenia often strikes its victims as they are completing their education and preparing to enter the workforce. Symptoms such as delusions, hallucinations, social withdrawal, and problems in emotional expression are often chronic and can have detrimental effects on a person's ability to function. Family members are often distraught when they hear the diagnosis and its typical prognosis. Although many of the symptoms can be controlled with drugs, a significant number of patients find the side effects of the drugs so troublesome that they stop taking them.

The wide array of symptoms in schizophrenia makes this a difficult disorder to study; two individuals with schizophrenia might not experience the same symptoms. Nevertheless, this perplexing and often misunderstood disorder (for example, schizophrenia is not the same as multiple personality) is the focus of continuing efforts to understand its cause (or causes) and to identify effective treatments.

The developer of the modern concept of schizophrenia described it as a group of related disorders. Today there seems to be a return to the notion that there are multiple forms of the disorder. One intriguing clue relevant to the search for possible causes comes from a previously neglected topic: sex differences. Men tend to develop schizophrenia at an earlier age than women do. This sex difference in the age of onset might suggest a possible sex difference in the cause; it may also suggest that some biological process is responsible for the difference in age of onset. Evidence such as this may also help researchers organize the various subtypes of schizophrenia into more meaningful groups for further research.

In the continuing search for the cause of schizophrenia, researchers are focusing their attention on brain abnormalities. Accumulating evidence points to the strong possibility that schizophrenia results from some abnormality in the brain's circuitry. Among the avenues for fruitful research are reductions in the size of certain parts of the brain, differences in the levels of activity in several brain areas, and problems related to various neurotransmitters (dopamine, for example). Some drugs that affect neurotransmitters other than dopamine have been shown to reduce some of the symptoms, which suggests that the dopamine hypothesis may be too simple.

For some time, researchers have known that there was an elevated incidence of schizophrenia among individuals born in the winter and spring. Now, one possible explanation for this finding seems to have received support. Babies born to mothers who suffered from influenza during pregnancy develop schizophrenia at an elevated rate. A possible mechanism for this effect is that the babies are more likely to be low birth weight and may be prone to some type of obstetric complication.

New and sophisticated brain imaging techniques have revealed differences between the brains of normal individuals and those suffering from schizophrenia. A recent study focused on the reduced size of the thalamus, which would go a long way toward explaining the array of symptoms.

Much has been learned about this disorder, but it is clear that we have a long way to go before we truly understand schizophrenia.

Looking Ahead: Challenge Questions

How might research on sex differences in the onset of schizophrenia help to organize the subtypes into groups that advance our understanding?

Explain why schizophrenia may not really be one disorder but instead may refer to several disorders with different causes.

Some research shows that certain brain areas in patients with schizophrenia differ from the same areas observed in normal individuals. Does this research explain the disorder? Discuss why or why not. What are some likely alternative explanations for the difference? How might researchers design their studies to rule out alternative explanations?

UNIT 3

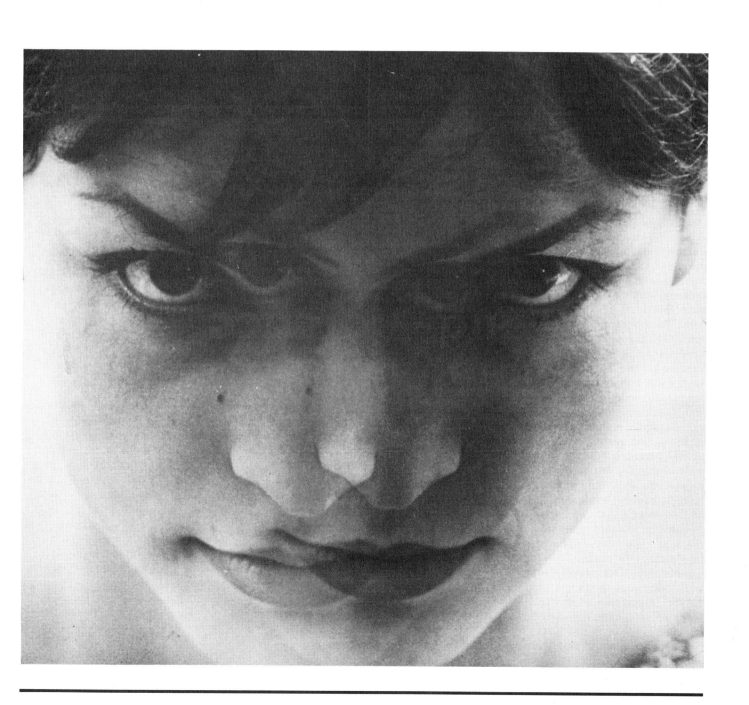

Age at Onset in Subtypes of Schizophrenic Disorders

**Stavroula Beratis,
Joanna Gabriel, and
Stavros Hoidas**

Stavroula Beratis, M.D., is Associate Professor of Psychiatry, Joanna Gabriel, M.D., is Assistant Professor of Psychiatry, and Stavros Hoidas, M.D., is Lecturer of Psychiatry, Department of Psychiatry, University of Patras Medical School, Patras, Greece.

Abstract

Age at onset and sex differences in the age at onset were investigated in the schizophrenic subtypes of 200 patients. Significant differences in the age at onset were observed among these subtypes; the disorganized subtype demonstrated the earliest and the paranoid the latest onset. The mean age at onset of all female patients was significantly greater than that of the male. Specifically, in the paranoid subtype the onset for men occurred earlier than for women. Conversely, in the disorganized subtype the disorder appeared earlier in women. There was no significant sex difference in the age at onset in the undifferentiated and the residual subtypes. In the paranoid subtype most men developed the disease before age 30 (72%), whereas women had an even distribution of the onset before and after 30. Ninety-six patients admitted for the first time demonstrated findings similar to those of the total sample. The data provide additional information on the phenotypic expression of the subtypes of schizophrenic disorders and indicate the necessity for further demographic and genetic studies to delineate the underlying defect.

Although the heterogeneity of schizophrenia's cause, clinical picture, and prognosis is well established (Cancro 1985), the underlying nature of this heterogeneity with respect to biological, psychological, and social aspects remains uncertain.

Among the factors that may contribute to our understanding of the heterogeneity in schizophrenia are the gender differences reported in the literature, which refer to brain morphology and functioning, to neurochemistry, to family transmission, to premorbid functioning, course and prognosis, and to clinical phenomenology (Goldstein and Tsuang 1990).

It has been hypothesized that the gender differences may be associated with or caused by the following: (1) hormonal differences between men and women, such as the "protective effect" of estrogens and the "triggering" of androgens, which may lead to a greater vulnerability in the male gender (Seeman 1985; Seeman and Lang 1990); (2) differences in brain morphology, conceptualized as a form of the existing sexual dimorphism (Lewine et al. 1990); and (3) diverse cultural and social factors that lead to stressful experiences earlier for men than for women (Loranger 1984). None of these hypotheses, however, has been widely accepted as the cause of the existing variability in schizophrenia.

One of the most consistent findings in the gender differences is the earlier onset of the schizophrenic disorders in men than women (Noreik and Ødegaard

1967; McCabe 1975; Lewine 1980; Loranger 1984; Goldstein et al. 1990; Gureje 1991). It has been estimated (Loranger 1984) that in Bleuler's (1911/1950) classic study of dementia praecox the mean age at onset of the male patients was 3.7 years earlier, whereas in the cases reported by Kraepelin (1919/1971) the mean age at onset of the male schizophrenia patients was 2.2 years earlier. Also, in the cases reported by Bleuler (1911/1950), more male patients became ill before the age of 30, whereas more female patients showed the disorder after that age.

A critique about the early studies was that the reported difference in the age at onset was due to diagnostic misclassification, in which affective disorders were included among schizophrenic disorders (Goldstein and Link 1988). More recent studies, however, using well-defined diagnostic criteria, verify the existence of a difference in the age at onset between male and female patients. Further, the sex differences in the age at onset cannot be attributed to an earlier hospitalization of the male patients (Raskin and Golob 1966), since the time of the first hospitalization for schizophrenia is very close to the time of first symptoms reported by the patients' relatives (Kramer 1978; Loranger 1984).

Among the more recent papers, Loranger (1984) reported that the

Reprint requests should be sent to Dr. S. Beratis, Dept. of Psychiatry, University of Patras Medical School, 265 00 Rion, Patras, Greece.

From *Schizophrenia Bulletin*, Vol. 20, No. 2, 1994, pp. 287-296. Reprinted by permission of the U.S. Department of Health and Human Services, Division of Clinical Treatment Research, National Institute of Mental Health (NIMH), National Institutes of Health.

mean age at onset of schizophrenia in men was approximately 5 years earlier than that of women. Also, in 17 percent of the women, but in only 2 percent of the men, the onset of psychosis occurred after age 35. The diagnosis of schizophrenia in these cases was made retrospectively according to *DSM–III* (American Psychiatric Association 1980) criteria. Goldstein et al. (1990), also used the *DSM–III* criteria, but without the criterion that limits the age at onset to 45 years, and found that the mean age at onset was 24.3 for men with schizophrenia and 27.9 for women with schizophrenia; 53 percent of the men and 32 percent of the women had become ill by the age of 25.

Applying the Research Diagnostic Criteria (Spitzer et al. 1978) to a Nigerian sample of schizophrenia patients, Gureje (1991) found that the mean age at onset of illness was 23.5 years for men and 26.4 years for women, with 83 percent of the male and 66 percent of the female patients becoming ill by age 30. He concluded that the gender difference in the age at onset of schizophrenia is present across cultures, implying a biological rather than a social etiology. However, in Gureje's study there was an uncertainty about some patients' birth years, and in some cases the data collection on the onset of illness was made by nonmedical personnel. In a better designed study of Nigerian schizophrenia patients, Ohaeri (1992) reported similar findings.

A later onset of schizophrenia for women has also been reported in a number of studies referring to patients with late-onset schizophrenia that is manifested after age 40 to 45 (Gold 1984; American Psychiatric Association 1987; Harris and Jeste 1988; Pearlson et al. 1989). Because most of these patients are female and show mainly paranoid symptomatology, the idea has been advanced that late-onset schizophrenia is a distinct entity (Gold 1984; Harris and Jeste 1988; Pearlson et al. 1989). Several of the studies on late-onset schizophrenia, however, are said to have methodologic problems, especially with the identification of cases and

the applied diagnostic criteria (Harris and Jeste 1988).

Although the clinical subtypes of schizophrenic disorders comprise well-accepted nosologic entities (American Psychiatric Association 1987; McGlashan and Fenton 1991), the investigation of their relationship to the age at onset is inadequate. Gruenberg et al. (1985), in a study of reliability and concordance of the subtypes of schizophrenia according to four major diagnostic systems, showed that the age at onset for the paranoid subtype was significantly later than for the disorganized and the undifferentiated subtypes. Likewise, Fenton and McGlashan (1991), rediagnosing patients according to the subtype criteria, concluded that the paranoid subtype has a later age at onset, while the hebephrenic and the undifferentiated subtypes are early and insidious in onset.

Investigation of early schizophrenia, such as the study of first-admission patients, can provide clues for a better characterization of the disorder. Studying early cases allows the following: (1) minimization of the confounding effects of chronicity and institutionalization; (2) study of drug-free patients; (3) the opportunity to perform prospective longitudinal studies; (4) a greater likelihood of detecting factors related to the etiology or pathophysiology of the disease; and (5) increased understanding of the variability in clinical morbidity observed in the first few years of the onset of the disorder (Keshavan and Schooler 1992).

None of the previous investigations has attempted to study the five schizophrenic subtypes as separate entities (American Psychiatric Association 1987) taking into consideration both gender and age at onset. If, however, the schizophrenic subtypes have different etiologies, or are different expressions of the same basic defect, the subtypes can be expected to have, in addition to the known specific clinical characteristics, differences in the age at onset as well as between the sexes. For this reason, we undertook to investigate the

following: (1) the age at onset in the five subtypes of schizophrenic disorders, namely, the disorganized, catatonic, paranoid, undifferentiated, and residual; and (2) differences in the age at onset between male and female patients in each of these subtypes. Information in these areas could help reveal factors associated with the etiology of schizophrenia.

Method

We investigated the medical records of 163 successive hospital admissions of schizophrenia patients diagnosed from the beginning according to *DSM–III–R* criteria (American Psychiatric Association 1987). Among this group, 100 were male and 63 were female. Thereafter, only successive female cases were studied until the number of women patients grew to 100 and the total sample, males and females, was 200. All patients were hospitalized for the first time in the Department of Psychiatry of the University of Patras Medical School, Patras, Greece, from January 1988 through December 1992. Ninety-six of them were admitted for the first time in any psychiatric inpatient service; the remainder had one or more earlier hospitalizations elsewhere.

Patras is the third largest population center of Greece, located in the southwestern part of the country. The psychiatry department's wards are the only inpatient service in a larger administrative area of approximately 1 million people, and the department accepts cases with a 3-month maximum time of hospitalization.

The original diagnosis was made by staff psychiatrists during the patients' hospital stay after assessment of their history, clinical symptomatology, and overall behavior. To test reliability of the diagnosis, the records of each patient were reviewed independently by the three authors. The reviewers were blind to patients' age at onset of schizophrenia because this information was excluded from the case charts before assessment. For the present study, the diagnosis of the three reviewers was used. In all cases there was agreement by at least two of the reviewers. The unweighted kappa for interrater agreement among the three reviewers was 0.942 ($z = 21.284$, $p < 0.00001$). The interrater reliability among the three reviewers for the diagnosis of schizophrenia versus nonschizophrenia was estimated by reviewing 60 randomly selected case charts. There was complete agreement in all cases (kappa = 1.00, $z = 6.213$, $p < 0.00001$).

Three male patients, two with the paranoid subtype and one with the catatonic subtype, presented with the residual subtype on readmission. For the purposes of this study, they were given the later diagnosis of the residual subtype. Five additional cases of schizophrenic disorders (a male and a female with the paranoid subtype, two males with the residual subtype, and a male with the undifferentiated subtype) for whom the age at onset was uncertain were excluded from the study.

The onset of the disease was determined by the report of the immediate family and, when possible, by the patient specifying the time when the first prodromal symptoms required for a DSM–III–R diagnosis of a schizophrenic disorder were observed.

In addition to the unweighted kappa for three raters, Student's t test and the chi-square test were applied for the statistical analysis of the data. When multiple comparisons were made, the p value with the Bonferroni correction was estimated (Hochberg 1988). In general, p values smaller than 0.05 were considered significant.

Results

Table 1 shows the distribution of the 200 patients in the five subtypes of schizophrenic disorders and the age at onset in both males and females. The paranoid subtype was diagnosed most frequently in 39 of the males and 46 of the females.

The mean age at onset ± standard deviation (SD) of 30.4 ± 9.3 years observed in the paranoid subtype was the latest onset, whereas the 17.0 ± 2.2 years of the disorganized subtype was the earliest of all subtypes. The differences between the mean age at onset of the paranoid subtype and the mean age at onset of the other four subtypes were significant (disorganized: $t = 12.45$, $df = 112$, $p < 0.00001$; undifferentiated: $t = 6.94$, $df = 133$, $p < 0.00001$; residual: $t = 5.77$, $df = 113$, $p < 0.00001$; catatonic: $t = 4.25$, $df = 89$, $p < 0.001$). The mean age at onset of the disorganized subtype was significantly earlier than that of the residual subtype ($t = 5.31$, $df = 57$, $p < 0.00001$) or the undifferentiated subtype ($t = 5.13$, $df = 77$, $p < 0.00001$). There was no significant difference in the mean age at onset between the undifferentiated and the residual subtypes ($t = 0.30$, $df = 78$, $p > 0.05$); the disorganized and the catatonic subtypes ($t = 1.86$, $df = 33$, $p > 0.05$); the undifferentiated and the catatonic subtypes ($t = 0.61$, $df = 54$, $p > 0.05$); or the residual and the catatonic subtypes ($t = 0.74$, $df = 34$, $p > 0.05$) (Student's t test with Bonferroni correction).

The mean age at onset of all female patients was significantly later than that of male patients ($t = 2.95$, $df = 198$, $p = 0.017$). Further analysis of the age at onset showed significant differences between male and female patients within the subtypes of schizophrenic disorders.

In the paranoid subtype, the mean age at onset for females was significantly later than that for males ($t = 3.72$, $df = 83$, $p = 0.00017$). However, in the disorganized subtype, the disorder started significantly earlier in the female patients than in the male patients ($t = 2.20$, $df = 27$, $p = 0.018$). The mean onset of the undifferentiated subtype was earlier in the male than in the female patients, but the difference was not significant ($t = 1.89$, $df = 48$, $p = 0.07$). There was no significant difference in the mean age at onset between male and female patients of the residual subtype ($t = 0.25$, $df = 28$, $p = 0.40$).

Table 2 lists the differences in the age at onset between the 39 male and the 46 female patients with the paranoid subtype. The number (28) of paranoid male patients with an age at onset before 30 was significantly greater than the 4 male patients who were diagnosed with the disorder after age 35 ($\chi^2 = 36$, $df = 1$, $p < 0.001$). On the contrary, there was no significant difference between the number of female subjects with age at onset before 30 (19 cases) and after 35 (21 cases) ($\chi^2 = 0.211$, $df = 1$, $p > 0.50$). Figure 1 illustrates the age at onset of the 200 patients in each of the five subtypes of schizophrenic disorders.

Table 1. Age at onset in schizophrenia patients according to subtype and sex (n = 200)

Subtype	Male		Female		Total	
	n	Onset mean (SD)	n	Onset mean (SD)	n	Onset mean (SD)
Paranoid	39	26.7 (6.7)	46	33.5 (10.1)	85	30.4 (9.3)
Undifferentiated	23	20.9 (3.7)	27	22.8 (5.3)	50	22.0 (4.7)
Residual	21	22.1 (4.6)	9	22.8 (6.8)	30	22.3 (5.2)
Disorganized	12	17.7 (1.6)	17	16.1 (2.4)	29	17.0 (2.2)
Catatonic	5	21.0 (5.5)	1	19.0 —	6	20.7 (5.0)
Total	100	23.0 (6.0)	100	26.6 (10.2)	200	24.8 (8.6)

Note.—SD = standard deviation.

Figure 1. Distribution of age at onset of paranoid, undifferentiated, disorganized, residual, and catatonic subtypes of 200 schizophrenia patients (100 male and 100 female)

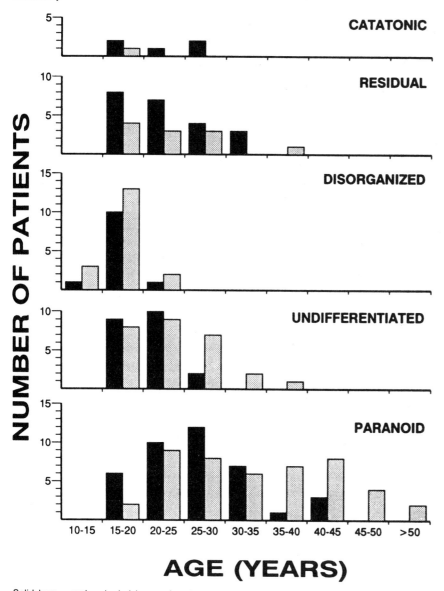

Solid bars = male; shaded bars = female.

Of the 85 patients with paranoid subtype, approximately 72 percent of the male and 41 percent of the female patients showed the disorder before age 30. The onset occurred after age 35 in 10 percent of the male and 46 percent of the female cases. In the 30 to 35 age group, the onset occurred in 18 percent of the male and in 13 percent of the female cases (table 2). Analysis of the distribution of the age at onset of the 39 male and the 46 female subjects with the paranoid subtype showed that the percentage of males with an onset before age 30 was significantly greater than the percentage of females ($\chi^2 = 19.55$, $df = 1$, $p < 0.001$), whereas the percentage of females with onset after age 35 was significantly greater than that of males ($\chi^2 = 32.143$, $df = 1$, $p < 0.001$). There was no significant difference between the percentage of the two sexes when the onset was between 30 and 35 years ($\chi^2 = 0.954$, $df = 1$, $p > 0.30$).

The mean age at onset ± SD for the male patients with undifferentiated, residual, disorganized, and catatonic subtypes was 20.7 ± 4.1 years; for the female patients with the same subtypes it was 20.6 ± 5.7 years. This difference is not significant ($t = 0.97$, $df = 113$, $p > 0.4$). On the other hand, the mean age at onset ± SD (26.7 ± 6.7 years) of the male patients with the paranoid subtype was significantly greater than that of the female patients with all other subtypes of schizophrenic disorders (20.6 ± 6.7 years) ($t = 4.54$, $df = 91$, $p < 0.0001$).

When only first admissions were considered ($n = 96$; see table 3), analysis of the data confirmed the findings obtained from the total sample of the 200 patients. However, in this case no analysis could be made of the catatonic or residual subtypes because of the small number of such first admissions. The mean age at onset of first-admission paranoid patients to any hospital was 29.9 ± 9.4 years, whereas that of the first-admission patients with the undifferentiated subtype was 22.9 ± 5.3 years ($t = 3.99$, $df = 69$, $p < 0.00001$). There was also a significant difference in the age at onset between the first-admission patients with the paranoid and those with the disorganized subtype (16.7 ± 2.5 years; $t = 8.75$, $df = 64$, $p < 0.00001$). Similarly, in first-admission patients, the onset of the disease occurred significantly earlier in the disorganized than in the undifferentiated subtype ($t = 5.13$, $df = 43$,

Table 2. Differences in age at onset between male and female paranoid patients ($n = 85$)

Age at onset (yrs)	Male ($n = 39$)		Female ($n = 16$)		Significance	
	n	(%)	n	(%)	χ^2	p
< 30	28	(72)	19	(41)	7.938	<0.01
30–35	7	(18)	6	(13)	0.392	>0.5
>35	4	(10)	21	(46)	12.737	<0.001

Table 3. Age at onset in 96 first-admission schizophrenia patients according to gender and subtype

| | Onset (yrs) | | | | Significance | |
| | Male | | Female | | | |
Subtype	n	mean (SD)	n	mean (SD)	t	p
Paranoid	22	26.4 (6.4)	24	33.0 (10.8)	2.57	<0.007
Undifferentiated	9	22.6 (4.5)	16	23.1 (5.8)	0.24	>0.400
Disorganized	8	17.9 (1.8)	12	16.0 (2.6)	1.89	<0.037
Catatonic	2	26.5 —	1	19.0 —	—	—
Residual	1	19.0 —	1	15.0 —	—	—
Total	42	23.8 (6.2)	54	26.0 (10.6)	1.27	>0.100

Note.—SD = standard deviation.

$p < 0.00001$) (Student's t test with Bonferroni correction).

Table 4 shows the differences in the age at onset between 22 male and 24 female first-admission paranoid patients. The number of the first-admission male paranoid patients with the age at onset before 30, was significantly greater than the male patients with onset of the disorder after age 35 ($\chi^2 = 18.427$, $df = 1$, $p < 0.001$). There was no difference in the number of the first-admission female patients with onset before age 30 or after age 35.

Discussion

These data demonstrate that there are not only sex differences in the age at onset of the schizophrenic disorders, but also differences in the mean age at onset among the various subtypes of schizophrenia. The subtype with the earliest appearance was the disorganized, for which the mean age at onset was approximately 5 years earlier than the undifferentiated and residual subtypes, and 13 years earlier than the paranoid subtype. The later appearance of the paranoid subtype was first recognized by Kraepelin (1919/1971).

In addition to the earliest onset, the disorganized subtype demonstrated the sharpest peak of incidence of the age at onset of all subtypes. For both men and women, all cases appeared in a 9-year span, between ages 11 and 20. The widest spread for age at onset was observed in the paranoid subtype, in which new cases appeared between 17 and 60 years of age. In this subtype, women had a much wider peak of incidence rates than men. For women the age at onset spread over a period of 42 years, whereas for men the spread was 26 years. Also, a wider peak of age at onset incidence rates was observed in women than in men with the undifferentiated subtype, except that the difference between the sexes was smaller (see figure 1). The small number of cases with the catatonic subtype does not permit meaningful comparisons of this subtype with the others.

Our observation that the mean age at onset in all subtypes of schizophrenic disorders we studied was 3.6 years earlier for men than for women is in accord with the findings of earlier reports (Noreik and Ødegaard 1967; McCabe 1975; Lewine 1980; Loranger 1984; Goldstein et al. 1990; Gureje 1991). This sex difference has been demonstrated regardless of the historical period, culture or diagnostic system applied (Bleuler 1911/1950); Kraepelin 1919/1971; Lewine 1981; Loranger 1984; Goldstein et al. 1990; Gureje 1991).

The significantly earlier onset of schizophrenia in female patients

with four of the five subtypes (disorganized, undifferentiated, residual, catatonic) when compared with male patients with the paranoid subtype demonstrates that men do not always have an earlier age at onset of the schizophrenic disorders than women and indicates the existence of differences among the subtypes of schizophrenia. Furthermore, this finding helps to explain the observation that age distributions of the two sexes do not consist of two isomorphic curves separated by a time interval (Loranger 1984), for there are female patients with an early onset as well. The existence of differences in the age at onset among the subtypes of schizophrenic disorders is also evidenced by the fact that the mean age at onset between all male and female cases in the present study was significantly greater in the female cases, whereas male and female cases of all other subtypes, except the paranoid, had an almost identical mean age at onset, differing only by a factor of 0.1 years.

The findings of the study indicate that the overall earlier onset of schizophrenia in men is caused by the impact of the significantly earlier onset of the disorder in men of the paranoid subtype. This observation does not support the hypothesis that estrogens or androgens, either as fetal hormones affecting the structure and functioning of the brain (organizational effects) or as circulating hormones (triggering effects), cause the gender differences in the age at onset of schizophrenia (Seeman 1985; Seeman and Lang 1990). If estrogens play a protective role or androgens a triggering role in the age at onset, this should be limited to the paranoid and, possibly, the undifferentiated subtypes.

Table 4. Differences in age at onset between first-admission male and female paranoid patients

| Age at onset (yrs) | Male (n = 22) | Female (n = 24) | Significance | |
	n (%)	n (%)	χ^2	p
<30	16 (73)	10 (42)	5.64	<0.02
30–35	4 (18)	3 (12)	0.29	>0.50
>35	2 (9)	11 (46)	7.64	<0.01

However, such a selective effect of these hormones is plausible only if the subtypes are the phenotypic expression of biological or genetic heterogeneity of schizophrenia.

The observation that 72 percent of the men with the paranoid subtype became ill before age 30, whereas only 10 percent developed the illness after age 35, demonstrates the tendency of men to develop the paranoid subtype of schizophrenia before the age of 30; the peak period of onset is between ages 25 and 29. On the contrary, the finding that women show a similar age at onset distribution before their 30th birthday (41%) and after their 35th (46%) leads to the conclusion that women have an equal risk for developing the disorder earlier or later in life. Actually, women appeared to have two peaks in the age at onset, one from ages 20 to 24, and the other from ages 40 to 44. It is of interest that even men showed a small increase in the frequency of the age at onset from ages 40 through 44. The lowest frequency of the age at onset in the age span of 20 to 45 years was found from ages 30 through 34. After age 45 the frequency of the onset of the disorder starts decreasing, with the latest onset observed at age 60 (see figure 2). These observations may indicate the presence of two peaks in the age at onset, suggesting the existence of two different forms of the disorder. This possibility is supported by the finding that patients with paranoid schizophrenia had a greater stability of the subtype when the onset occurred after age 30 (Kendler et al. 1985). Further investigation of this aspect is warranted.

The differences in the age at onset among the subtypes of schizophrenic disorders observed in this study appear to be real, as they are highly unlikely to have resulted from the selection criteria used for the admission of patients. If such a factor had operated, a similar trend should exist in all subtypes. The patients included in the study were unselected, with the exception of the successive female patients only selected after 100 male cases were obtained. Only 5 cases were excluded, because their age at onset was uncertain.

The fact that the 96 schizophrenia patients admitted for the first time to any hospital demonstrated findings similar to those in the total sample of 200 patients supports the position that the study data reflect the real phenotypic expression of the subtypes and do not result from the confounding effects of chronicity, drug treatment, or institutionalization.

Also, since the number of studies examining first-episode schizophrenia is relatively small (Keshavan and Schooler 1992), the data on the first hospitalization sample can be used for comparisons with the multiple-episode cases.

The earlier onset of the disorganized subtype in the female when compared with the male patients should be looked at as representing one extreme of the spectrum of the gender differences in the age at onset among the subtypes of the schizophrenic disorders. The paranoid subtype has an earlier onset of 6.8 years in the male patients, followed by an earlier onset of 1.9 years in the undifferentiated subtype (again in the male patients), a nonsignificant difference between the sexes of 0.7 years for the residual subtype and an earlier onset by 1.6 years in the female patients for the disorganized subtype. This gradual transition of the age at onset between the sexes in the subtypes, observed in both the multiple and first-admission patients, suggests that it does not result from a cultural ascertainment bias, but rather that it is an intrinsic characteristic of the subtypes.

Figure 2. Age at onset for 85 schizophrenia patients, paranoid subtype

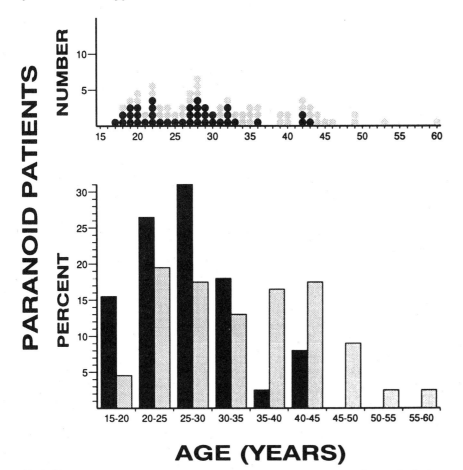

Vertical bars = percentage of age at onset in each sex per 5-year period. Dots = distribution of age at onset of 85 patients. Solid symbols = male; shaded symbols = female. Each dot corresponds to one individual.

Age at onset is an important clinical finding of schizophrenia that could be helpful in shedding light on the primary defect of the disorder. The findings of this study provide evidence of both gender and subtype differences in the age at onset of the schizophrenic disorders and may help to clarify the clinical spectrum and etiology of the subtypes.

The division of schizophrenia into subtypes has been controversial, and Blashfield (1973) claimed that the subtypes cannot be reliably diagnosed. However, more recent studies have demonstrated adequate to excellent reliability of the subtyping of schizophrenia (Gruenberg et al. 1985). In a review article, McGlashan and Fenton (1991) addressed the question of whether or not there is a reason to maintain the subtypes of schizophrenia in *DSM–IV* and concluded that all of them should be retained. The data presented in this article provide additional support for the validity of the schizophrenic subtypes as distinct clinical entities.

It has been suggested (DeLisi et al. 1987; Crow 1988) that one of the genes of schizophrenia, perhaps that which determines time of onset, could be sex linked. This hypothesis, however, seems unlikely for the entire group of schizophrenic disorders in light of the findings of the present study showing both variable gender differences and differences in the age at onset among the subtypes regardless of sex.

A genetic predisposition for schizophrenia is widely accepted, but segregation analyses of pedigrees have failed to identify a classic single gene pattern of inheritance. However, the variable clinical picture of the disorder could be attributed to underlying genetic heterogeneity. When we are considering a disease, we need to be sure that we are talking about the same entity. In genetic heterogeneity the same clinical picture can be caused by more than one mutation at different loci. On the other hand, pleiotropism, the multiple effects of a single mutant gene, can lead to different phenotypes. The question, therefore, as

to whether or not all or some of the subtypes of the schizophrenic disorders are the result of genetic heterogeneity or pleiotropism remains unsettled.

In seeking to better understand the etiology of schizophrenic disorders one can rely on clinical, genetic, and biochemical data. Biochemical evidence is the most reliable category of evidence. Although the biological basis of schizophrenia remains unknown, it seems that genetic studies may provide clues to the primary defect of the disorder.

The differences in the age at onset of the schizophrenic disorders we described may indicate biological differences among the subtypes or groups of subtypes. If these differences had an environmental origin, such as social pressures, we would expect to find a similar trend in the age at onset of the two sexes among the subtypes. Therefore, genetic studies, which will take into consideration the phenotype of the schizophrenic disorders, are needed. If such studies can provide evidence of genetic heterogeneity, phenotypic differences will attain their proper perspective, and earlier unnoticed differences, similar to those reported in this article, may emerge to serve as truly diagnostic phenotypic features.

References

American Psychiatric Association. *DSM–III: Diagnostic and Statistical Manual of Mental Disorders.* 3rd ed. Washington, DC: The Association, 1980.

American Psychiatric Association. *DSM–III–R: Diagnostic and Statistical Manual of Mental Disorders.* 3rd ed., revised. Washington, DC: The Association, 1987.

Blashfield, R. An evaluation of the *DSM–II* classification of schizophrenia as a nomenclature. *Journal of Abnormal Psychology,* 82:382–389, 1973.

Bleuler, E. *Dementia Praecox or the Group of Schizophrenias.* (1911) Translated by J. Zinkin. New York, NY: International Universities Press, 1950.

Cancro, R. History and overview of schizophrenia. In: Kaplan, H.I., and Sadock, B.J., eds. *Comprehensive Textbook of Psychiatry IV.* Vol. I. Baltimore, MD: Williams & Wilkins Company, 1985. pp. 631–643.

Crow, T.J. Sex chromosomes and psychosis: The case for a pseudoautosomal locus. *British Journal of Psychiatry,* 153:675–683, 1988.

DeLisi, L.E.; Goldin, L.R.; Maxwell, M.E.; Kazuba, D.M.; and Gershon, E.S. Clinical features of illness in siblings with schizophrenia or schizoaffective disorder. *Archives of General Psychiatry,* 44:891–896, 1987.

Fenton, W.S., and McGlashan, T.H. Natural history of schizophrenia subtypes: I. Longitudinal study of paranoid, hebephrenic, and undifferentiated schizophrenia. *Archives of General Psychiatry,* 48:969–977, 1991.

Gold, D.D. Late age of onset schizophrenia: Present but unaccounted for. *Comprehensive Psychiatry,* 25:225–237, 1984.

Goldstein, J.M., and Link, B.J. Gender differences in the clinical expression of schizophrenia. *Journal of Psychiatric Research,* 22:141–155, 1988.

Goldstein, J.M.; Santagelo, S.L.; Simpson, J.C.; and Tsuang, M.T. The role of gender in identifying subtypes of schizophrenia: A latent class analytic approach. *Schizophrenia Bulletin,* 16:263–275, 1990.

Goldstein, J.M., and Tsuang, M.T. Gender and schizophrenia: An introduction and synthesis of findings. *Schizophrenia Bulletin,* 16:179–183, 1990.

Gruenberg, A.M.; Kendler, K.S.; and Tsuang, M.T. Reliability and concordance in the subtyping of schizophrenia. *American Journal of Psychiatry,* 142:1355–1358, 1985.

Gureje, O. Gender and schizophrenia: Age-at-onset and sociodemographic attributes. *Acta Psychiatrica Scandinavica,* 83:402–405, 1991.

Harris, M.J., and Jeste, D.V. Late-onset schizophrenia: An overview. *Schizophrenia Bulletin,* 14:39–55, 1988.

Hochberg, Y. A sharper Bonferroni for multiple tests of significance. *Biometrica*, 75:800–802, 1988.

Kendler, K.S.; Gruenberg, A.M.; and Tsuang, M.T. Subtype stability in schizophrenia. *American Journal of Psychiatry*, 142:827–832, 1985.

Keshavan, M.S., and Schooler, N.R. First-episode studies in schizophrenia: Criteria and characterization. *Schizophrenia Bulletin*, 18:491–513, 1992.

Kraepelin, E. *Dementia Praecox and Paraphrenia.* (1919) Translated by Barclay, R.M., and Robertson, G.M. New York, NY: Robert E. Krieger Publishing Company, 1971.

Kramer, M. Population changes and schizophrenia 1970–1975. In: Wynne, L.C.; Cromwell, R.L.; and Matthysse, S., eds. *The Nature of Schizophrenia—New Approaches to Research and Treatment.* New York, NY: John Wiley & Sons, 1978. pp. 545–571.

Lewine, R.R.J. Sex differences in age of symptom onset and first hospitalization in schizophrenia. *American Journal of Orthopsychiatry*, 50:316–322, 1980.

Lewine, R.R.J. Sex differences in schizophrenia: Timing or subtypes? *Psychological Bulletin*, 90:432–444, 1981.

Lewine, R.R.J.; Gulley, L.R.; Risch, S.C.; Jewart, R.; and Houpt, J.L. Sexual dimorphism, brain morphology, and schizophrenia. *Schizophrenia Bulletin*, 16:195–203, 1990.

Loranger, A.W. Sex differences in age-at-onset of schizophrenia. *Archives of General Psychiatry*, 41:157–161, 1984.

McCabe, M. Demographic differences in functional psychoses. *British Journal of Psychiatry*, 127:320–323, 1975.

McGlashan, T.H., and Fenton, W.S. Classical subtypes for schizophrenia: Literature review for *DSM–IV*. *Schizophrenia Bulletin*, 17:609–623, 1991.

Noreik, K., and Ødegaard, Ø. Age at onset of schizophrenia in relation to socioeconomic factors. *British Journal of Social Psychiatry*, 1:243–249, 1967.

Ohaeri, J.U. Age at onset in a cohort of schizophrenics in Nigeria.

Acta Psychiatrica Scandinavica, 86:332–334, 1992.

Pearlson, G.D.; Kreger, L.; Rabins, P.V.; Chase, G.A.; Cohen, B.; Wirth, J.B.; Schlaepfer, T.B.; and Tune, L.E. A chart review study of late-onset and early-onset schizophrenia. *American Journal of Psychiatry*, 146:1568–1574, 1989.

Raskin, A., and Golob, R. Occurrence of sex and social class differences in premorbid competence, symptom and outcome measures in acute schizophrenia. *Psychological Reports*, 18:11–22, 1966.

Seeman, M.V. Sex and schizophrenia. *Canadian Journal of Psychiatry*, 30:313–315, 1985.

Seeman, M.V., and Lang, M. The role of estrogens in schizophrenia gender differences. *Schizophrenia Bulletin*, 16:185–194, 1990.

Spitzer, R.L.; Endicott, J.; and Robins, E. Research Diagnostic Criteria: Rationale and reliability. *Archives of General Psychiatry*, 35:773–782, 1978.

Maternal Influenza, Obstetric Complications, and Schizophrenia

Padraig Wright, M.R.C.Psych., Noriyoshi Takei, M.D., M.Sc.,
Larry Rifkin, M.R.C.Psych., and Robin M. Murray, D.Sc., F.R.C.Psych.

Objective: Epidemiologic studies have reported an association between prenatal exposure to influenza and adult schizophrenia. The authors studied this association in individual patients with schizophrenia and also investigated the relationship of obstetric complications, another postulated risk factor, to adult schizophrenia. Method: Using a structured interview instrument, the authors assessed infections during pregnancy, obstetric complications, gestational age, and birth weight by interviewing the mothers of 121 patients with DSM-III-R schizophrenia. Results: Significantly more infections were reported in the second trimester of the patients' gestations than in the combined first and third trimesters. Influenza accounted for 70% of second-trimester infections. Patients with schizophrenia whose mothers reported having influenza during the second trimester were almost five times more likely to experience at least one definite obstetric complication than were patients who were not exposed to influenza during the second trimester; the exposed patients weighed a mean of 210 g less at birth than the unexposed patients. Conclusions: Maternal influenza during the second trimester may impair fetal growth and predispose to obstetric complications and lower birth weight in a proportion of individuals destined to develop schizophrenia.

The overwhelming majority of studies that have investigated the birth dates of individuals who later developed schizophrenia reported that these individuals are 7%–15% more likely to be born in late winter or spring (1, 2). Methodological artifacts caused by measuring age in whole years and failing to correct for the longer period at risk that patients born in the early months of any year have experienced were put forward as possible explanations of this finding (3–5). However, more recent studies using rigorous techniques to exclude such errors (6, 7) confirmed that individuals who later develop schizophrenia are indeed more likely to be born during late winter and spring than at other times of the year.

What causes this excess of births of future schizophrenic patients in late winter and spring? Many infectious diseases have a seasonally varying prevalence, and several studies have examined the birth dates of patients with schizophrenia in relation to epidemics of influenza. Some found no association (8–10), but the majority of studies that have examined single epidemics of influenza and, perhaps more importantly, its varying prevalence over several decades, reported an association between prenatal exposure to influenza, particularly during the second trimester of gestation, and adult schizophrenia (11–21). No consistent relationship has been found between schizophrenia and prenatal exposure to any other infectious disease, with the exception of bronchopneumonia, which, of course, often follows influenza infection (22).

These studies did not demonstrate a link between prenatal influenza exposure and schizophrenia for any individual patient. Stober et al. (23), however, found that influenza during the second trimester was reported by 30.8% of the mothers of schizophrenic patients, compared with 7.8% who reported having influenza at other times during the schizophrenic patient's gestation. Similarly, using contemporaneous obstetric records, Mednick et al. (24) reported that influenza was recorded in the antenatal medical records during the second trimester of pregnancy in 86.7% of a small number of women who gave birth to schizophrenic children following the 1957 A2 influenza epidemic in Helsinki; influenza was recorded

Received Jan. 13, 1995; revision received June 23, 1995; accepted July 19, 1995. From the Genetics Section, Department of Psychological Medicine, Institute of Psychiatry and King's College Hospital. Address reprint requests to Professor Murray, Genetics Section, Department of Psychological Medicine, Institute of Psychiatry, De Crespigny Park, London, SE5 8AF, UK.

Supported in part by the Wellcome Trust and the Stanley Foundation.

The authors thank the patients, families, and National Schizophrenia Fellowship members who participated in this study and Drs. E. O'Callaghan and M. Gill for helpful comments.

From *The American Journal of Psychiatry,* December 1995, pp. 1714-1720. © 1995 by the American Psychiatric Association. Reprinted by permission.

TABLE 1. Gestational Infections Reported by the Mothers of 121 Schizophrenic Patients

Infection	First N	First %	Second N	Second %	Third N	Third %	Total N	Total %	p[a]
Influenza[b]	0	0.0	14	11.6	2	1.7	16	13.2	0.004[c]
Respiratory infection	0	0.0	4	3.3	0	0.0	4	3.3	0.12[d]
Pyelonephritis	0	0.0	2	1.7	0	0.0	2	1.7	0.50[d]
Gastroenteritis	0	0.0	0	0.0	1	0.8	1	0.8	1.00[d]
Candidiasis (oral)	1	0.8	0	0.0	0	0.0	1	0.8	1.00[d]
Rubella	0	0.0	0	0.0	1	0.8	1	0.8	1.00[d]
Dental abscess	1	0.8	0	0.0	0	0.0	1	0.8	1.00[d]
Total	2	1.7	20	16.5	4	3.3	26	21.5	0.005[e]
Other[f]	4	3.3	4	3.3	0	0.0	7	5.8	0.70[d]

[a]Comparison of number of women infected during the second trimester with those infected during the combined first and third trimester.
[b]Sixteen influenza cases account for 61.5% of all infections; 14 influenza cases account for 70.0% of second-trimester infections.
[c]$\chi^2=8.1$, df=1.
[d]Fisher's exact test.
[e]$\chi^2=8.45$, df=1.
[f]Includes a woman given rubella vaccine, one given thalidomide, one whose sister had measles during the first trimester, one given smallpox vaccine, one given Asian influenza vaccine, one whose husband had influenza during the second trimester, and one who handled sera at an influenza research laboratory during the first and second trimesters. The figures in this row are not included in the calculation of the total number of infections.

during the other two trimesters for only 20% of the women who had schizophrenic children.

Although McCreadie et al. (25) and Done et al. (26) found no association between pregnancy and perinatal difficulties (collectively termed obstetric complications) and schizophrenia, most studies reported an excess of obstetric complications in schizophrenia (27–30). Some studies also suggested that schizophrenic patients weigh less than comparison subjects at birth (31, 32); Rifkin et al. (33) reported that a birth weight below 2500 g is more common in schizophrenic patients than in patients with affective psychosis. Rifkin et al. (33) also reported that a lower birth weight correlated significantly with impaired premorbid social adjustment and poor cognitive performance in adulthood.

The question of whether obstetric complications cause some cases of schizophrenia or are themselves caused by an earlier insult that also leads to schizophrenia remains unanswered (34). To our knowledge, no study has yet explored the potential relationship between schizophrenia and prenatal exposure to influenza, obstetric complications, or birth weight.

We now report such a study, undertaken to test the hypotheses that, in schizophrenia, 1) maternal infection, especially influenza, is more common during the second trimester of gestation than in the combined first and third trimesters and 2) maternal infection, especially influenza, is associated with obstetric complications and low birth weight.

METHOD

As part of a program of studies investigating immune function in schizophrenia, white patients of British parentage who had the diagnosis of schizophrenia were recruited at two south London hospitals (N=81) and from southeast England through the National Schizophre-

nia Fellowship (N=40). The study protocol required that the patients satisfied DSM-III-R criteria for schizophrenia, agreed that their mothers could be interviewed, and were born between either February and May or between August and November. There is marked seasonal variation in the prevalence of influenza, and these two periods were chosen to enable further division of the patients into subgroups at high (born April to May) and low (born August to November) risk of exposure to prenatal influenza in mid-gestation, as required for our immunological studies. After the study had been described completely to the patient subjects and to their mothers, written informed consent was obtained.

The mothers of the 121 patients were interviewed by using a structured instrument (available on request). The interviewer (P.W.) first collected demographic data and detailed information about psychiatric illness in first-degree relatives using Family History Research Diagnostic Criteria (35) and then asked the mother about her health during the patient's gestation and birth. Questioning proceeded from the general (e.g., "Do you recall anything in particular of the pregnancy") to the particular (e.g., "Did you have any infections during pregnancy"). Cues (e.g., events the woman reported in her own life, annual holidays or feast days, topical news items, etc.) were given to the mother to accurately time the occurrence of reported events. If an obstetric complication or infectious disease was reported, the mother was questioned closely about duration, symptoms, and treatment to determine the most likely diagnosis. Finally, the interviewer read out the list of obstetric complications from the scale of Lewis et al. (29) and a list of infections (rubella; syphilis; respiratory tract infection/common cold; influenza; gastroenteritis; cold sores/herpes; urinary tract infection; jaundice; infections of the skin/eyes/ears/nose, mouth/gut, throat/chest, bladder/kidneys, or blood; vaccinations; medicines or drugs; fever/temperature/pyrexia; and medical care other than antenatal care), using both medical and nontechnical terminology, and asked the woman to indicate if any of these had occurred during any trimester of the patient's gestation. Definite and possible obstetric complications according to the scale of Lewis et al. (29) were recorded but only definite obstetric complications were counted in the analysis. To avoid recording common colds as influenza, the interviewer recorded a diagnosis of influenza only when the mother reported typical symptoms of influenza (fever, cough, headache, and one or more of lethargy, myalgia, or arthralgia) or stated that such a diagnosis had been made at the time by a physician. Gestational infections, preterm (gestational age less than 37 weeks), or postterm (gestational age greater than 42 weeks) birth or a birth weight below 2500 g were not counted as obstetric complications because they were analyzed separately.

Statistical analysis was based on chi-square tests with appropriate corrections when comparing proportional distributions, t tests for comparison of means, and odds ratios for associations between schizophrenia and obstetric complications, birth weight, and exposure to gestational infection. Obstetric complications were subdivided into those occurring during the first, second, and third trimesters; intrapartum obstetric complications arising between the onset of labor and 24 hours after the schizophrenic patient's birth; and disorders arising in the newborn during the first 24 hours of life. A multivariate analysis was performed to control for the effects of confounding by sex and gestational age on birth weight.

RESULTS

Significantly more of the mothers of patients with schizophrenia reported infections during the second trimester of their offsprings' gestations than during the combined first and third trimesters (table 1). In addition to the 14 women who reported influenza infections during the second trimester, a further three women were exposed to influenza virus in some form at this time during pregnancy—one was given a smallpox and Asian influenza vaccine, the husband of one had influ-

enza, and one handled sera at an influenza research laboratory.

Eighty-seven (71.9%) of the patients were male and 34 (28.1%) were female. The proportions of male and female patients who were or were not exposed to infection during gestation were similar (tables 2 and 3).

Of the 121 mothers interviewed, 38 (31.4%) reported at least one definite obstetric complication on the scale of Lewis et al. (29) during the schizophrenic patient's gestation. Significantly more of the women who reported gestational infections than of those who did not also reported at least one definite obstetric complication (tables 2 and 3). The mean birth weight of the children of the women who reported gestational infections was 244 g lighter than that of the children of women with no gestational infections (table 2). When the 14 women who reported having influenza in the second trimester were compared with the rest of the women, the statistical significance of the difference between groups in the proportion who experienced at

TABLE 2. Sex, Obstetric Complications, Gestational Age, Birth Weight, and Family History of Schizophrenia in Schizophrenic Patients Who Were or Were Not Exposed to Gestational Infections During First, Second, or Third Trimester

Variable	Patients Exposed to Infection (N=26)		Patients Not Exposed to Infection (N=95)		Analysis			
	N	%	N	%	Odds Ratio	95% Confidence Interval	χ^2 (df=1)	p
Sex					1.39	0.47–4.69	0.16	0.69
Male	20	76.9	67	70.5				
Female	6	23.1	28	29.5				
Obstetric complications present	15	57.7	23	24.2	4.27	1.58–11.72	10.62	<0.01
Family history of schizophrenia	2	7.7	16	16.8	0.41	0.04–1.97		0.4[a]
	Mean	SD	Mean	SD	Mean Difference	95% Confidence Interval	t (df=119)	p
Gestation (weeks)	39.5	2.1	39.7	1.6	−0.2	−0.90–0.59	−0.41	0.69
Birth weight (g)	3134.4	521.1	3378.0	529.0	−243.6	−474.8–12.4	−2.09	0.04

[a]Fisher's exact test.

TABLE 3. Sex, Obstetric Complications, Gestational Age, Birth Weight, and Family History of Schizophrenia in Schizophrenic Patients Who Were or Were Not Exposed to Gestational Influenza During Second Trimester

Variable	Patients Exposed to Influenza (N=14)		Patients Not Exposed to Influenza (N=107)		Analysis		
	N	%	N	%	Odds Ratio	95% Confidence Interval	p[a]
Sex					1.50	0.36–8.89	0.75
Male	11	78.6	76	71.0			
Female	3	21.4	31	29.0			
Obstetric complications present	9	64.3	29	27.1	4.84	1.31–19.70	0.01
Family history of schizophrenia	0	0.0	18	16.8	0.00	0.00–1.67	0.13
	Mean	SD	Mean	SD	Mean Difference	95% Confidence Interval	t (df=119)	p
Gestation (weeks)	39.8	1.3	39.6	1.7	−0.2	−0.77–1.14	0.39	0.70
Birth weight (g)	3140.0	370.0	3350.0	549.3	−210.0	−509.8–89.8	−1.39	0.17

[a]Fisher's exact test.

least one definite obstetric complication was increased (table 3). The greater number of obstetric complications in women with influenza during the second trimester was not associated with a significantly lower mean birth weight.

There were too few first-trimester infections and ob-

DISCUSSION

This study investigated any association between second-trimester gestational influenza, obstetric complications, and low birth weight in newborns who later developed schizophrenia. More mothers of schizo-

TABLE 4. Obstetric Complications,[a] Gestational Age, and Birth Weights Reported by 15 of 26 Women Who Reported Influenza Infection While Pregnant With Schizophrenic Patients

Patient and Time of Infection	Complication	Gestational Age (weeks)	Birth Weight (g)
Second trimester			
1	Induced because of eclampsia; precipitate birth	40	3000
2	Undiagnosed twin pregnancy; first-born; breech presentation; mid-forceps birth	40	3000
3	Breech presentation; induced as postterm; in incubator for 10 days	42	2270
4	Threatened abortion at 16 weeks; cesarean section for cephalopelvic disproportion	38	3500
5	Pre-eclampsia treated with bed rest and induction; low-forceps birth	39	3060
6	Threatened abortion; failure to progress in labor; difficult forceps birth	40	3400
7	Difficult high-forceps birth (reason unknown)	40	2800
8	Anemia treated with parenteral iron in first and second trimesters; breech birth	40	3500
9	Threatened abortion at 14 weeks	38	3100
First or third trimester			
10	Induced because of eclampsia; intrapartum hemorrhage	40	3400
11	Fetal distress; emergency cesarean section	42	3340
12	First-born of twins; difficult forceps birth; incubator for 4 weeks	32	1420
13	Induced preterm (reason unknown)	36	2270
14	Induced because of eclampsia; neonate apneic; neonate intubated/ventilated	39	3405
15	Severe anemia in first and second trimesters; hospitalized for iron injections	40	3200

[a]Only definite obstetric complications on the scale of Lewis et al. (29) were used in the analyses.

stetric complications as well as postpartum complications in the mother or neonate to allow for the assessment of any possible interaction between gestational infections and obstetric complications during early pregnancy or the immediate postpartum period. Thirteen (50.0%) of the 26 women who reported second-trimester infections, compared with 21 (22.1%) of the 95 who did not, recalled one or more third-trimester or intrapartum obstetric complications (p=0.005, Fisher's exact test). Eight (57.1%) of the 14 women who reported second-trimester influenza, compared with 26 (24.3%) of the 107 who did not, recalled one or more third-trimester or intrapartum obstetric complications (p=0.02, Fisher's exact test).

The obstetric complications experienced by the 15 women who reported both obstetric complications and gestational infection are listed in table 4.

Patients whose mothers did or did not report gestational infections did not differ significantly in sex or gestational age, and although none of the patients whose mothers reported second-trimester influenza had a schizophrenic first-degree relative, this finding did not reach statistical significance (table 3). Because there were no overall differences in sex or gestational age between the patients who were or were not exposed to infections, it is unlikely that these factors confounded our results. To ensure this, we carried out analyses of covariance allowing for sex and gestational age and found that the lower birth weight in the exposed group remained significant (F=4.28, df=119, p=0.04). When we used logistic regression to allow for sex in the analysis of association between infection and obstetric complications, there was no modification of effect.

phrenic patients reported infections during the second trimester of gestation than in the combined first and third, and influenza accounted for the great majority of these infections. Schizophrenic patients exposed to gestational infections had a significantly lower mean birth weight, and significantly more of these patients experienced obstetric complications than did patients who were not exposed to gestational infections. The mean birth weight of schizophrenic patients exposed to influenza in the second trimester was 210 g lower than that of patients not so exposed, and the exposed patients were almost five times more likely to have experienced at least one definite obstetric complication (odds ratio=4.8).

Methodological issues must be considered before attempting any interpretation of our results. First, a third of the women studied were recruited through the National Schizophrenia Fellowship, and we selectively studied patients born from February to May and from August to November. It is possible that National Schizophrenia Fellowship members are not representative of schizophrenic patients and their families, and that this factor, as well as the selection of patients by season of birth, led to ascertainment or recall biases. However, although infectious diseases (12) and perhaps obstetric complications (28, 36) show seasonal variations, we found no significant differences in sex, family history of schizophrenia, birth weight, or gestational infections and obstetric complications when National Schizophrenia Fellowship and non-National Schizophrenia Fellowship, or subjects born from February to May or August to November, were compared. It is possible that this indicates that our subjects were not a representative sample, but a more likely explanation is that a study group of 121 subjects is simply too small to detect seasonal variation for these items.

Because data were obtained retrospectively by maternal interview, selective maternal recall of all adverse events occurring during the gestations of offspring who later developed schizophrenia must be considered. However, there is evidence that mothers are reliable informants about major obstetric events that occurred several decades previously, and maternal recall has been found to correlate closely with contemporaneous medical records in several studies (37–39; personal communication from E. Franzek and G. Stober to R.M.M.). It is also very unlikely that any systematic recall bias could account for either the higher number of infections reported in the second trimester or the association between infections and both obstetric complications and lower birth weight.

Furthermore, only definite obstetric complications were analyzed and infections were recorded conservatively so that, for example, three second-trimester infections that might well have been categorized as influenza were placed in the respiratory infection group because fever was not reported. This research was conducted before the considerable publicity that now surrounds the prenatal influenza hypothesis in the United Kingdom, and the rate of reported infections or obstetric complications in the National Schizophrenia Fellowship subgroup was not higher than the rate in the London hospital subgroup, even though the subjects in the National Schizophrenia Fellowship subgroup would more likely be familiar with the influenza hypothesis. Finally, the same set of questions were used when recording data on infections for each trimester, thus serving to further minimize bias.

Other possible shortcomings of the study are that we did not have a control group consisting of mothers of nonschizophrenic offspring and that we compared the reported number of infections during the second trimester with the combined number reported for the first and third trimesters because much of the first trimester can pass before pregnancy is confirmed and the third trimester may be of variable duration. However, obstetric complications were found in 31% of the patients we studied, and this figure is in keeping with most other retrospectively reported rates of obstetric complications in schizophrenia. For example, Gunther-Genta et al. (40) found obstetric complications in 45% of schizophrenic patients, DeLisi et al. (41) in 29%, and Foerster et al. (42) in 40%. Reported rates of second-trimester influenza in several series of schizophrenic patients ranged from 4.8% (1992 master's thesis by D. Fishleigh-Eaton) to 30.8% (23), compared with our rate of 11.6%. Mednick et al. (24) studied contemporaneous obstetric records and reported a rate of 86.7%, but this was in a small number of schizophrenic patients born in Helsinki during the months following the 1957 A2 influenza pandemic. Finally, our comparison of the combined data from the first and third trimesters with those for the second trimester would serve to reduce rather than to enhance our results.

Our findings may be explained in two ways. First, it is possible that our diagnoses of gestational infections are incorrect. They depend on maternal recall of events that took place several decades previously, and one could imagine, for example, that many systemic and respiratory viral infections are included under the general rubric of influenza. Although there must remain some doubt as to the exact nature of the infections we recorded, it is difficult to see how recall errors (either not recalling what did happen or thinking something happened that did not) could account for the concentration of infections in the second trimester (especially when these are compared with the total number of infections for the combined first and third trimesters), the fact that the majority of these infections were influenza, the association with obstetric complications and lower birth weight, and the significant excess of third-trimester and intrapartum obstetric complications in mothers who reported infections.

Second, the gestational infections we report may have caused impaired intrauterine growth, as evidenced by lower birth weight, and smaller fetuses may be at greater risk for obstetric complications and subsequent schizophrenia. There is evidence that influenza during pregnancy can lead to low birth weight (43), preterm birth (44), early neonatal mortality (45), and congenital central nervous system deformities (46, 47) in offspring. This model is in keeping with suggestions that obstetric complications may be the result rather than the cause of earlier prenatal insult (34, 39). It is also consistent with our finding that women who reported second-trimester infection or influenza were almost twice as likely to experience at least one definite third trimester or intrapartum obstetric complication when compared with women who did not. Thus, our findings can be interpreted to mean that maternal infection during the second trimester of pregnancy may cause neurodevelopmental damage and result in lower birth weight and obstetric complications. This chain of events may represent the pre- and perinatal components of a congenital disorder that has both childhood (premorbid social and cognitive abnormalities) and adult (social and cognitive abnormalities and schizophrenia) sequelae (33).

Finally, our results provide no evidence that the most potent risk factor for schizophrenia—that of having a schizophrenic first-degree relative—interacts etiologically with prenatal influenza, obstetric complications, or lower birth weight. It remains possible, however, that the genetic predisposition for a proportion of schizophrenia is determined by genes controlling the maternal immune response to gestational influenza (48, 49).

This study is preliminary and needs to be replicated by using both maternal recall and contemporaneous medical records to determine the prevalence of infections during pregnancy. There is ample reason for such research because confirmation of the prenatal influenza/schizophrenia hypothesis would imply that a proportion of schizophrenia is preventable and would generate a pathophysiological paradigm on which further research could be based.

REFERENCES

1. Bradbury TN, Miller GA: Season of birth in schizophrenia: a review of evidence, methodology and etiology. Psychol Bull 1985; 98:569–594
2. Boyd JH, Pulver AE, Stewart W: Season of birth: schizophrenia and bipolar disorder. Schizophr Bull 1986; 12:173–186
3. Hare EH, Price JS, Slater E: Mental disorder and season of birth: a national survey compared with the general population. Br J Psychiatry 1974; 152:460–465
4. Lewis MS, Griffin TA: An explanation for the season of birth effect in schizophrenia and certain other diseases. Psychol Bull 1981; 89:589–596
5. Lewis MS: Age incidence and schizophrenia, part I: the season of birth controversy. Schizophr Bull 1989; 15:59–73
6. O'Callaghan E, Gibson T, Colohan HA, Walsh D, Buckley P, Larkin C, Waddington JL: Season of birth in schizophrenia: evidence for confinement of an excess of winter births to patients without a family history of mental disorder. Br J Psychiatry 1991; 158:764–769
7. Pallast EGM, Jongbloet PH, Straatman HM, Zielhuis GA: Excess seasonality of births among patients with schizophrenia and seasonal ovopathy. Schizophr Bull 1994; 20:269–276
8. Torrey EF, Bowler AE, Rawlings R: An influenza epidemic and the seasonality of schizophrenic births, in Psychiatry and Biological Factors. New York, Plenum, 1991, pp 106–116
9. Crow TJ, Done DJ: Prenatal exposure to influenza does not cause schizophrenia. Br J Psychiatry 1992; 161:390–393
10. Susser E, Lin SP, Brown AS, Lumey LH, Erlenmeyer-Kimling L: No relation between risk of schizophrenia and prenatal exposure to influenza in Holland. Am J Psychiatry 1994; 151:922–924
11. Mednick SA, Machon RA, Huttunen MO, Bonett D: Adult schizophrenia following prenatal exposure to an influenza epidemic. Arch Gen Psychiatry 1988; 45:189–192
12. O'Callaghan E, Sham P, Takei N, Glover G, Murray RM: Schizophrenia after prenatal exposure to 1957 A2 influenza epidemic. Lancet 1991; 337:1248–1250
13. Barr CE, Mednick SA, Munk-Jorgensen P: Exposure to influenza epidemics during gestation and adult schizophrenia: a 40-year study. Arch Gen Psychiatry 1990; 47:869–874
14. Sham PC, O'Callaghan E, Takei N, Murray GK, Hare EH, Murray RM: Schizophrenia following pre-natal exposure to influenza epidemics between 1939 and 1960. Br J Psychiatry 1992; 160:461–466
15. Fahy TA, Jones PB, Sham PC: Schizophrenia in Afro-Caribbeans in the UK following prenatal exposure to the 1957 A2 influenza epidemic. Schizophr Res 1992; 6:98–99
16. Adams W, Kendell RE, Hare EH, Munk-Jorgensen P: Epidemiological evidence that maternal influenza contributes to the aetiology of schizophrenia: an analysis of Scottish, English and Danish data. Br J Psychiatry 1993; 163:522–534
17. Kunugi H, Nanko S, Takei N: Influenza and schizophrenia in Japan. Br J Psychiatry 1992; 161:274–275
18. Takei N, Van Os J, Murray RM: Maternal exposure to influenza and risk of schizophrenia: a 22 year study from the Netherlands. J Psychiatr Res (in press)
19. Takei N, Mortensen MD, Klaening U, Murray RM, Sham PC, O'Callaghan E, Munk-Jorgensen P: Relationship between in utero exposure to influenza epidemics and risk of schizophrenia in Denmark (abstract). Schizophr Res 1994; 11:95
20. Takei N, Sham P, O'Callaghan E, Murray GK, Glover G, Murray RM: Prenatal exposure to influenza and the development of schizophrenia: is the effect confined to females? Am J Psychiatry 1994; 151:117–119
21. McGrath JJ, Pemberton MR, Welham JL, Murray RM: Schizophrenia and the influenza epidemics of 1954, 1957 and 1959: a Southern Hemisphere study. Schizophr Res 1994; 14:1–8
22. O'Callaghan E, Sham PC, Takei N, Murray G, Glover G, Hare EH, Murray RM: The relationship of schizophrenic births to 16 infectious diseases. Br J Psychiatry 1994; 165:353–356
23. Stober G, Franzek E, Beckmann H: The role of maternal infectious diseases during pregnancy in the etiology of schizophrenia in offspring. Eur Psychiatry 1992; 7:147–152
24. Mednick SA, Huttunen MO, Machon RA: Prenatal influenza infections and adult schizophrenia. Schizophr Bull 1994; 20:263–276
25. McCreadie RG, Hall DJ, Berry IJ, Robertson LJ, Ewing JI, Geals MF: The Nithsdale schizophrenia surveys: obstetric complications, family history and abnormal movements. Br J Psychiatry 1992; 160:799–805
26. Done J, Johnstone EC, Frith CD, Golding J, Shepherd PM, Crow TJ: Complications of pregnancy and delivery in relation to psychosis in adult life: data from the British perinatal mortality survey sample. Br Med J 1991; 302:1576–1580
27. Lewis SW, Murray RM: Obstetric complications, neurodevelopmental deviance and risk of schizophrenia. J Psychiatr Res 1987; 21:413–421
28. McNeil TF: Obstetric factors and perinatal injuries, in Handbook of Schizophrenia, vol 3: Nosology, Epidemiology and Genetics of Schizophrenia. Edited by Tsuang MT, Simpson FC. Amsterdam, Elsevier, 1988, pp 319–344
29. Lewis SW, Owen MJ, Murray RM: Obstetric complications and schizophrenia: methodology and mechanisms, in Schizophrenia: Scientific Progress. Edited by Schulz SC, Tamminga CA. New York, Oxford University Press, 1989, pp 56–68
30. McGrath J, Murray RM: Risk factors for schizophrenia: from conception to birth, in Schizophrenia. Edited by Hirsch SR, Weinberger DR. Cambridge, Mass, Blackwell Science, 1995, pp 187–205
31. Lane EA, Albee GW: Comparative birth weight of schizophrenics and their siblings. J Psychol 1966; 64:227–231
32. McNeil TF, Cantor-Graae E, Nordstrom LG, Roselund T: Head circumference in "preschizophrenic" and control neonates. Br J Psychiatry 1993; 162:517–523
33. Rifkin L, Lewis S, Jones P, Toone B, Murray R: Low birth weight and schizophrenia. Br J Psychiatry 1994; 165:357–362
34. Goodman R: Are complications of pregnancy and birth causes of schizophrenia? Dev Med Child Neurol 1988; 30:391–395
35. Andreasen NC, Rice J, Endicott J, Reich T, Coryell W: The family history approach to diagnosis: how useful is it? Arch Gen Psychiatry 1986; 43:421–429
36. Pasamanick B, Knobloch H: Seasonal variation in complications of pregnancy. J Obst Gyn NY 1958; 12:110–112
37. Tilley BC, Barnes AB, Bergstrath E: A comparison of pregnancy history recall and medical records. Am J Epidemiol 1985; 121:269–281
38. O'Callaghan E, Larkin C, Waddington JL: Obstetric complications in schizophrenia and the validity of maternal recall. Psychol Med 1990; 20:89–94
39. Cook JTE, Levy JC, Page RCL: Association of low birth weight with beta cell function in adult first degree relatives of non-insulin dependent diabetic subjects. Br Med J 1993; 306:302–306
40. Gunther-Genta F, Bovet P, Hohlfeld P: Obstetric complications and schizophrenia: a case control study. Br J Psychiatry 1994; 164:165–170
41. DeLisi LE, Boccio AM, Riordan H, Hoff AL, Dorfman A, McClelland J, Kushner M, Van Eyl O, Oden N: Familial thyroid disease and delayed language development in first admission patients with schizophrenia. Psychiatry Res 1991; 38:39–50
42. Foerster A, Lewis SW, Owen MJ, Murray RM: Low birth weight and a family history of schizophrenia predict poor premorbid functioning in psychosis. Schizophr Res 1991; 5:13–20
43. Coffey VP, Jessop WJE: Congenital abnormalities—6th series. Ir J Med Sci 1955; 349:30–46
44. Hardy JMB, Azarowicz EN, Mannini A: The effect of Asian influenza on the outcome of pregnancy. Am J Public Health 1961; 51:1182–1188
45. Wynne Griffith G, Adelstein AM, Lambert PM: Influenza and infant mortality. Br Med J 1972; 3:553–556
46. Coffey VP, Jessop WJE: Maternal influenza and congenital deformities. Lancet 1972; 2:935–938
47. Lynberg MC, Khoury MJ, Lu X, Cociañ T: Maternal flu, fever, and the risk of neural tube defects: a population based case control study. Am J Epidemiol 1994; 140:244–255
48. Wright P, Murray RM: Schizophrenia: prenatal influenza and autoimmunity. Ann Med 1993; 25:497–502
49. Wright P, Gill M, Murray RM: Schizophrenia: genetics and the maternal immune response to viral infection. Am J Med Genet 1993; 48:40–46

The wizards of genetics keep closing in on the biological roots of personality. It's not your imagination that one baby seems born cheerful and another morose. But that's not the complete picture. DNA is not destiny; experience plays a powerful role, too.

Shyness, Sadness, Curiosity, Joy.

Is It Nature or Nurture?

By Marc Peyser and Anne Underwood

IF ANY CHILD SEEMED DESTINED TO GROW UP AFRAID OF her shadow and just about anything else that moved, it was 2-year-old Marjorie. She was so painfully shy that she wouldn't talk to or look at a stranger. She was even afraid of friendly cats and dogs. When Jerome Kagan, a Harvard professor who discovered that shyness has a strong genetic component, sent a clown to play with Marjorie, she ran to her mother. "It was as if a cobra entered that room," Kagan says. His diagnosis: Marjorie showed every sign of inherited shyness, a condition in which the brain somehow sends out messages to avoid new experiences. But as Kagan continued to examine her over the years, Marjorie's temperament changed. When she started school, she gained confidence from ballet classes and her good grades, and she began to make friends. Her parents even coaxed her into taking horseback-riding lessons. Marjorie may have been born shy, but she has grown into a bubbly second grader.

For Marjorie, then, biology—more specifically, her genetic inheritance—was not her destiny. And therein lies our tale. In the last few years scientists have identified genes that appear to predict all sorts of emotional behavior, from happiness to aggressiveness to risk-taking. The age-old question of whether nature or nurture determines temperament seems finally to have been decided in favor of Mother Nature and her ever-deepening gene pool. But the answer may not be so simple after all. Scientists are beginning to discover that genetics and environment work together to determine personality as intricately as Astaire and Rogers danced. "If either Fred or Ginger moves too fast, they both stumble," says Stanley Greenspan, a pediatric psychiatrist at George Washington University and the author of "The Growth of the Mind." "Nature affects nurture affects nature and back and forth. Each step influences the next." Many scientists now believe that some experiences can actually alter

61% of all parents believe that differences in behavior between girls and boys are not inborn but a result of the way they're raised

the structure of the brain. An aggressive toddler, under the right circumstances, can essentially be rewired to channel his energy more constructively. Marjorie can overcome her shyness—forever. No child need be held captive to her genetic blueprint. The implications for child rearing—and social policy—are profound.

While Gregor Mendel's pea plants did wonders to explain how humans inherit blue eyes or a bald spot, they turn out to be an inferior model for analyzing something as complex as the brain. The human body contains about 100,000 genes, of which 50,000 to 70,000 are involved in brain function. Genes control the brain's neurotransmitters and receptors, which deliver and accept mental messages like so many cars headed for their assigned parking spaces. But there are billions of roads to each parking lot, and those paths are highly susceptible to environmental factors. In his book "The New View of Self," Dr. Larry Siever, a psychiatry professor at Mount Sinai Medical Center, writes about how the trauma of the Holocaust caused such intense genetic scrambling in some survivors that their children inherited the same stress-related abnormalities. "Perhaps the sense of danger and uncertainty associated with living through such a time is passed on in the family milieu and primes the biological systems of the children as well," says Siever. He added that that might explain why pianist David Helfgott, the subject of the movie "Shine," had his mental breakdown.

A gene is only a probability for a given trait, not a guarantee. For that trait to be expressed, a gene often must be "turned on" by an outside force before it does its job. High levels of stress apparently activate a variety of genes, including those suspected of being involved in fear, shyness and some mental illnesses. Children conceived during a three-month famine in the Netherlands during a Nazi blockade in 1945 were later found to have twice the rate of schizophrenia

From *Newsweek*, Spring/Summer 1997, pp. 60–63. © 1997 by Newsweek, Inc. All rights reserved. Reprinted by permission.

Scientists estimate that genes determine only about 50 percent of a child's personality

as did Dutch children born to parents who were spared the trauma of famine. "Twenty years ago, you couldn't get your research funded if you were looking for a genetic basis for schizophrenia, because everyone knew it was what your mother did to you in the first few years of life, as Freud said," says Robert Plomin, a geneticist at London's Institute of Psychiatry. "Now you can't get funded *unless* you're looking for a genetic basis. Neither extreme is right, and the data show why. There's only a 50 percent concordance between genetics and the development of schizophrenia."

SCIENTISTS HAVE BEEN DE-voting enormous energy to determining what part of a given character trait is "heritable" and what part is the result of socialization. Frank Sulloway's book "Born to Rebel," which analyzes the influence of birth order on personality, opened a huge window on a universal—and largely overlooked—environmental factor. But that's a broad brush-stroke. Most studies focus on remarkably precise slivers of human emotions. One study at Allegheny University in Pennsylvania found that the tendency for a person to throw dishes or slam doors when he's angry is 40 percent heritable, while the likelihood a person will yell in anger is only 28 percent heritable. The most common method for determining these statistics is studying twins. If identical twins are more alike in some way than are fraternal twins, that trait is believed to have a higher likelihood of being inherited. But the nature-nurture knot is far from being untied.

The trick, then, is to isolate a given gene and study the different ways environment interacts with it. For instance, scientists believe that people with the longer variety of a dopamine-4 receptor gene are biologically predisposed to be thrill seekers. Because the gene appears to make them less sensitive to pain and physical sensation, the children are more likely to, say, crash their tricycles into a wall, just to see what it feels like. "These are the daredevils," says Greenspan. But they need not be. Given strict boundaries,

78% of those polled who are in two-parent families say that they share equally when it comes to setting rules for their young child

Greenspan says, thrill-seeking kids can be taught to modulate and channel their over-active curiosity. A risk-taking child who likes to pound his fist into hard objects can be taught games that involve hitting softly as well. "If you give them constructive ways to meet their needs," says Greenspan, "they can become charismatic, action-oriented leaders."

Shyness has been studied perhaps more than any other personality trait. Kagan, who has monitored 500 children for more than 17 years at Harvard, can detect telltale signs of shyness in babies even before they're born. He's found that the hearts of shy children in the womb consistently beat faster than 140 times a minute, which is much faster than the heartbeats of other babies. The shy fetus is already highly reactive, wired to overmonitor his environment. But he can also outgrow this predisposition if his parents gently but firmly desensitize him to the situations that cause anxiety, such as encouraging him to play with other children or, as in Marjorie's fear of animals, taking her to the stables and teaching her to ride a horse. Kagan has found that by the age of 4, no more than 20 percent of the previously shy children remain that way.

Will the reprogramming last into adulthood? Because evidence of the role of genes has been discovered only recently, it's still too early to tell. But studies of animals give some indication. Stephen Suomi at the National Institute of Child Health and Human Development works with rhesus monkeys that possess the same genetic predisposition to shyness that affects humans. He's shown that by giving a shy monkey to a foster mother who is an expert caregiver, the baby will outgrow the shyness. Even more surprising, the once shy monkey will become a leader among her peers and an unusually competent parent, just like the foster mom. Though she will likely pass along her shyness genes to her own child, she will teach it how to overcome her predisposition, just as she was taught. And the cycle continues—generations of genetically shy monkeys become not just normal, but superior, adults and parents. The lesson, says Suomi: "You

can't prejudge anyone at birth. No matter what your genetic background, a negative characteristic you're born with may even turn out to be an advantage."

But parents aren't scientists, and it's not always easy to see how experience can influence a child's character. A baby who smiles a lot and makes eye contact is, in part, determining her own environment, which in turn affects her temperament. As her parents coo and smile and wrinkle their noses in delighted response, they are reinforcing their baby's sunny disposition. But what about children who are born with low muscle tone, who at 4 months can barely hold up their own heads, let alone smile? Greenspan has discovered that mothers of these kids smile at the baby for a while, but when the affection isn't returned, they give up. And so does the baby, who over time fails to develop the ability to socialize normally. "If you move in the wrong patterns, the problem is exacerbated," Greenspan says. He has found that if parents respond to nonsmiling babies by being superanimated—like Bob Barker hosting a game show—they can engage their child's interest in the world.

The ramifications of these findings clearly have the potential to revolutionize child-rearing theory and practice. But to an uncertain end. "Our society has a strong belief that what happens in childhood determines your fate. If you have a happy childhood, everything will be all right. That's silly," says Michael Lewis, director of the Institute for the Study of Child Development in New Jersey and the author of "Altering Fate." Lewis estimates that experience ultimately rewrites 90 percent of a child's personality traits, leaving an adult with only one tenth of his inborn temperament. "The idea that early childhood is such a powerful moment to see individual differences in biology or environment is not valid," he says. "We are too open to and modifiable by experience." Some scientists warn that attempting to reprogram even a narrow sliver of childhood emotions can prove to be a daunting task, despite research's fascinating new insights. "Children are not a 24-hour controlled experiment," says C. Robert Cloninger, a professor of psychiatry and genetics at the Washington University School of Medicine in St. Louis. "If you put a child in a Skinner box, *then* maybe you could have substantial influence." So, mindful of the blinding insights of geneticists and grateful for the lingering influences of environment, parents must get on with the business of raising their child, an inexact science if ever there was one.

The Release of the Mentally Ill From Institutions: a Well-Intentioned Disaster

"It is imperative that we focus attention on what we have done to the severely mentally ill so that we may learn what went wrong and why."

By E. Fuller Torrey

THE PRACTICE, over the past four decades, of releasing people with severe mental illnesses from institutions has been one of the largest social experiments in 20th-century America. Research shows that if state psychiatric hospitals today housed the same proportion of the population as they did in 1955, almost 900,000 people would be in such institutions now. Instead, such facilities house fewer than 70,000 patients. Thus, more than 800,000 people are living outside of hospitals who would have been hospitalized 40 years ago.

Where are these people? Approximately half of them are living with their families, in group homes or boarding houses, or on their own. Many of these people are doing well. Among the other half, however, approximately 150,000 are homeless on any given day, and another 150,000 are in jails and prisons, most charged with crimes directly attributable to their mental illnesses. The remainder are confined to nursing homes, many of which—because they lack recreational programs designed for mentally ill residents or are located in urban areas where it is unsafe for residents to walk outside—are substantially bleaker and more restrictive than the state psychiatric hospitals used to be.

What price has the average American citizen paid for this experiment? One cannot go into any city without confronting severely mentally ill people living in parks or on the street. Many public libraries and bus and train stations have become *de facto* psychiatric shelters. Police officers routinely spend more time responding to psychiatric crises than to robberies or burglaries. And a small number of the severely mentally ill who are not receiving treatment become violent, leading to crimes that include an estimated 1,000 homicides a year—or approximately 4 per cent of all homicides.

The disaster of "deinstitutionalization" is, in fact, a perfect case study of a well-intentioned public policy gone wrong. The policy originated as a reaction against public exposés of state psychiatric hospitals as "snake pits" in the 1940s and 1950s; it was reinforced by the introduction of the first effective medications for treating psychoses in the mid-to-late 1950s. At the time the movement got under way in the late 1950s, we had no pilot programs and virtually no data with which to predict what would happen.

Rather than starting to release patients in a few locales and measuring the outcome, officials implemented the policy in cities and counties across the United States virtually simultaneously, based on the widespread hope that the new drugs would cure people and the widespread belief in state legislatures that the policy would save taxpayers money. In addition, with the publication of Thomas Szasz's *The Myth of Mental Illness* in 1961 and Ken Kesey's *One Flew Over the Cuckoo's Nest* the following year, the idea gained currency that there really wasn't

From *The Chronicle of Higher Education*, June 13, 1997, pp. B1, B5. © 1997 by E. Fuller Torrey. Reprinted by permission.

much wrong with those folks in the psychiatric hospitals. Deinstitutionalization quickly became the "humane" thing to do. Without adequate follow-up of the discharged patients, however, it was doomed to failure.

Changes in who paid for the treatment of mentally ill people also guaranteed that deinstitutionalization would fail. Until the early 1960s, almost all of the costs of programs for the mentally ill were borne by the states. However, in the early 1960s, Congress realized that the people who were being discharged would need financial support. It made seriously mentally ill people eligible for such federal programs as Supplemental Security Income, food stamps, and certain housing and Medicaid and Medicare programs. States thus could shift the cost of care for the mentally ill to the federal government simply by discharging patients from state hospitals or transferring them to nursing homes. The states reaped all their savings right away; they had no financial incentive to insure that patients received adequate follow-up care.

The result was a giant fiscal carrot, which the states eagerly devoured. The federal share of total costs for care of the mentally ill climbed to 62 per cent by 1994 from 2 per cent in 1963. With no fiscal incentive to do so, the states provided little, if any, care for the discharged patients, and any student in Public Policy 101 could have successfully predicted the result.

The legal profession and law schools compounded the failure of deinstitutionalization. The 1960s was the decade of civil rights, and many legal activists categorized the mentally ill with blacks, Hispanics, and other ethnic groups as legitimate targets for liberation. The American Civil Liberties Union, the privately supported Mental Health Law Project, and some law schools devoted significant resources to establishing legal precedents to force states to discharge psychiatric patients from hospitals and to make it increasingly difficult to rehospitalize them involuntarily. The lawyers' efforts were abetted by the Citizens Commission on Human Rights, an arm of the Church of Scientology, which has opposed involuntary hospitalization and use of medications for the mentally ill.

Lawyers made fundamental errors in categorizing severely mentally ill people with blacks and other minority groups and in opposing all involuntary treatment. They assumed that severely mentally ill people, like those who are not mentally ill, are able to think logically about their own needs and to seek help voluntarily if and when they need it. In fact, studies by Xavier Amador, a psychologist at the New York State Psychiatric Institute, and other researchers have shown that approximately half of those with severe mental illnesses have markedly impaired insight into their illnesses and personal needs. This impaired insight is part of the brain dysfunction causing their illnesses. About half of the severely mentally ill people who were "liberated" from psychiatric hospitals never sought treatment, because they did not—and do not—believe there is anything wrong with them.

The lawyers involved would have become aware of this problem if they had asked what was happening to the people being released from institutions. As early as 1972, Marc Abramson, a psychiatrist with the San Mateo County Department of Mental Health in California, noted that "mentally disordered persons are being increasingly subjected to arrest and criminal prosecution" as a result of leaving institutions. By the early 1980s, psychiatrists and other experts had published studies showing that one-third of discharged psychiatric patients were homeless within six months. But the lawyers and the law schools did not ask such questions, for they were driving on the automatic pilot of ideology.

Academic departments of psychiatry, psychology, and social work also share some blame for the disaster. Beginning with the "mental-hygiene movement" of the 1920s, these departments promoted the idea that severe mental illnesses are merely one end of the spectrum of mental health, different in degree but not in kind from the panoply of normal reaction to life's disappointments and vicissitudes. The corollary of this was that one could nip mental illness in the bud by providing counseling and psychotherapy to the "worried well," so that today's unhappiness would not become tomorrow's schizophrenia.

OVER THE PAST DECADE, it has become clear that this view of mental illness is profoundly wrong. Severe psychiatric disorders are no more linked to minor mental perturbations than are multiple sclerosis, Parkinson's disease, or Alzheimer's disease. The severe psychiatric disorders—including schizophrenia, bipolar disorder, severe depression, and obsessive-compulsive disorder—have been, like other neurologically caused diseases such as Parkinson's and Alzheimer's, clearly proved to be diseases of the brain. Their proper treatment demands expertise in brain physiology and pharmacology, rather than in human relationships. We have trained literally hundreds of thousands of mental-health professionals—psychiatrists, psychologists, and psychiatric social workers—to provide counseling when what we really need are a few thousand professionals such as neurologists, who are trained to treat diseases of the brain.

What should be done now? First, a formal divorce of "mental health" from mental illness is overdue. What this would mean is that existing psychologists, social workers, and counselors would continue to focus on helping people to deal with the problems of everyday life. Psychiatry, on the other hand, would merge with neurology to produce researchers and clinicians who possess expertise on the full spectrum of brain diseases. This would place neuropsychiatry as a single entity exactly where it was 100 years ago, before the Freudian revolution and the mental-hygiene movement led it to focus on general mental health rather than the most severe mental disorders.

Second, it is incumbent on the legal profession and law schools to revisit the consequences of their well-meaning but misguided efforts, which have made it extremely difficult to involuntarily hospitalize or treat people with severe mental illnesses. Lawyers are public-interest-law projects should take the lead in trying to modify state laws so that mentally ill people who lack insight into their condition can be treated.

Finally, schools of public policy should study how to structure government programs to include financial incentives to provide services for the mentally ill—rather than incentives *not* to provide them, as is now the case. For example, states could offer bonuses to local governments that reduced the number of severely mentally ill people in local jails, or that increased the number of such people who hold jobs. Given the major changes under way in the delivery of medical services in this country, this is a propitious time to set up small pilot programs with different incentive systems and to examine a variety of ways to measure their success, including the quality of life of the people being served.

In his *Collected Essays,* Aldous Huxley wrote: "That men do not learn very much from the lessons of history is the most important of all the lessons that history has to teach." It is imperative that we focus attention on the disaster of what we have done to the severely mentally ill so that we may learn what went wrong and why—and avoid such well-meaning disasters in the future. The exercise is not merely academic, however; it directly affects the lives of hundreds of thousands of individuals and their families.

E. Fuller Torrey, a research psychiatrist in Washington, is the author of Out of the Shadows: Confronting America's Mental Illness Crisis *(Wiley, 1996).*

Schizophrenia: A Disorder of Brain Circuitry

William T. O'Connor Ph.D.*

Things fall apart, the center cannot hold, Mere anarchy is loosed upon the world.

W. B. YEATS

Research into schizophrenia is slowly beginning to gather momentum. Imaging techniques are helping to identify physical abnormalities in schizophrenic brains, and now scientists are trying to link these abnormalities with specific symptoms of the disease. The main message is becoming clear: schizophrenia is a disorder of brain circuitry, not some mysterious demon. Increasing evidence points to abnormalities that arise very early in life, probably before birth, which disrupt the normal development of the brain.

Of all the disorders of the human condition, none is more devastating than schizophrenia. About one percent of the population, or approximately 20 million people worldwide, suffer from this particularly cruel illness, which claims its victims at a youthful age and results in severe psychosocial disability. For each sufferer, a string of relatives is also affected, so that at least 100 million people have to deal with the consequences of this disorder.

The word *schizophrenia* was first coined in 1911 by Eugen Bleuler, and today the syndrome is characterized by psychotic symptoms that typically include hallucinations and delusions. Hallucinations are commonly experienced as noises, music or more typically "voices"; and delusions involve disturbances in thought rather than perception. Schizophrenics also have a lack of emotional drive, which they often report as a feeling of being dead inside or even of someone else occupying their bodies. There is also guilt, which is of a particularly crushing and severe kind.

Schizophrenics do not, as popular myth holds, have split personalities. Rather, the disease causes a wider fragmentation of their intellect and social selves, attacking the very qualities that make us human. They often have difficulty with sustaining attention to a specific task and communicating through language and facial expression. They are generally unable to put themselves in someone else's shoes, or to judge others' intentions towards them.

In neuropsychological terms, schizophrenia may be described as a disorder of A) spatial attention, B) language, and C) thought processes. There is strong evidence that an area of the frontal cortex called the anterior cingulate gyrus is involved in mediating all three of these functions. Indeed neurons in this area may form a central processing unit of sorts. Recent brain imaging (PET) studies in normal subjects have targeted this area of the frontal cortex as being involved in the process of attention to language and visual targets via neuronal connections with another area of the cortex known as the posterior parietal lobe. In fact, the anterior cingulate appears to be part of a more extensive attention system, the anterior attention system. With regard to language, there is evidence that the cingulate is involved in the control of language processing via connections with the dorsolateral prefrontal cortex. The cingulate also plays an important role in thought processes. For example, people with schizophrenia are similar to patients with lesions (such as a stroke) in the frontal lobe region of the brain including the anterior cingulate. They both find it difficult to inhibit learned concepts; in other words, they find it difficult to get rid of certain patterns of thoughts and ideas.

According to some theories, attention is used to inhibit the activation of meanings that do not fit the general context of the discourse. Thus the activation of

From *The Decade of the Brain*, Winter 1994, pp. 1-4. © 1994 by the National Alliance for the Mentally Ill. Reprinted by permission.

the anterior cingulate—which is observed in attention tasks in normal human subjects—results in selective inhibition of inappropriate stimuli via connections to other areas of the cortex or in "relays" deeper down in the brain. If this inhibitory control were reduced due to a faulty connection(s), language would go off in tangents and lose its meaning. The result is fluent and incoherent speech.

There are clear structural and functional differences in the brains of people with schizophrenia, including an abnormally high blood flow in the left globus pallidus of newly diagnosed, never-medicated patients. This is an interesting finding in terms of the disturbances in attention, language, and thought process associated with schizophrenia because the globus pallidus is part of a circuit that influences nervous activity in the anterior cingulate. In fact, the globus pallidus can be divided into upper and lower parts—the so-called "dorsal" and "ventral" pallidus. This distinction has been made on the basis of the fact that two sets of neurons project in a parallel fashion from the dorsal and ventral pallidus to carry information further "upstream" to the anterior cingulate and the motor cortex respectively. What is particularly exciting about the finding of an abnormality in the function of the globus pallidus of never-medicated persons with schizophrenia is that both sets of neurons in this brain region are only one synapse "upstream" from neurons that carry dopamine as their neurotransmitter. Dopamine has been implicated in schizophrenia for the past 25 years.

The evidence suggesting the involvement of the neurotransmitter dopamine in schizophrenia is derived from two main sources—first, from the clinical effects of the drug amphetamine, which activates dopamine transmission in the brain and produces schizophrenia-like behaviors; and second, from the pharmacology of the antipsychotic drugs, which all to a greater or lesser extent block dopamine receptors. Antipsychotics ameliorate the hallucinations, delusions, disorganized thinking, and inappropriate emotion—the "positive" symptoms of schizophrenia that are most evident during acute psychotic episodes. However, they all produce subtle abnormal movements when administered to treat acute episodes of illness (hence the name *neuroleptics*). Moreover, when administered for a long time, they often cause a devastating disorder called tardive dyskinesia. Involuntary and at times incessant writhing of the limbs and trunk characterize this disorder which can persist long after the drug is discontinued.

Why would a drug that affects mental function also produce motor symptoms? The answer lies in the fact that conventional antipsychotics prevent the binding of dopamine to its postsynaptic receptors on those two sets of neurons that project to the dorsal and ventral pallidus. To appreciate the importance of this insight, one must know that the dopamine-containing nerve cell bodies gathered deep in the midbrain, like the

neurons in the pallidus, can also be divided into two main sets. The two sets are the dorsal and ventral projection pathways that are targeted on those neurons that project to the dorsal and ventral pallidus. In fact, these dorsal and ventral pathways form links in two separate yet parallel circuits that ultimately influence nervous activity "upstream" in the motor and cingulate cortices respectively. A major function of dopamine appears to be the control of these parallel dorsal and ventral projections to the dorsal and ventral pallidus. Indeed the different abilities of neuroleptics to selectively block the postsynaptic dopamine receptors on the dorsal and ventral projections to the pallidus may ultimately underlie the differences in their ability to induce motor and/or antipsychotic effects.

A new drug, clozapine, differs from the conventional antipsychotics such as haloperidol, in that it does not cause tardive dyskinesia. Clozapine may selectively block dopamine receptors on the ventral pathway and thus influence nervous activity in the anterior cingulate without interfering with the dopamine regulation of the dorsal (motor) circuit.

The finding of an abnormal increase in blood flow in the globus pallidus of drug-free, newly diagnosed people with schizophrenia is consistent with the concept of a dysregulation of the ventral dopamine input into those GABA neurons that are targeted on the ventral pallidum. The result is a disturbance in nervous activity in the cingulate cortex. Thus the ventral pallidum may be the critical link relating the specific deficits found in attention tasks with the dysregulation of the input from the ventral dopamine pathway. This approach allows the description of schizophrenia in both cognitive and neuroscience terms.

At this stage, a central question arises for the neuroscientist; What is the functional consequence of dopamine receptor activation on those neurons that project to the dorsal and ventral pallidum? Such neurons are thought to use GABA as their transmitter substance. Over the past seven years I have been working in the Department of Pharmacology at The Karolinska Institute, Stockholm, Sweden, where I use the technique of *in vivo* brain microdialysis to study the chemical communication between neurons. Brain microdialysis is essentially a miniaturized version of kidney dialysis in that small regions within the brain of experimental animals can be studied. This technique allows one to continuously monitor chemical changes in the brain by monitoring the "overflow" of neurotransmitter into the extracellular space. Thanks to the generous support from the National Alliance for the Mentally Ill and The Stanley Foundation we are able to use this technique to investigate the nature of the dopamine regulation of those GABA pathways that project to the dorsal and ventral pallidus in awake, freely moving animals. In this approach microdialysis probes can be used to simultaneously infuse substances (e.g. dopamine receptor activators and blockers) and to recover substances (e.g. neurotransmitters such as dopamine and GABA) from the extracellular space. In addition, by placing one probe at the cell body region where the neuron receives incoming chemical signals from its neighbors and another probe in the terminal region where the neuron passes on a chemical signal *via* release of transmitter substance to the next neuron, one can study how neurotransmitters modulate each pathway in the circuit.

If schizophrenia is a disorder in brain circuitry, how can we hope to cure it? We are still at an early stage in understanding the dynamics of brain circuitry. However, with the aid of highly selective ligands—molecules that bind to receptors—it will be possible to activate and deactivate specific pathways and thus influence the activity of individual circuits in the brain.

The present approach allows us to follow up on the emerging findings of physical and functional abnormalities in the brains of persons with schizophrenia by investigating how neurotransmitters modulate the relevant brain circuits. This will provide an understanding of how disruptions in these circuits underlie the symptoms of schizophrenia and will also result in the development of new strategies for the treatment and eventual cure of this disease.

*About the Author: Dr. Billy O'Connor is Associate Professor at the Department of Physiology and Pharmacology, Division of Pharmacology, Karolinska Institute, Stockholm, Sweden. In 1986, he was awarded a Ph.D. in Psychopharmacology from University College, Galway, Ireland, for his work on a behavioral, physiological and neurochemical investigation of an animal model of depression. Dr. O'Connor has pioneered the application of the *in vivo* microdialysis technique to the study of the functional neuroanatomy of pathways and circuits in the brain. He has published over 70 papers in the area of neuroscience.

Thalamic Abnormalities in Schizophrenia Visualized Through Magnetic Resonance Image Averaging

Nancy C. Andreasen,* Stephan Arndt, Victor Swayze II,
Ted Cizadlo, Michael Flaum, Daniel O'Leary, James C. Ehrhardt,
William T. C. Yuh

N. C. Andreasen, S. Arndt, V. Swayze II, T. Cizadlo, M. Flaum, D. O'Leary, The Mental Health Clinical Research Center and Department of Psychiatry, College of Medicine and University of Iowa Hospitals and Clinics, Iowa City, IA 52242, USA.
J. C. Ehrhardt and W. T. C. Yuh, Department of Radiology, College of Medicine and University of Iowa Hospitals and Clinics, Iowa City, IA 52242, USA.

Schizophrenia is a complex illness characterized by multiple types of symptoms involving many aspects of cognition and emotion. Most efforts to identify its underlying neural substrates have focused on a strategy that relates a single symptom to a single brain region. An alternative hypothesis, that the variety of symptoms could be explained by a lesion in midline neural circuits mediating attention and information processing, is explored. Magnetic resonance images from patients and controls were transformed with a "bounding box" to produce an "average schizophrenic brain" and an "average normal brain." After image subtraction of the two averages, the areas of difference were displayed as an effect size map. Specific regional abnormalities were observed in the thalamus and adjacent white matter. An abnormality in the thalamus and related circuitry explains the diverse symptoms of schizophrenia parsimoniously because they could all result from a defect in filtering or gating sensory input, which is one of the primary functions of the thalamus in the human brain.

Schizophrenia is a disorder characterized by a multiplicity of signs and symptoms, no single one of which is present in all patients. Patients have a mixture of cognitive and emotional disturbances in a variety of functional systems such as perception, language, inferential thinking, and emotional expression and experience. Nevertheless, the fact that this illness is recognized throughout the world suggests that there must be some central feature that gives the disorder conceptual unity. When Bleuler named the disorder "schizophrenia" early in the 20th century, he identified such a feature: the fragmenting or splitting apart of the cognitive and emotional functions of the mind (1). Although not all patients given this diagnosis have delusions, hallucinations, or disorganized speech, all share a fragmentation of the mind: a catastrophic experience involving the loss of control over thoughts and emotions, the capacity to integrate experience and expression, and the sense of personal autonomy.

In the search for the neural substrates of the symptoms of schizophrenia, links have been noted between hallucinations and temporal lobe abnormalities, thought disorder and hippocampal abnormalities, and negative symptoms and prefrontal abnormalities (2). A central problem with this work has been the use of small samples, owing to the labor-intensiveness of the methods used, and a related difficulty in finding abnormalities consistent across studies.

We propose a parsimonious explanation for the multiplicity of signs and symptoms: abnormalities in midline structures that mediate attention and information processing, particularly the thalamus and related midline circuitry. To support this explanation, we provide evidence from magnetic resonance (MR) imaging. Fully automated techniques for image analysis of MR scans were used to generate an "average brain" from a sample of normal individuals and a sample of patients suffering from schizophrenia (3). The "average brain" is used to compare the two groups and to identify regions where they differ. This strategy provides an efficient alternative to current methods for analysis of MR imaging data, which involve manually tracing structures on prespecified areas of each individual scan.

MR data were collected with a 1.5-T GE Signa Scanner. The three-dimensional SPGR sequence was used with the following scanning parameters: 1.5-mm coronal slices, flip angle 40°, repetition time 24 ms, echo time 5 ms, two excitations, field of view 26 cm, matrix 256 × 192. Postacquisition processing was done with locally developed software (4).

*To whom correspondence should be addressed.

Reprinted with permission from *Science,* October 14, 1994, pp. 294-298. © 1994 by the American Association for the Advancement of Science.

The imaged brains were then linearly transformed with a "bounding box" technique that included six points: the most anterior and posterior, the most right and left lateral, and the most superior and inferior (5). Each imaged brain was stretched or compressed in three dimensions, creating three scaling factors: S_x, S_y, and S_z. After each brain was transformed to the same three-dimensional space, brains were subsequently averaged on a pixel by pixel basis. Before averaging, signal intensity was normalized with a histogram equalization process (6). Signal intensity values were then averaged separately for each of the two groups, normal controls and schizophrenic patients, by calculation of the mean and standard deviation for each equivalent pixel within the bounding box. Thus, an "average brain" was generated for the schizophrenic group and for the normal group. This average brain can be visualized and resampled three-dimensionally in the same manner as an individual MR data set. It has the advantage, however, of providing a concise numeric and visual summary of the group as a whole.

In order to submit the average brains to statistical analysis, we used the strategy of comparing groups by examining differences between the schizophrenic and normals as displayed in subtracted images. This approach to determining whether the two groups differ anatomically and to identifying the specific regions where they differ is analogous to methods used for many years for the analysis of positron emission tomography (PET) data (7). A variety of techniques are currently in use for the analysis of differences in PET images; most rely on some type of "t statistic" (8). In this case, we chose instead to display the differences as an effect size (ES) map, considering it a better indicator of the extent to which the two groups actually differ in a biologically significant way. An image-based ES shows the extent of difference between images in terms of the average intersubject variability. Thus, the image presents a descriptive picture of the size of group differences (9). The statistical image was built from the ES for group differences voxel by voxel.

Before the image subtraction analyses, the total volume of tissue and cerebrospinal fluid (CSF) was compared for the schizophrenic patients and normal control subjects. The patients had a mean brain tissue volume of 1263 ± 91 cm³, as compared to 1327 ± 114 cm³ in controls ($t = 2.90$, $P < 0.006$); CSF volume in patients was 131 ± 32 cm³, as compared to 108 ± 29 cm³ in controls ($t = 3.48$, $P < 0.001$). Thus, patients have more CSF and less brain tissue; results remained the same after covarying height. These results confirm earlier reports

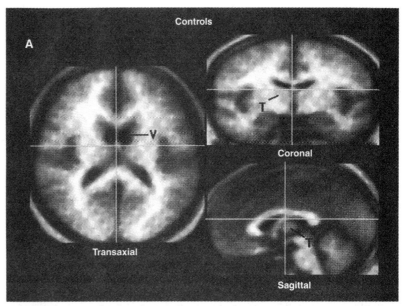

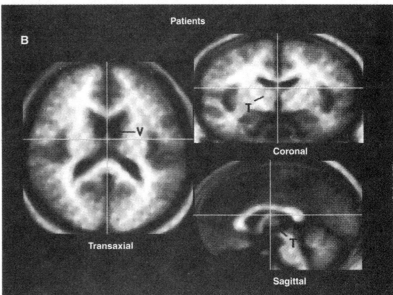

Fig. 1. Three orthogonal views of the "average brains" from (**A**) 47 healthy male volunteers and (**B**) 39 male patients suffering from schizophrenia. [C]ross hairs display the coordinates of the location three-dimensionally. T, thalamus: V, ventricles.

indicating reduced brain size and increased ventricular size in schizophrenia (10). A fundamental question raised by these studies is whether the reduced brain size and increased area of CSF-filled space results from a diffuse abnormality or whether it is a consequence of specific regional abnormalities. There appears to be a subtle but visually detectable difference in ventricular size, seen especially on the transaxial view (Fig. 1). The most noticeable regional difference is in the thalamus, which appears to be smaller, especially as visualized on the midsagittal view.

The major abnormalities identified when the images are subtracted and portrayed as ES maps are in two areas: the thalamus, and white matter tracts adjacent to it. These abnormalities are primarily in the right hemisphere and are seen on all three orthogonal planes. Differences in signal intensity occur primarily in lateral thalamic regions, but may also be seen in medial areas. Differences are also present in white matter regions in the frontal lobe and to a lesser extent in the parietal and temporal lobes. An area of difference is also seen in the posterior (occipital) regions: this reflects the differences in brain size, which produces an aliasing ("nose wrap") artifact in the controls because of their larger amount of brain tissue. Thus, this type of image analysis appears to be sensitive to group differences and may offer an efficient and empirical method for analysis of MR data.

As a check on the possibility that these

results could be due to some unknown artifact, the 48 normal males in this study were subtracted from a sample of 44 normal females, collected in an ongoing study of gender differences in the normal brain (*11*). In contrast to the control-patient images, no major differences are seen, apart from the rim of color in the skull and scalp, which reflects larger male head size. No differences are seen in brain parenchyma, apart from the posterior region, which reflects an aliasing artifact in the males because of their larger heads.

Decreased thalamic size has been our most consistently replicated finding in earlier studies, in addition to increased ventricular size (*12*). Thalamic abnormalities in schizophrenia have been previously reported in the neuropathological literature; five previous studies have shown either decreased size or neuronal loss (*13*). The thalamic abnormalities noted in this study cannot be localized specifically, owing to the inherent limits of resolution of the MR sequences used. While they may involve the medial dorsal regions of thalamus (which have been most frequently studied in neuropathological literature), the abnormalities seen in the lateral thalamus are more prominent. The medial dorsal nucleus is of interest because it projects to the prefrontal cortex, whereas lateral nuclei project to parietal and temporal association regions (*14*). Other studies have also reported abnormalities in midline attentional circuits either downstream or upstream of the thalamus, such as the cingulate gyrus or the pontine reticular activating system (*15*).

These findings are consistent with the role that the thalamus plays in modulating overall brain function and its possible relation to schizophrenia. The thalamus serves as the major way station that receives input from the reticular activating system, structures involved in emotion and memory such as the amygdala, and cortical association areas. Thus, it plays a significant role in filtering, gating, processing, and relaying information. An abnormality in this structure could explain most of the psychopathology in schizophrenia, which can be readily understood as the result of abnormalities in filtering stimuli, focusing attention, or sensory gating (*16*). A person with a defective thalamus is likely to be flooded with information and overwhelmed with stimuli. That person may consequently experience the striking misperceptions that we refer to as delusions or hallucinations or may withdraw and retreat and display negative symptoms such as avolition.

The thalamic abnormalities are coupled with an area of difference in the white matter that may implicate tracts connecting the thalamus with the prefrontal cortex, a finding consistent with a large literature documenting frontal abnormalities in schizophrenia (*17*). An abnormality in temporal and parietal projections may also be present. The abnormalities occur primarily in the right hemisphere. A right-sided abnormality appears to run counter to the substantial literature suggesting deficits in left hemisphere brain regions, particularly those dedicated to language functions. Nevertheless, an abnormality in the right thalamus, and particularly in the lateral nuclei that project to temporoparietal association areas, is also consistent with both the clinical picture of the illness and with some existing literature. Several studies have indicated linked circuitry between frontal and right parietal regions, particularly when higher level cognitive tasks are performed (*18*). Right temporoparietal regions are also crucial for spatial orientation. An individual who cannot correctly link multimodal information in a spatial context is likely to feel confused, overwhelmed, and almost literally "lost in space."

REFERENCES AND NOTES

1. E. Bleuler, *Dementia Praecox of the Group of Schizophrenias* J. Zinkin, Transl. (1911) (International Universities Press, New York, 1950).

2. E. Kraepelin, R. M. Barclay, G. M. Robertson, *Dementia Praecox and Paraphrenia* (Livingstone, Edinburgh, 1919); K. Kleist, *J. Ment. Sci.* **106**, 246 (1960); P. E. Barta, G. D. Pearlson, R. E. Powers, S. S. Richards, L. E. Tune, *Am. J. Psychiatry* **147**, 1457 (1990); N. D. Volkow *et al.*, *J. Cereb. Blood Flow Metab.* **5**, 199 (1985); M. E. Shenton *et al.*, *N. Engl. J. Med.* **327**, 604 (1992); P. F. Liddle *et al.*, *Br. J. Psychiatry* **60**, 179 (1992); N. C. Andreasen *et al.*, *Arch. Gen. Psychiatry* **49**, 943 (1992).

3. Subjects included 47 healthy normal male volunteers recruited from the community and 39 male patients suffering from schizophrenia recruited for admission to the University of Iowa Mental Health Clinical Research Center and diagnosed by DSM-IIIR criteria according to the Comprehensive Assessment of Symptoms and History [N. C. Andreasen, M. Flaum, S. Arndt, *Arch. Gen. Psychiatry* **49**, 615 (1992)]. The mean age of the patients was 30.3 years. The majority had been chronically ill (mean duration of illness, 51.5 months), although five were first admissions. Lifetime duration of hospitalization was 7.7 months, and mean age of onset was 21.4 years. Most had received neuroleptic treatment at some time in the past, but eight were neuroleptic naïve or nearly so (that is, had not received more than the equivalent of 20 mg of haloperidol over their lifetime). None had been receiving medications known to affect MR scans, such as steroids, or had any recent alcohol or drug abuse. Patients were excluded if they had a lifetime history of serious head trauma, neurological illness, or a serious medical or surgical illness. Mean parental educational level was 12.7 years. The comparison group consisted of healthy volunteers recruited from the community by newspaper advertising and matched on relevant measures such as age,

height, and parental education. Subjects were excluded if there was any history of psychiatric, neurologic, or medical illness, or a family history of schizophrenia. Their mean parental educational level was 13.8 years. All subjects gave informed consent.

4. This software, BRAINS (Brain Research: Analysis of Images, Networks, and Systems), is described in the following: N. C. Andreasen *et al.*, *J. Neuropsychiatry Clin. Neurosci.* **4**, 125 (1992); N. C. Andreasen *et al.*, *ibid.* **5**, 121 (1993); N. C. Andreasen *et al.*, *Proc. Natl. Acad. Sci. U.S.A.* **91**, 93 (1994). The BRAINS package includes utilities for tissue classification, surface and volume rendering, edge detection, volume measurement, resampling with simultaneous visualization in multiple planes, and automated measurement of sulcal-gyral surface anatomy. The initial step in image analysis involved removing the brain from the skull by edge detection techniques and manual tracing. Data were then converted to a three-dimensional data set by volume rendering. The pixels representing CSF were "washed off" with the use of a threshold based on training classes and histograms. The data for each subject were then realigned and resampled with the anterior commissure–posterior commissure line in the transaxial plane and the interhemispheric fissure coronally, in order to ensure comparability of head position across all subjects.

5. J. Talairach and P. Tournoux, *Co-Planar Stereotaxic Atlas of the Human Brain*, (Thieme, New York, 1988); A. C. Evans *et al.*, *NeuroImage* **1**, 43 (1992); A. C. Evans, C. Beil, S. Marrett, C. J. Thompson, A. Hakim, *J. Cereb. Blood Flow Metab.* **8**, 513 (1988).

6. J. C. Russ, *Image Processing Handbook* (CRC Press, Boca Raton, FL 1992).

7. R. J. Zatorre, A. C. Evans, E. Meyer, A. Gjedde, *Science* **256**, 846 (1992); C. D. Frith, K. J. Friston, P. F. Liddle, R. S. J. Frackowiak, *Neuropsychologia* **29**, 1137 (1991); S. E. Petersen, P. T. Fox, M. I. Posner, M. Mintun, M. E. Raichle, *Nature* **331**, 585 (1988).

8. K. J. Friston, C. D. Frith, P. F. Liddle, R. S. J. Frackowiak, *J. Cereb. Blood Flow Metab.* **13**, 5 (1993); K. Worsley, A. Evans, S. Marrett, P. A. Neelin, *ibid.* **12**, 900 (1992).

9. J. Cohen, *Statistical Power Analysis for the Behavioral Sciences* (Erlbaum, Hillsdale, NJ, 1988). The ES values were computed with the standard formula that reflects the difference in group averages in pooled standard deviation units (SD_{pooled}). Thus, an ES value of 1.0 for a given voxel indicates a mean difference corresponding to 1 SD. The SD_{pooled} is the weighted average of the standard deviation from the two groups. For each voxel, X, in the brain region at location i,

$$ES_i = \frac{\bar{X}_{iP} - \bar{X}_{iC}}{SD_{pooled\,i}}$$

where $\bar{X}$ is the group mean for patients (P) or controls (C). Because the ES is closely tied to the amount of variance, it is more sensitive to detection of differences in areas of low variance and less sensitive in areas of high variance. Consequently, in Fig. 2 no areas of effect size are seen in the lateral ventricles because of the large variance in their boundaries in both groups. The sample size of the voxels used in ES calculations also varied around tissue-CSF borders, because only voxels containing brain tissue (that is, not CSF) were used in these calculations, and the exact brain tissue–CSF boundaries varied from subject to subject.

10. The BRAINS software provides automated estimates of intracranial components (that is, brain tissue, CSF) in cubic centimeters, on the basis of principles of tissue classification and pixel counting [G. Cohen *et al.*, *Psychiatric Research: Neuroimaging* **45**, 33 (1992); S. Arndt *et al.*, *NeuroImage* **1**, 191 (1994). Earlier reports of ventricular enlargement are summarized in R. E. Gur and G. D. Pearlson [*Schizophr. Bull.* **19**, 337 (1993)].

11. N. C. Andreasen, B. S. McEwen, R. A. Gorski, E. Frank, paper presented at the Society for Neurosciences 23nd Annual Meeting, Washington, DC, 7–12 November 1993 (abstr. 3).

12. N. C. Andreasen *et al.*, *Arch. Gen. Psychiatry* **43**, 136 (1986) (unpublished data); N. C. Andreasen *et*

al., ibid. **47**, 35 (1990); M. Flaum, *et al., Am. J. Psychiatry,* in press.

13. B. Bogerts, *Schizophr. Bull.* **19**, 431 (1993); H. Baumer, *Journal fuer Hirnforschung* **1**, 157 (1954); W. M. Treff and K. J. Hempel, *ibid.* **4**, 314 (1958); A. Lesch and B. Bogerts, *Eur. Arch. Psychiatry Neurol. Sci.* **23**, 212 (1984); J. R. Stevens, *Arch. Gen. Psychiatry* **29**, 177 (1973); B. Pakkenberg, *Acta Neurol. Scand.* **137**, 20 (1992).

14. E. G. Jones, *The Thalamus* (Plenum, New York, 1985); E. G. Jones and T. P. S. Powell, *Brain* **93**, 793 (1970).

15. F. M. Benes, J. McSparren, E. D. Bird, J. P. San-Giovanni, S. L. Vincent, *Arch. Gen. Psychiatry* **48**, 996 (1991); F. M. Benes and E. D. Bird, *ibid.* **44**, 608 (1987); C. N. Karson, M. F. Casanova, J. E. Kleinman, W. S. T. Griffin, *Am. J. Psychiatry* **150**, 454 (1993).

16. D. E. Broadbent, *Perception and Communication,* (Pergamon, London, 1958); A. McGhie and J. Chapman, *Br. J. Med. Psychol.* **34**, 103 (1961); P. S. Holzman, D. L. Levy, L. R. Proctor, *Arch. Gen. Psychiatry* **33**, 1415 (1976); D. L. Braff, *Schizophr. Bull.* **19**, 233 (1993); M. Carlsson and A. Carlsson, *ibid.* **16**, 425 (1990);

17. J. M. Fuster, *The Prefrontal Cortex: Anatomy, Physiology, and Neuropsychology of the Prefrontal Cortex* (Raven, New York, 1989); M. S. Buchsbaum, *Schizophr. Bull.* **16**, 379 (1990); D. R. Weinberger, K. F. Berman, R. F. Zec, *Arch. Gen. Psychiatry* **43**, 114 (1986).

18. M. Petrides and D. N. Pandya, *J. Comp. Neurol.* **228**, 105 (1984); M. I. Posner, J. A. Walker, F. J. Friedrich, R. D. Rafal, *J. Neurosci.* **4**, 1863 (1984); P. S. Goldman-Rakic, *Brain Research: The Prefrontal Cortex—Its Structure, Function, and Pathology,* H. B. M. Uylings, C. G. Van Eden, J. P. C. DeBruin, M. A. Corner, M. G. Feensta, Eds. (Elsevier, New York, 1990), pp. 325–335.

19. Supported in part by National Institute of Mental Health grants MH31593, MH40856, and MHCRC 43271; The Nellie Ball Trust Fund, Iowa State Bank and Trust Company, Trustee; Research Scientist Award MH00625; and an award from the National Alliance for Research on Schizophrenia and Depression.

20 April 1994; accepted 10 August 1994

Drug/Alcohol Abuse
and Violence

Currently, much attention is focused on the problem of drugs in this country, yet it is legal to consume alcohol—a widely abused drug. This obvious fact seems to be a constant reminder to those who argue that a "just say no" approach is the proper way to deal with problems associated with drug use. Controversy concerning drug use will continue. For example, a current debate involves the possible use of marijuana to alleviate the pain associated with a number of medical conditions. Society has a great stake in trying to deal with problems related to drugs, but there is little agreement on which drugs to control and how.

The majority of people in this country drink alcoholic beverages at least occasionally. Thus, it is not surprising that college students drink alcohol. A significant number of them, however, engage in what is termed binge drinking. A recent survey of 140 college campuses reveals the extent of this practice and describes the negative consequences of drinking four to five drinks on a single occasion.

Rather than view drug problems as separate, depending on the drug, researchers are turning their attention to trying to find the common root of drug addictions. Prominent among the possible explanations are biological factors, especially involving the neurotransmitter dopamine. These findings hold great promise for increasing our understanding of addiction and for offering better and more effective treatments in the future.

Do you know someone who is glib, egocentric, irresponsible, and impulsive? If so, you may know someone who fits Robert Hare's description of a psychopath in the article "Predators: The Disturbing World of the Psychopaths among Us." Hare has spent his professional life studying these individuals, whom he also calls predators because of their tendency to take advantage of others. The concept of a psychopath overlaps with criminal behavior and the *Diagnostic and Statistical Manual of Mental Disorders* (*DSM-IV*) diagnosis called antisocial personality disorder. However, there are also some important differences that Hare outlines. One of his key points is sobering: a significant number of psychopaths are not found in prisons; they can be found in our everyday lives.

Looking Ahead: Challenge Questions

How should society determine which drugs should be legal and which ones should be illegal?

Why do people continue to use alcohol in spite of its potential negative consequences?

What are the common behavioral components of drug addictions?

After reading "Predators: The Disturbing World of the Psychopaths among Us," discuss whether or not some of the characteristics of Robert Hare's psychopathic individual are actually desirable in some cases. How do we differentiate desirable characteristics from those that are not desirable?

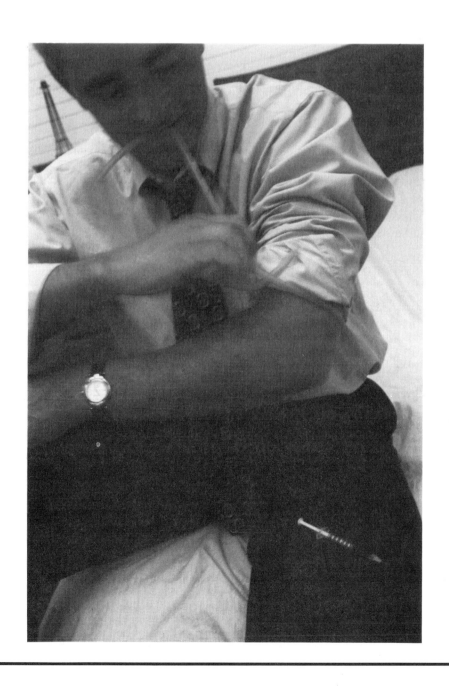

NATIONAL AFFAIRS

It can be a seductive argument: why not let sick people ease their pain by smoking pot? But drug warriors say 'medical marijuana' could lead to legalization—and the country does not seem ready for that. BY TOM MORGANTHAU

The War Over Weed

CONSIDERED SOLELY AS AN EXAMPLE OF practical politics, the campaign for Proposition 215 was brilliant. It was fought and won in California, a bellwether state whose law on ballot initiatives makes it uniquely open to grass-roots political movements. It attacked a policy, the U.S. drug war, about which many opinion leaders have large doubts. It mobilized a politically potent interest group—doctors—to defend their right to practice their profession as they see fit, and it appealed to voters' compassion for people with cancer, AIDS and other deadly diseases. It used the federal government as a scapegoat and made cops and prosecutors look like dolts. On Election Day, Prop 215 scored a clean kill, 56 percent to 44. Now the fun begins.

Simply put, Prop 215 and Proposition 200, a similar measure passed in Arizona last fall, pose a frontal challenge to the American prohibition against drugs—which is exactly what some, though not all, backers of these initiatives wanted to do. By convincing voters there are humane reasons to relax current laws against marijuana use, a Hungarian-born billionaire named George Soros and his helpers created a muddle that may take years to sort out. Like many political controversies, this one is headed for the courts. After the initiative passed, Gen. Barry McCaffrey,

the drug czar, publicly warned doctors not to break federal law by prescribing marijuana. That prompted a group of California physicians to file suit claiming that their rights to advise their patients were being infringed. The policy is, who controls America's drug laws—the federal government or the voters of California and Arizona? The political issue is whether we Americans, fighting what seems to be an endless war, want to move toward greater tolerance of marijuana and other drugs. That is not overstatement: the Arizona law permits the use of heroin, LSD and methamphetamines if a user gets prescriptions from two doctors.

Marijuana is the soft spot in the national opposition to drugs. Millions have tried it at some point in their lives and found that it was pleasurable and not particularly addictive. To that reservoir of latent tolerance, the backers of Prop 215 shrewdly added the irresistible notion of helping people in pain—people like 77-year-old Hazel Rodgers of San Francisco, who regularly smokes pot to relieve the symptoms of glaucoma and her anxiety about having been diagnosed with breast cancer. Drug warriors like McCaffrey (see box "We're on a Perilous Path") are thus forced into the no-win position of trying to deny the weed to thousands of patients who say it makes them feel better. Never mind

the fact that current medical research suggests pot doesn't do anything for glaucoma, or that other prescription drugs alleviate pain and anxiety. And never mind the fact that the fine print in the California law makes it a sham. Though sold to the voters as a way of helping people with terrible illnesses, the law specifically permits pot use for almost any complaint—even migraine headaches. It sidesteps federal law by specifying that pot use is legal if a doctor merely "recommends" it orally. That may mean doctors will not lose their licenses because they didn't *prescribe* the drug. It also means there will be no paper trail for narcs to follow.

Considering the fact that poll after poll reveals no sign that U.S. voters want to legalize pot or any other drug, this outcome is arguably perverse. It greatly disturbs groups like the Partnership for a Drug-Free America, which points out that marijuana use among teenagers is rising steadily and that the California law contains no age restrictions. The theory here is that marijuana is a "gateway" to harder drugs. That isn't Reefer Madness alarmism: reliable research shows that virtually all heroin and cocaine addicts started out with pot.

What worries drug warriors now is the possibility that would-be users will find friendly doctors to give them oral approval

From *Newsweek*, February 3, 1997, pp. 20, 22, 27. © 1997 by Newsweek, Inc. All rights reserved. Reprinted by permission.

We're on a Perilous Path

The drug czar says there's no proof marijuana is the best treatment for anything.
BY BARRY R. MCCAFFREY

WHY IS IT DANGEROUS for Americans to use marijuana as medicine? The answer is: it may not be. It may surprise you to hear the national drug-policy director say this, but I don't think we should automatically reject the possibility that marijuana may have some medicinal benefits. In fact, a synthetic version of THC, the main active ingredient in marijuana, is already approved by the FDA and available with a doctor's prescription. Called Marinol, it's used to ease nausea in cancer patients and help people with AIDS keep up their appetites.

Does that mean the new California law legalizing marijuana as medicine is a good idea? Absolutely not. The truth is, despite the insistence of legalization activists, there is no proof that smoked marijuana is the most effective available treatment for anything. Don't take my word for it. The National Institutes of Health recently examined all of the existing clinical evidence about smoked marijuana. Its conclusion: "There is no scientifically sound evidence that smoked marijuana is medically superior to currently available therapies." This isn't an argument between advocates for legalizing marijuana and the federal government. It's an argument between the legalizers and the American Medical Association, and the American Cancer Society, and the American Ophthalmological Society—all of which oppose the California marijuana initiative.

It seems to me entirely sensible that before we go rushing to embrace the medicinal use of marijuana—or LSD, heroin or any other illicit drug—we ought to find out if it is safe and effective. Every other drug on the market was required to undergo exhaustive testing by the FDA before it was made available to the public. As far as I'm concerned, the door is wide open to marijuana or any other substance—but first it has to pass scientific scrutiny and be subject to peer-group review. (It surprises many people to learn that methamphetamines and even cocaine have been approved for specific medical purposes.)

We have made $1 million available to the Institute of Medicine at the National Academy of Sciences to ask physicians and scientists for all that is known about smoked pot, and what questions need to be asked about it. And I have asked Dr. Harold Varmus, the Nobel laureate and head of the National Institutes of Health, to examine the potential benefits of marijuana. If researchers find there are compounds in marijuana that may have medicinal benefits (cannabis is made up of more than 400 different substances), we must immediately make them available to the American medical community. If they can demonstrate that they are safe and effective, then let's approve them.

Until then, though, it is inconceivable to allow anyone of any age to have uncontrolled use of marijuana for any alleged illness—without a doctor's examination or even prescription. But that is precisely what the California law lets people do. Can you think of any other untested, home-made, mind-altering medicine that you self-dose, and that uses a burning carcinogen as a delivery vehicle?

I think it's clear that a lot of the people arguing for the California proposition and others like it are pushing the legalization of drugs, plain and simple. It sends a very mixed and confusing message to the young. We've got 68 million kids age 18 and below. They're using drugs in enormously increasing numbers. Drug use among eighth graders alone has more than tripled in the last five years. Pretending pot is just another choice makes their decision to stay off drugs that much harder.

McCAFFREY, a retired army general, is the director of the Office of National Drug Control Policy.

---

and then buy the weed on the black market or at so-called cannabis buyers' clubs, which serve as middlemen between illicit growers and their middle-class clientele. That will surely create large problems for cops trying to suppress the underground pot trade, and it could produce a new class of criminal defendants who could claim their doctors said pot was a good thing to do. Ultimately, it may lead to a test case in which some prosecutor will press charges against an old lady like Hazel Rodgers. "The sense of frustration here is just huge," says a U.S. Justice Department official. "The dilemma is that in trying to look tough [to deter pot use], we wind up looking draconian."

What we have here, thanks to the voters of California and Arizona, is a nightmare of drug warriors everywhere—and a small but potentially significant breach in the national resolve against drugs. Earnest appeals by McCaffrey and many others failed to stop these slippery proposals at the ballot box, and it is time for clear leadership from the top—from Bill Clinton, the man who didn't inhale. Should we legalize pot, or not? That question is clearly implied in the controversy over medicinal marijuana. It is an issue that all Americans, ready or not, must confront honestly and resolve.

With MATT BAI and PATRICIA KING in San Francisco and DANIEL KLAIDMAN in Washington

Health and Behavioral Consequences of Binge Drinking in College

A National Survey of Students at 140 Campuses

Henry Wechsler, PhD; Andrea Davenport, MPH; George Dowdall, PhD; Barbara Moeykens, MS; Sonia Castillo, PhD

Objective.—To examine the extent of binge drinking by college students and the ensuing health and behavioral problems that binge drinkers create for themselves and others on their campus.

Design.—Self-administered survey mailed to a national representative sample of US 4-year college students.

Setting.—One hundred forty US 4-year colleges in 1993.

Participants.—A total of 17 592 college students.

Main Outcome Measures.—Self-reports of drinking behavior, alcohol-related health problems, and other problems.

Results.—Almost half (44%) of college students responding to the survey were binge drinkers, including almost one fifth (19%) of the students who were frequent binge drinkers. Frequent binge drinkers are more likely to experience serious health and other consequences of their drinking behavior than other students. Almost half (47%) of the frequent binge drinkers experienced five or more different drinking-related problems, including injuries and engaging in unplanned sex, since the beginning of the school year. Most binge drinkers do not consider themselves to be problem drinkers and have not sought treatment for an alcohol problem. Binge drinkers create problems for classmates who are not binge drinkers. Students who are not binge drinkers at schools with higher binge rates were more likely than students at schools with lower binge rates to experience problems such as being pushed, hit, or assaulted or experiencing an unwanted sexual advance.

Conclusions.—Binge drinking is widespread on college campuses. Programs aimed at reducing this problem should focus on frequent binge drinkers, refer them to treatment or educational programs, and emphasize the harm they cause for students who are not binge drinkers.

HEAVY episodic or binge drinking poses a danger of serious health and other consequences for alcohol abusers and for others in the immediate environment. Alcohol contributes to the leading causes of accidental death in the United States, such as motor vehicle crashes and falls.[1] Alcohol abuse is seen as contributing to almost half of motor vehicle fatalities, the most important cause of death among young Americans.[2] Unsafe sex—a growing threat with the spread of acquired immunodeficiency syndrome (AIDS) and other sexually transmitted diseases—and unintentional injuries have been associated with alcohol intoxication.[3-5] These findings support the view of college presidents who believe that alcohol abuse is the No. 1 problem on campus.[6]

Despite the fact that alcohol is illegal for most undergraduates, alcohol continues to be widely used on most college campuses today. Since the national study by Straus and Bacon in 1949,[7] numerous subsequent surveys have documented the overwhelming use of alcohol by college students and have pointed to problem drinking among this group.[8-10] Most previous studies of drinking by college students have been conducted on single college campuses and have not used random sampling of students.[9-12] While these studies are in general agreement about the prevalence and consequences of binge drinking, they do not provide a national representative sample of college drinking.

A few large-scale, multicollege surveys have been conducted in recent years. However, these have not selected a representative national sample of colleges, but have used colleges in one state[3] or those participating in a federal program,[5] or have followed a sample of high school seniors through college.[13]

In general, studies of college alcohol use have consistently found higher rates of binge drinking among men than women. However, these studies used the same definition of binge drinking for men and women, without taking into account sex differences in metabolism of ethanol or in body mass.[3,5,9-12,14-17]

The consequences of binge drinking often pose serious risks for drinkers and for others in the college environment. Binge drinking has been associated with unplanned and unsafe sexual activity, physical and sexual assault, unintentional injuries, other criminal violations, interpersonal problems, physical or cognitive impairment, and poor academic performance.[3-5]

This study examines the nature and extent of binge drinking among a representative national sample of students

From the Departments of Health and Social Behavior (Drs Wechsler and Dowdall and Mss Davenport and Moeykens) and Biostatistics (Dr Castillo), Harvard School of Public Health, Boston, Mass.

Reprint requests to the Department of Health and Social Behavior, Harvard School of Public Health, 677 Huntington Ave, Boston, MA 02115 (Dr Wechsler).

From *JAMA: The Journal of the American Medical Association*, December 7, 1994, pp. 1672-1677. © 1994 by the American Medical Association. Reprinted by permission.

at 140 US 4-year colleges and details the problems such drinking causes for drinkers themselves and for others on their college campus. Binge drinking is defined through a sex-specific measure to take into account sex differences in the dosage effects of ethanol.

METHODS

The Colleges

A national sample of 179 colleges was selected from the American Council on Education's list of 4-year colleges and universities accredited by one of the six regional bodies covering the United States. The sample was selected using probability proportionate to enrollment size sampling. All full-time undergraduate students at a university were eligible to be chosen for this study, regardless of the college in which they were enrolled. This sample contained few women-only colleges and few colleges with less than 1000 students. To correct for this problem, an oversample of 15 additional colleges with enrollments of less than 1000 students and 10 all-women's colleges were added to the sample. Nine colleges were subsequently dropped because they were considered inappropriate. These included seminary schools, military schools, and allied health schools.

One hundred forty (72%) of the final sample of 195 colleges agreed to participate. The primary reason stated for nonparticipation by college administrators was inability to provide a random sample of students and their addresses within the time requirements of the study. The 140 participating colleges are located in 40 states and the District of Columbia. They represent a cross-section of US higher education. Two thirds of the colleges sampled are public and one third are private. Approximately two thirds are located in a suburban or urban setting and one third in a small town/rural setting. Four percent are women-only, and 4% are predominantly black institutions.

When the 55 nonparticipating schools were compared with the 140 in the study, the only statistically significant difference found was in terms of enrollment size. Proportionately fewer small colleges (fewer than 1000 students) participated in the study. Since these were oversampled, sufficient numbers are present for statistical analysis.

Sampling Procedures

Colleges were sent a set of specific guidelines for drawing a random sample of students based on the total enrollment of full-time undergraduates. Depending on enrollment size, every xth student was selected from the student registry using a random starting point. A sample of undergraduate students was provided by each of the 140 participating colleges: 215 students at each of 127 colleges, and 108 at each of 13 colleges (12 of which were in the oversample). The final student sample included 28 709 students.

The Questionnaire

The 20-page survey instrument asked students a number of questions about their drinking behavior as well as other health issues. Whenever possible, the survey instrument included questions that had been used previously in other national or large-scale epidemiological studies.[13,14] A drink was defined as a 12-oz (360-mL) can (or bottle) of beer, a 4-oz (120-mL) glass of wine, a 12-oz (360-mL) bottle (or can) of wine cooler, or a shot (1.25 oz [37 mL]) of liquor straight or in a mixed drink. The following four questions were used to assess binge drinking: (1) sex; (2) recency of last drink ("never," "not in past year," "within last year but more than 30 days ago," "within 30 days but more than 1 week ago," or "within week"); (3) "Think back over the last two weeks. How many times have you had five or more drinks in a row?" (The use of this question, without specification of time elapsed in a drinking episode, is consistent with standard practice in recent research on alcohol use among this population.[3,5,13,18]); and (4) "During the last two weeks, how many times have you had four drinks in a row (but no more than that) (for women)?" Missing responses to any of these four questions excluded the student from the binging analyses.

Students were also asked the extent to which they had experienced any of the following 12 problems as a consequence of their drinking since the beginning of the school year: have a hangover; miss a class; get behind in schoolwork; do something you later regretted; forget where you were or what you did; argue with friends; engage in unplanned sexual activity; not use protection when you had sex; damage property; get into trouble with campus or local police; get hurt or injured; or require medical treatment for an alcohol overdose. They were also asked if, since the beginning of the school year, they had experienced any of the following eight problems caused by other students' drinking: been insulted or humiliated; had a serious argument or quarrel; been pushed, hit, or assaulted; had your property damaged; had to "babysit" or take care of another student who drank too much; had your studying or sleep interrupted; experienced an unwanted sexual advance; or

had been a victim of sexual assault or date rape.

The Mailing

The initial mailing of questionnaires to students began on February 5, 1993. By the end of March, 87% of the final group of questionnaires had been received, with another 10% in April and 2% in May and June. There are no discernible differences in binging rates among questionnaires received in each of the 5 months of the survey. Mailings were modified to take into account spring break, so that students would be responding about their binge drinking behavior during a 2-week time on campus. Responses were voluntary and anonymous. Four separate mailings, usually 10 days apart, were sent at each college: a questionnaire, a reminder postcard, a second questionnaire, and a second reminder postcard. To encourage students to respond, the following cash awards were offered: one $1000 award to a student whose name was drawn from among students responding within 1 week, and one $500 award and ten $100 awards to students selected from all those who responded.

The Response Rate

The questionnaires were mailed to 28 709 students. Overall, 3082 students were eliminated from the sample because of school reports of incorrect addresses, withdrawal from school, or leaves of absence, reducing the sample size to 25 627. A total of 17 592 students returned questionnaires, yielding an overall student response rate of approximately 69%. The response rate is likely to be underestimated since it does not take into account all of the students who may not have received questionnaires. At 104 of the colleges, response rates were between 60% and 80%, and only six colleges had response rates less than 50%. Response rate was not associated with the binging rate (ie, the Pearson correlation coefficient between the binge drinking rate at the college and the response rate was 0.06 with a P value of .46).

When responses of early and late responders to the survey were compared, there were no significant differences in the percent of nondrinkers, nonbinge drinkers, and binge drinkers. In the case of 11 557 students who could be classified as early or late responders, there was no significant difference in terms of binge drinking (43% for the early responders vs 42% for the late responders). An additional short form of the questionnaire was mailed to a segment of students who had failed to return the questionnaire. The rate of binge drink-

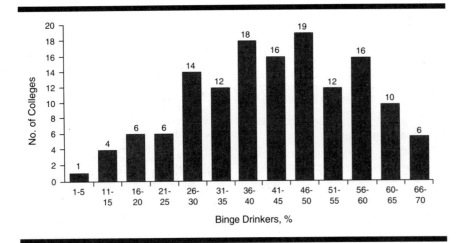

Distribution of colleges by percentage of binge drinkers.

Table 1.—Drinking Styles of Students Who Were Nonbinge Drinkers, Infrequent Binge Drinkers, or Frequent Binge Drinkers*

Drinking Styles	Nonbinge Drinkers, %†		Infrequent Binge Drinkers, %‡		Frequent Binge Drinkers, %§	
	Men (n=2539)	Women (n=4400)	Men (n=1968)	Women (n=2130)	Men (n=1630)	Women (n=1684)
Drank on 10 or more occasions in the past 30 d‖	3	1	11	6	61	39
Usually binges when drinks	4	4	43	45	83	82
Was drunk three or more times in the past month	2	1	17	13	70	55
Drinks to get drunk¶	22	18	49	44	73	68

*Chi-square comparisons of students who were nonbinge drinkers, infrequent binge drinkers, and frequent binge drinkers and each of the four drinking styles were significant for men and women separately at $P<.001$. Sample sizes vary slightly for each question because of missing values. Binging is defined as four or more drinks for women and five or more drinks for men.
†Students who consumed alcohol in the past year, but did not binge.
‡Students who binged one or two times in a 2-week period.
§Students who binged three or more times in a 2-week period.
‖Question asked, "On how many occasions have you had a drink of alcohol in the past 30 days?" Response categories were 1 to 2 occasions, 3 to 5 occasions, 6 to 9 occasions, 10 to 19 occasions, 20 to 39 occasions, and 40 or more occasions.
¶Says that to get drunk is an important reason for drinking.

ing of these nonresponders did not differ from that of responders to the original student survey.

Data Analysis

All statistical analyses were carried out using the current version of SAS.[19] Comparisons of unweighted and weighted sample results suggested little difference between them, so unweighted results are reported here. Chi-square analyses among students who had a drink in the past year were used to compare nonbinge drinkers, infrequent binge drinkers, and binge drinkers. Binge drinking was defined as the consumption of five or more drinks in a row for men and four or more drinks in a row for women during the 2 weeks prior to the survey. An extensive analysis showed that this sex-specific measure accurately indicates an equivalent likelihood of alcohol-related problems. In this article, the term "binge drinker" is used to refer to students who binged at least once in the previous 2 weeks. Frequent binge

drinkers were defined as those who binged three or more times in the past 2 weeks and infrequent binge drinkers as those who binged one or two times in the past 2 weeks. Nonbinge drinkers were those who had consumed alcohol in the past year, but had not binged.

Logistic regression analyses were used to examine how much more likely frequent binge drinkers were to experience an alcohol-related problem or driving behavior compared with nonbinge drinkers, and to compare infrequent binge drinkers with nonbinge drinkers. Odds ratios were adjusted for age, sex, race, marital status, and parents' college education.

In examining secondary binge effects, schools were divided into three groups on the basis of the percentage of students who were binge drinkers at each school. The responses of students who had not binged in the past 2 weeks (including those who had never had a drink) and who resided in dormitories, fraternities, or sororities were compared through χ^2 analy-

ses across the three school types. High-level binge schools (where 51% or more students were binge drinkers) included 44 schools with 6084 students; middle-level binge schools (36% to 50% of students were binge drinkers) included 53 schools with 6455 students; and low-level binge schools (35% or less of students were binge drinkers) included 43 schools with 5043 students (for 10 students, information regarding school of attendance was missing). For two of the problems that occurred primarily or almost exclusively to women (sexual assault and experiencing an unwanted sexual advance), only women were included in the analyses.

RESULTS

Characteristics of the Student Sample

This analysis is based on data from 17 592 undergraduate students at 140 US 4-year colleges. The student sample includes more women (58%) than men (42%), due in part to the inclusion of six all-women's institutions. This compares with national 1991 data that report 51% of undergraduates at 4-year institutions are women.[20] The sample is predominantly white (81%). This coincides exactly with national 1991 data that report 81% of undergraduates at 4-year institutions are white.[20] Minority groups included Asian/Pacific Islander (7%), Spanish/Hispanic (7%), black/African American (6%), and Native American (1%). The age of the students was distributed as follows: 45% younger than 21 years, 38% aged 21 to 23 years, and 17% aged 24 years or more. There were slightly more juniors (25%) and seniors (26%) in the sample than freshmen (20%) and sophomores (19%), probably because 30% of the students were transfers from other institutions. Ten percent of the students were in their fifth undergraduate year of school or beyond. Religious affiliation was discerned by asking students in which of the following religions they were raised: Protestant (44%), Catholic (36%), Jewish (3%), Muslim (1%), other (4%), and none (12%). Religion was cited as an important to very important activity among 36% of the students. Approximately three of five students (59%) worked for pay. Approximately half (49%) of the students had a grade-point average of A, A−, or B+.

Extent of Binge Drinking

Because of missing responses, there were 496 students excluded from binging analyses (ie, 17 096 were included). Most students drank alcohol during the past year. Only about one of six (16%) were nondrinkers (15% of the men and 16% of the women). About two of five students (41%) drank but were nonbinge

Table 2.—Risk of Alcohol-Related Problems Comparing Students Who Were Infrequent Binge Drinkers or Frequent Binge Drinkers With Students Who Were Nonbinge Drinkers Among College Students Who Had a Drink in the Past Year*

Reporting Problem	Nonbinge Drinkers, % (n=6894)	Infrequent Binge Drinkers		Frequent Binge Drinkers	
		% (n=4090)	Adjusted OR (95% CI)†	% (n=3291)	Adjusted OR (95% CI)‡
Have a hangover	30	75	6.28 (5.73-6.87)	90	17.62 (15.50-20.04)
Do something you regret	14	37	3.31 (3.00-3.64)	63	8.98 (8.11-9.95)
Miss a class	8	30	4.66 (4.15-5.24)	61	16.58 (14.73-18.65)
Forget where you were or what you did	8	26	3.62 (3.22-4.06)	54	11.23 (10.05-12.65)
Get behind in school work	6	21	3.70 (3.26-4.20)	46	11.43 (10.09-12.94)
Argue with friends	8	22	3.06 (2.72-3.46)	42	7.77 (6.90-8.74)
Engage in unplanned sexual activity	8	20	2.78 (2.46-3.13)	41	7.17 (6.37-8.06)
Get hurt or injured	2	9	3.65 (3.01-4.43)	23	10.43 (8.70-12.52)
Damage property	2	8	3.09 (2.53-3.77)	22	9.48 (7.86-11.43)
Not use protection when having sex	4	10	2.90 (2.45-3.42)	22	7.11 (6.07-8.34)
Get into trouble with campus or local police	1	4	2.50 (1.92-3.26)	11	6.92 (5.44-8.81)
Require medical treatment of alcohol overdose	<1	<1	NS	1	2.81 (1.39-5.68)
Have five or more alcohol-related problems since the beginning of the school year§	3	14	4.95 (4.17-5.89)	47	25.10 (21.30-29.58)

*Problem occurred not at all or one or more times. Chi-square comparisons of nonbinge drinkers, infrequent binge drinkers, and frequent binge drinkers and each of the problems are significant at $P<.001$, except for alcohol overdose ($P=.002$). Sample sizes vary slightly for each problem because of missing values. OR indicates odds ratio; CI, confidence interval. See Table 1 for explanation of drinking classification.
†Adjusted ORs of infrequent binge drinkers vs nonbinge drinkers are significant at $P<.001$.
‡Adjusted ORs of frequent binge drinkers vs nonbinge drinkers are significant at $P<.001$, except for alcohol overdose, $P<.01$.
§Excludes hangover and includes driving after drinking as one of the problems.

Table 3.—Alcohol-Related Driving Behavior for a 30-Day Period Comparing Students Who Were Infrequent Binge Drinkers or Frequent Binge Drinkers With Students Who Were Nonbinge Drinkers*

Driving Behavior	Nonbinge Drinkers		Infrequent Binge Drinkers			Frequent Binge Drinkers		
	Men, % (n=2531)	Women, % (n=4393)	Men, % (n=1975)	Women, % (n=2132)	Adjusted OR (95% CI)†	Men, % (n=1630)	Women, % (n=1684)	Adjusted OR (95% CI)‡
Drove after drinking alcohol	20	13	47	33	5.13 (4.67-5.64)	62	49	10.33 (9.34-11.42)
Drove after having five or more drinks	2	1	18	7	22.23 (16.89-29.26)	40	21	74.30 (56.56-97.58)
Rode with a driver who was high or drunk	7	7	23	22	4.73 (4.20-5.32)	53	48	15.97 (14.22-17.95)

*Chi-square comparisons of nonbinge drinkers, infrequent binge drinkers, and frequent binge drinkers and each of the three driving behaviors were all significant for men and women separately at $P<.001$. Sample sizes vary slightly for each question because of missing values. OR indicates odds ratio; CI, confidence interval. See Table 1 for explanation of drinking classification.
†Adjusted OR of infrequent binge drinkers vs nonbinge drinkers (sex combined) are significant at $P<.001$.
‡Adjusted OR of frequent binge drinkers vs nonbinge drinkers (sex combined) are significant at $P<.001$.

drinkers (35% of the men and 45% of the women). Slightly fewer than half (44%) of the students were binge drinkers (50% of the men and 39% of the women). About half of this group of binge drinkers, or about one in five students (19%) overall, were frequent binge drinkers (overall, 23% of the men and 17% of the women).

Binge Drinking Rates at Colleges

The Figure shows that binge drinking rates vary extensively among the 140 colleges in the study. While 1% of the students were binge drinkers at the school with the lowest rate of binge drinkers, 70% of students were binge drinkers at the school with the highest rate. At 44 schools, more than half of the responding students were binge drinkers.

When the 140 colleges were divided into levels of binging rate, χ^2 analyses showed that several college characteristics were individually associated (at $P<.05$) with binging rate. Colleges located in the Northeast or North Central regions of the United States (compared with those in the West or South) or those that were residential (compared with

commuter schools, where 90% or more of the students lived off campus)[21] tended to have higher rates of binging. In addition, traditionally black institutions and women's colleges had lower binge rates than schools that were not traditionally black or were coeducational colleges. Other characteristics, such as whether the college was public or private and its enrollment size, were not related to binge drinker rates.

Examination of whether college alcohol programs and policies have any association with binge drinking will be presented in a separate publication. There is little evidence to conclude that current policies have had strong impacts on overall drinking levels. Preliminary analyses suggest that individual binge drinking is less likely if the institution does not have any alcohol outlets within 1 mile of campus, or if it prohibits alcohol use for all persons (even those older than 21 years) on campus.

Drinking Patterns of Binge Drinkers

Table 1 indicates that our designations of binge drinker and frequent binge

drinker are strongly indicative of a drinking style that involves more frequent and heavier drinking. Furthermore, intoxication (often intentional) is associated with binge drinking in men and women.

Binge drinking is related to age. Students who are in the predominant college age group (between 17 and 23 years) have much higher binging rates than older students. However, within the predominant college age group, students who are younger than the legal drinking age of 21 years do not differ in binging rates from students aged 21 to 23 years. In contrast to the modest effects of age, there is no relationship between year in school and binging, with rates of binge drinking virtually identical among students across the years of college attendance.

Alcohol-Related Health and Other Problems

There is a strong, positive relationship between the frequency of binge drinking and alcohol-related health and other problems reported by the students (Table 2). Among the more serious alcohol-related

Table 4.—Students Experiencing Secondary Binge Effects (Based on Students Who Were Not Binge Drinkers and Living in Dormitories, Fraternities, or Sororities)*

| | | School's Binging Level | | | |
| | | Middle | | High | |
Secondary Binge Effect	Low, % (n=801)	% (n=1115)	Adjusted OR (95% CI)†	% (n=1064)	Adjusted OR (95% CI)‡
Been insulted or humiliated	21	30	1.6 (1.3-2.1)	34	1.9 (1.5-2.3)
Had a serious argument or quarrel	13	18	1.3 (1.0-1.7)	20	1.5 (1.1-2.0)
Been pushed, hit, or assaulted	7	10	1.4 (1.0-2.1)	13	2.0 (1.4-2.8)
Had your property damaged	6	13	2.0 (1.4-2.8)	15	2.3 (1.6-3.2)
Had to take care of drunken student	31	47	1.9 (1.6-2.3)	54	2.5 (2.0-3.0)
Had your studying/sleep interrupted	42	64	2.3 (1.9-2.8)	68	2.6 (2.2-3.2)
Experienced an unwanted sexual advance§	15	21	1.7 (1.2-2.3)	26	2.1 (1.5-2.8)
Been a victim of sexual assault or date rape§	2	1	NS	2	NS
Experienced at least one of the above problems	62	82	2.8 (2.3-3.5)	87	4.1 (3.2-5.2)

*OR indicates odds ratio; CI, confidence interval.
†Adjusted ORs of students at schools with middle levels of binging vs students at schools with low levels are significant at P<.05.
‡Adjusted ORs of students at schools with high levels of binging vs students at schools with low levels are significant at P<.05.
§Based on women only.

problems, the frequent binge drinkers were seven to 10 times more likely than the nonbinge drinkers to not use protection when having sex, to engage in unplanned sexual activity, to get into trouble with campus police, to damage property, or to get hurt or injured. A similar comparison between the infrequent binge drinkers and nonbinge drinkers also shows a strong relationship.

Men and women reported similar frequencies for most of the problems, except for damaging property or getting into trouble with the campus police. Among the frequent binge drinkers, 35% of the men and 9% of the women reported damaging property, and 16% of the men and 6% of the women reported getting into trouble with the campus police.

Drinking and Driving

There is also a positive relationship between binge drinking and driving under the influence of alcohol (Table 3). A large proportion of the student population reported driving after drinking alcohol. Binge drinkers, particularly frequent binge drinkers, reported significantly (P<.001) higher frequencies of dangerous driving behaviors than nonbinge drinkers.

Number of Problems

Nearly half (47%) of the frequent binge drinkers reported having experienced five or more of the 12 problems listed in Table 2 (omitting hangover and including driving after drinking) since the beginning of the school year, compared with 14% of infrequent binge drinkers and 3% of nonbinge drinkers. The adjusted odds ratios indicate that frequent binge drinkers were 25 times more likely than nonbinge drinkers to experience five or more of these

problems, while the infrequent binge drinkers were five times more likely than nonbinge drinkers to experience five or more problems.

Self-assessment of Drinking Problem

Few students describe themselves as having a drinking problem. When asked to classify themselves in terms of their current alcohol use, less than 1% of the total sample (0.2%), including only 0.6% of the frequent binge drinkers, designated themselves as problem drinkers. In addition, few students have ever sought treatment for a problem with alcohol.

A somewhat larger proportion of students indicated that they had ever had a drinking problem. Slightly more than one fifth (22%) of the frequent binge drinkers thought that they ever had a drinking problem, compared with 12% of the infrequent binge drinkers and 7% of the nonbinge drinkers.

Secondary Binge Effects

Table 4 reports on the percentage of nonbinging students who experienced "secondary binge effects," each of eight types of problems due to other students' drinking at each of the three different school types (ie, schools with high, middle, and low binge levels). For seven of the eight problems studied, students at schools with high and middle binge levels were more likely than students at schools with low binge levels to experience problems as a result of the drinking behaviors of others. Odds ratios (adjusted for age, sex, race, marital status, and parents' college education) indicated that nonbinging students at schools with the high binge levels were more likely than nonbinging students at schools with low binge levels to experience secondary binge effects.

The odds of experiencing at least one of the eight problems was roughly 4:1 when students at schools with high binge levels were compared with students at schools with low binge levels.

Binge Drinking in High School

Most students reported the same drinking behavior in high school as in college. Almost half (47%) had not been binge drinkers in high school and did not binge in college, while one fifth (22%) binged in high school and in college. One fifth (22%) of the students were binge drinkers in college but not in high school, while 10% were not binge drinkers at the time of the survey in college, but reported having been binge drinkers in high school.

COMMENT

To our knowledge, this is the first study that has used a representative national sample, and the first large-scale study to measure binge drinking under a sex-specific definition. Forty-four percent of the college students in this study were classified as binge drinkers. This finding is consistent with the findings of other national studies such as the University of Michigan's Monitoring the Future Project, which found that 41% of college students were binge drinkers,[13] and the Core Alcohol and Drug Survey, which found that 42% of college students were binge drinkers.[5] All three studies used a definition of binging over a 2-week period, but the other studies used the same five-drink measure for both sexes. Binge drinking was defined in terms of the number of drinks consumed in a single episode. No attempt was made to specify the duration of time for each episode. Future research might examine whether subgroup differences exist in duration and whether such differences are linked to outcomes.

A possible limitation of surveys using self-reports of drinking behavior pertains to the validity of responses; however, a number of studies have confirmed the validity of self-reports of alcohol and substance use.[22-24] Findings indicate that if a self-report bias exists, it is largely limited to the heaviest use group[25] and should not affect such a conservative estimate of heavy volume as five drinks.

The results confirm that binge drinking is widespread on college campuses. Overall, almost half of all students were binge drinkers. One fifth of all students were frequent binge drinkers (had three or more binge drinking occasions in the past 2 weeks) and were deeply involved in a lifestyle characterized by frequent and deliberate intoxication. Frequent binge drinkers are much more likely to experience serious health and other consequences of their drinking behavior than other students. Almost half of them have experienced five or more alcohol-related problems since the beginning of the school year, one of three report they were hurt or injured, and two in five engaged in unplanned sexual activity. Frequent binge drinkers also report drinking and driving: Three of five male frequent binge drinkers drove after drinking some alcohol in the 30 days prior to the survey, and two of five drove after having five or more drinks. A recent national report that reviewed published studies concluded that alcohol was involved in two thirds of college student suicides, in 90% of campus rapes, and in 95% of violent crime on campus.[26]

Almost a third of the colleges in the study have a majority of students who binge. Not only do these binge drinkers put themselves at risk, they also create problems for their fellow students who are not binge drinking. Students who did not binge and who reside at schools with high levels of binge drinkers were up to three times as likely to report being bothered by the drinking-related behaviors of other students than students who did not binge and who reside at schools with lower levels of binge drinkers. These problems included being pushed, hit, or assaulted and experiencing an unwanted sexual advance.

Effective interventions face a number of challenges. Drinking is not typically a behavior learned in college and often continues patterns established earlier. In fact, one of three students in the present study was already a binge drinker in the year before college.

The prominence of drinking on college campuses reflects its importance in the wider society, but drinking has traditionally occupied a unique place in campus life. Despite the overall decline in drinking in US society, recent time-trend studies have failed to show a corresponding decrease in binge drinking on college campuses.[3,13] The variation in binge drinking rates among the colleges in this study suggest that colleges may create and unwittingly perpetuate their own drinking cultures through selection, tradition, policy, and other strategies. On many campuses, drinking behavior that would elsewhere be classified as alcohol abuse may be socially acceptable, or even socially attractive, despite its documented implication in automobile crashes, other injury, violence, suicide, and high-risk sexual behavior.

The scope of the problem makes immediate results of any interventions highly unlikely. Colleges need to be committed to large-scale and long-term behavior change strategies, including referral of alcohol abusers to appropriate treatment. Frequent binge drinkers on college campuses are similar to other alcohol abusers elsewhere in their tendency to deny that they have a problem. Indeed, their youth, the visibility of others who drink the same way, and the shelter of the college community may make them less likely to recognize the problem. In addition to addressing the health problems of alcohol abusers, a major effort should address the large group of students who are not binge drinkers on campus who are adversely affected by the alcohol-related behavior of binge drinkers.

This study was supported by the Robert Wood Johnson Foundation. We wish to thank the following persons who assisted with the project: Lloyd Johnston, PhD, Thomas J. Mangione, PhD, Anthony M. Roman, MD, Nan Laird, PhD, Jeffrey Hansen, Avtar Khalsa, MSW, and Marianne Lee, MPA.

References

1. US Dept of Health and Human Services. *Alcohol and Health*. Rockville, Md: National Institute on Alcohol Abuse and Alcoholism; 1990.
2. Robert Wood Johnson Foundation. *Substance Abuse: The Nation's Number One Health Problem, Key Indicators for Policy*. Princeton, NJ: Robert Wood Johnson Foundation; October 1993.
3. Wechsler H, Isaac N. 'Binge' drinkers at Massachusetts colleges: prevalence, drinking styles, time trends, and associated problems. *JAMA*. 1992;267:2929-2931.
4. Hanson DJ, Engs RC. College students' drinking problems: a national study, 1982-1991. *Psychol Rep*. 1992;71:39-42.
5. Presley CA, Meilman PW, Lyerla R. *Alcohol and Drugs on American College Campuses: Use, Consequence, and Perceptions of the Campus Environment, Volume I: 1989-1991*. Carbondale, Ill: The Core Institute; 1993.
6. The Carnegie Foundation for the Advancement of Teaching. *Campus Life: In Search of Community*. Princeton, NJ: Princeton University Press; 1990.
7. Straus R, Bacon SD. *Drinking in College*. New Haven, Conn: Yale University Press; 1953.
8. Berkowitz AD, Perkins HW. Problem drinking among college students: a review of recent research. *J Am Coll Health*. 1986;35:21-28.
9. Saltz R, Elandt D. College student drinking studies: 1976-1985. *Contemp Drug Probl*. 1986;13:117-157.
10. Haworth-Hoeppner S, Globetti G, Stem J, Morasco F. The quantity and frequency of drinking among undergraduates at a southern university. *Int J Addict*. 1989;24:829-857.
11. Liljestrand P. Quality in college student drinking research: conceptual and methodological issues. *J Alcohol Drug Educ*. 1993;38:1-36.
12. Hughes S, Dodder R. Alcohol consumption patterns among college populations. *J Coll Student Personnel*. 1983;20:257-264.
13. Johnston LD, O'Malley PM, Bachman JG. *Drug Use Among American High School Seniors, College Students, and Young Adults, 1975-1990, Volume 2*. Washington, DC: Government Printing Office; 1991. US Dept of Health and Human Services publication ADM 91-1835.
14. Wechsler H, McFadden M. Drinking among college students in New England. *J Stud Alcohol*. 1979;40:969-996.
15. O'Hare TM. Drinking in college: consumption patterns, problems, sex differences, and legal drinking age. *J Stud Alcohol*. 1990;51:536-541.
16. Engs RC, Hanson DJ. The drinking patterns and problems of college students: 1983. *J Alcohol Drug Educ*. 1985;31:65-83.
17. Brennan AF, Walfish S, AuBuchon P. Alcohol use and abuse in college students, I: a review of individual and personality correlates. *Int J Addict*. 1986;21:449-474.
18. Room R. Measuring alcohol consumption in the US: methods and rationales. In: Clark WB, Hilton ME, eds. *Alcohol in America: Drinking Practices and Problems*. Albany: State University of New York Press; 1991:26-50.
19. SAS Institute Inc. *SAS/STAT User's Guide, Release 6.03 ed*. Cary, NC: SAS Institute Inc; 1988.
20. US Dept of Education. *Digest of Educational Statistics*. Washington, DC: National Center of Educational Statistics; 1993:180,205.
21. *Barron's Profiles of American Colleges*. Hauppauge, NY: Barron's Educational Series Inc; 1992.
22. Midanik L. Validity of self-reported alcohol use: a literature review and assessment. *Br J Addict*. 1988;83:1019-1030.
23. Cooper AM, Sobell MB, Sobell LC, Maisto SA. Validity of alcoholics' self-reports: duration data. *Int J Addict*. 1981;16:401-406.
24. Reinisch OJ, Bell RM, Ellickson PL. *How Accurate Are Adolescent Reports of Drug Use?* Santa Monica, Calif: RAND; 1991. RAND publication N-3189-CHF.
25. Room R. Survey vs sales data for the US. *Drink Drug Pract Surv*. 1971;3:15-16.
26. CASA Commission on Substance Abuse at Colleges and Universities. *Rethinking Rites of Passage: Substance Abuse on America's Campuses*. New York, NY: Columbia University; June 1994.

A D D I C T E D

Why do people get hooked? Mounting evidence points to a powerful brain chemical called dopamine

By J. MADELEINE NASH

IMAGINE YOU ARE TAKING A SLUG OF WHIS-key. A puff of a cigarette. A toke of mari-juana. A snort of cocaine. A shot of heroin. Put aside whether these drugs are le-gal or illegal. Concentrate, for now, on the chemistry. The moment you take that slug, that puff, that toke, that snort, that shot, tril-lions of potent molecules surge through your bloodstream and into your brain. Once there, they set off a cascade of chemical and elec-trical events, a kind of neurological chain re-action that ricochets around the skull and rearranges the interior reality of the mind.

Given the complexity of these events—and the inner workings of the mind in gen-eral—it's not surprising that scientists have struggled mightily to make sense of the mechanisms of addiction. Why do certain substances have the power to make us feel so good (at least at first)? Why do some peo-ple fall so easily into the thrall of alcohol, cocaine, nicotine and other addictive sub-stances, while others can, literally, take them or leave them?

The answer, many scientists are con-vinced, may be simpler than anyone has dared imagine. What ties all these mood-al-tering drugs together, they say, is a remark-able ability to elevate levels of a common substance in the brain called dopamine. In fact, so overwhelming has evidence of the link between dopamine and drugs of abuse

become that the distinction (pushed primar-ily by the tobacco industry and its support-ers) between substances that are addictive and those that are merely habit-forming has very nearly been swept away.

The Liggett Group, smallest of the U.S.'s Big Five cigarette makers, broke ranks in March and conceded not only that tobacco is addictive but also that the company has known it all along. While RJR Nabisco and the others continue to battle in the courts-in-sisting that smokers are not hooked, just ex-ercising free choice—their denials ring increasingly hollow in the face of the grow-ing weight of evidence. Over the past year, several scientific groups have made the case that in dopamine-rich areas of the brain, nicotine behaves remarkably like cocaine. And late last week a federal judge ruled for the first time that the Food and Drug Ad-ministration has the right to regulate to-bacco as a drug and cigarettes as drug-delivery devices.

Now, a team of researchers led by psychiatrist Dr. Nora Volkow of the Brook-haven National Labo-ratory in New York has published the

strongest evidence to date that the surge of dopamine in addicts' brains is what triggers a cocaine high. In last week's edition of the journal *Nature* they described how powerful brain-imaging technology can be used to track the rise of dopamine and link it to feelings of euphoria.

Like serotonin (the brain chemical affected by such antidepressants as Prozac), dopamine is a neurotransmitter—a molecule that ferries messages from one neuron within the brain to another. Serotonin is associated with feelings of sadness and well-being, dopamine with pleasure and elation. Dopamine can be elevated by a hug, a kiss, a word of praise or a winning poker hand—as well as by the potent pleasures that come from drugs.

The idea that a single chemical could be associated with everything from snorting co-caine and smoking tobacco to getting good

PRIME SUSPECT

They don't yet know the precise mechanism by which it works, but scientists are increasingly convinced that dopamine plays a key role in a wide range of addictions, including those to heroin, nicotine, alcohol and marijuana

From *Time*, May 5, 1997, pp. 68-76. © 1997 by Time Inc. Magazine Company. Reprinted by permission.

DOPAMINE MAY BE LINKED TO GAMBLING, CHOCOLATE AND EVEN SEX

grades and enjoying sex has electrified scientists and changed the way they look at a wide range of dependencies, chemical and otherwise. Dopamine, they now believe, is not just a chemical that transmits pleasure signals but may, in fact, be the master molecule of addiction.

This is not to say dopamine is the only chemical involved or that the deranged thought processes that mark chronic drug abuse are due to dopamine alone. The brain is subtler than that. Drugs modulate the activity of a variety of brain chemicals, each of which intersects with many others. "Drugs are like sledgehammers," observes Dr. Eric Nestler of the Yale University School of Medicine. "They profoundly alter many pathways."

Nevertheless, the realization that dopamine may be a common end point of all those pathways represents a signal advance. Provocative, controversial, unquestionably incomplete, the dopamine hypothesis provides a basic framework for understanding how a genetically encoded trait—such as a tendency to produce too little dopamine—might intersect with environmental influences to create a serious behavioral disorder. Therapists have long known of patients who, in addition to having psychological problems, abuse drugs as well. Could their drug problems be linked to some inborn quirk? Might an inability to absorb enough dopamine, with its pleasure-giving properties, cause them to seek gratification in drugs?

Such speculation is controversial, for it suggests that broad swaths of the population may be genetically predisposed to drug abuse. What is not controversial is that the social cost of drug abuse, whatever its cause, is enormous. Cigarettes contribute to the death toll from cancer and heart disease. Alcohol is the leading cause of domestic violence and highway deaths. The needles used to inject heroin and cocaine are spreading AIDS. Directly or indirectly, addiction to drugs, cigarettes and alcohol is thought to account for a third of all hospital admissions, a quarter of all deaths and a majority of serious crimes. In the U.S. alone the combined medical and social costs of drug abuse are believed to exceed $240 billion.

FOR NEARLY A QUARTER-CENTURY the U.S. has been waging a war on drugs, with little apparent success. As scientists learn more about how dopamine works (and how drugs work on it), the evidence suggests that we may be fighting the wrong battle. Americans tend to think of drug addiction as a failure of character. But this stereotype is beginning to give way to the recognition that drug dependence has a clear biological basis. "Addiction," declares Brookhaven's Volkow, "is a disorder of the brain no different from other forms of mental illness."

That new insight may be the dopamine hypothesis' most important contribution in the fight against drugs. It completes the loop between the mechanism of addiction and programs for treatment. And it raises hope for more effective therapies. Abstinence, if maintained, not only halts the physical and

HIGH AND LOWS
Number who used in the past month

Heroin — 200,000
Triggers release of dopamine; acts on other neurotransmitters

Amphetamines — 800,000
Stimulate excess release of dopamine

Cocaine/Crack — 1.5 million
Blocks dopamine absorption

Marijuana — 10 million
Binds to areas of brain involved in mood and memory; triggers release of dopamine

Alcohol — 11 million abusers
Triggers dopamine release; acts on other neurotransmitters

Nicotine — 61 million
Triggers release of dopamine

Caffeine — 130 million*
May trigger release of dopamine

Sources: SAMHSA, National Coffee Association   *coffee drinkers

psychological damage wrought by drugs but in large measure also reverses it.

Genes and social forces may conspire to turn people into addicts but do not doom them to remain so. Consider the case of Rafael Rios, who grew up in a housing project in New York City's drug-infested South Bronx. For 18 years, until he turned 31, Rios, whose father died of alcoholism, led a double life. He graduated from Harvard Law School and joined a prestigious Chicago law firm. Yet all the while he was secretly visiting a shooting gallery' once a day. His favored concoction: heroin spiked with a jolt

WHAT ELSE?

Preliminary evidence suggests that dopamine may be involved even when we form dependencies on things—like coffee or candy—that we don't think of as drugs at all

of cocaine. Ten years ago, Rios succeeded in kicking his habit—for good, he hopes. He is now executive director of A Safe Haven, a Chicago-based chain of residential facilities for recovering addicts.

How central is dopamine's role in this familiar morality play? Scientists are still trying to sort that out. It is no accident, they say, that people are attracted to drugs. The major drugs of abuse, whether depressants like heroin or stimulants like cocaine, mimic the structure of neurotransmitters, the most mind-bending chemicals nature has ever concocted. Neurotransmitters underlie every thought and emotion, memory and learning; they carry the signals between all the nerve cells, or neurons, in the brain. Among some 50 neurotransmitters discovered to date, a good half a dozen, including dopamine, are known to play a role in addiction.

The neurons that produce this molecular messenger are surprisingly rare. Clustered in loose knots buried deep in the brain, they number a few tens of thousands of nerve cells out of an estimated total of 100 billion. But through long, wire-like projections known as axons, these cells influence neurological activity in many regions, including the nucleus accumbens, the primitive structure that is one of the brain's key pleasure centers. At a purely chemical level, every experience humans find enjoyable—whether listening to music, embracing a lover or savoring chocolate—amounts to little more than an explosion of dopamine in the nucleus accumbens, as exhilarating and ephemeral as a firecracker.

Dopamine, like most biologically important molecules, must be kept within strict bounds. Too little dopamine in certain areas of the brain triggers the tremors and paralysis of Parkinson's disease. Too much causes the hallucinations and bizarre thoughts of schizophrenia. A breakthrough in addiction research came in 1975, when psychologists Roy Wise and Robert Yokel at Concordia University in Montreal reported on the remarkable behavior of some drug-addicted rats. One day the animals were placidly dispensing cocaine and amphetamines to themselves by pressing a lever attached to their cages. The next they were angrily banging at the lever like someone trying to summon a stalled elevator. The reason? The scientists had injected the rats with a drug that blocked the action of dopamine.

In the years since, evidence linking dopamine to drugs has mounted. Amphetamines stimulate dopamine-producing cells to pump out more of the chemical. Cocaine keeps dopamine levels high by inhibiting the activity of a transporter molecule that would ordinarily ferry dopamine back into the cells that produce it. Nicotine, heroin and alcohol trigger a complex chemical cascade that raises dopamine levels. And a still unknown chemical in cigarette smoke, a group led by Brookhaven chemist Joanna Fowler reported last year, may extend the activity of dopamine by blocking a mopping-up enzyme, called MAO B, that would otherwise destroy it.

The evidence that Volkow and her colleagues present in the current issue of *Nature* suggests that dopamine is directly responsible for the exhilarating rush that reinforces the desire to take drugs, at least in cocaine addicts. In all, 17 users participated in the study, says Volkow, and they experienced a high whose intensity was directly related to how extensively cocaine tied up available binding sites on the molecules that transport dopamine around the brain. To produce any high at all, she and her colleagues found, cocaine had to occupy at least 47% of these sites; the "best" results occurred when it took over 60% to 80% of the sites, effectively preventing the transporters from latching onto dopamine and spiriting it out of circulation.

SCIENTISTS BELIEVE THE DOPAMINE system arose very early in the course of animal evolution because it reinforces behaviors so essential to survival. "If it were not for the fact that sex is pleasurable," observes Charles Schuster of Wayne State University in Detroit, "we would not engage in it." Unfortunately, some of the activities humans are neurochemically tuned to find agreeable—eating foods rich in fat and sugar, for instance—have backfired in modern society. Just as a surfeit of food and a dearth of exercise have conspired to turn heart disease and diabetes into major health problems, so the easy availability of addictive chemicals has played a devious trick. Addicts do not crave heroin or cocaine or alcohol or nicotine per se but want the rush of dopamine that these drugs produce.

Dopamine, however, is more than just a feel-good molecule. It also exercises extraordinary power over learning and memory. Think of dopamine, suggests P. Read Montague of the Center for Theoretical Neuroscience at Houston's Baylor College of Medicine, as the proverbial carrot, a reward the brain doles out to networks of neurons for making survival-enhancing choices. And while the details of how this system works are not yet understood, Montague and his colleagues at the Salk Institute in San Diego, California, and M.I.T. have proposed a model that seems quite plausible. Each time the outcome of an action is better than expected, they predicted, dopamine-releasing neurons should increase the rate at which they fire. When an outcome is worse, they should

decrease it. And if the outcome is as expected, the firing rate need not change at all.

As a test of his model, Montague created a computer program that simulated the nectar-gathering activity of bees. Programmed with a dopamine-like reward system and set loose on a field of virtual "flowers," some of which were dependably sweet and some of which were either very sweet or not sweet at all, the virtual bees chose the reliably sweet flowers 85% of the time. In laboratory experiments real bees behave just like their virtual counterparts. What does this have to do with drug abuse? Possibly quite a lot, says Montague. The theory is that dopamine-enhancing chemicals fool the brain into thinking drugs are as beneficial as nectar to the bee, thus hijacking a natural reward system that dates back millions of years.

The degree to which learning and memory sustain the addictive process is only now being appreciated. Each time a neurotransmitter like dopamine floods a synapse, scientists believe, circuits that trigger thoughts and motivate actions are etched onto the brain. Indeed, the neurochemistry supporting addiction is so powerful that the people, objects and places associated with drug taking are also imprinted on the brain. Stimulated by food, sex or the smell of tobacco, former smokers can no more control the urge to light up than Pavlov's dogs could stop their urge to salivate. For months Rafael Rios lived in fear of catching a glimpse of bare arms—his own or someone else's. Whenever he did, he remembers, he would be seized by a nearly unbearable urge to find a drug-filled syringe.

Indeed, the brain has many devious tricks for ensuring that the irrational act of taking drugs, deemed "good" because it enhances dopamine, will be repeated. PET-scan images taken by Volkow and her colleagues reveal that the absorption of a cocaine-like chemical by neurons is profoundly reduced in cocaine addicts in contrast to normal subjects. One explanation: the addicts' neurons, assaulted by abnormally high levels of dopamine, have responded defensively and reduced the number of sites (or receptors) to which dopamine can bind. In the absence of drugs, these nerve cells probably experience a dopamine deficit, Volkow speculates, so while addicts begin by taking drugs to feel high, they end up taking them in order not to feel low.

PET-scan images of the brains of recovering cocaine addicts reveal other striking changes, including a dramatically impaired ability to process glucose, the primary energy source for working neurons. Moreover, this impairment—which persists for up to 100 days after withdrawal—is greatest in the

prefrontal cortex, a dopamine-rich area of the brain that controls impulsive and irrational behavior. Addicts, in fact, display many of the symptoms shown by patients who have suffered strokes or injuries to the prefrontal cortex. Damage to this region, University of Iowa neurologist Antonio Damasio and his colleagues have demonstrated, destroys the emotional compass that controls behaviors the patient knows are unacceptable.

Anyone who doubts that genes influence behavior should see the mice in Marc Caron's lab. These tireless rodents race around their cages for hours on end. They lose weight because they rarely stop to eat, and then they drop from exhaustion because they are unable to sleep. Why? The mice, says Caron, a biochemist at Duke University's Howard Hughes Medical Institute

CRACK

Prolonged cocaine use deadens nerve endings in the brain's pleasure-regulation system. A brain scan of a cocaine abuser shows a marked drop in the number of functioning dopamine receptors

laboratory, are high on dopamine. They lack the genetic mechanism that sponges up this powerful stuff and spirits it away. Result: there is so much dopamine banging around in the poor creatures' synapses that the mice, though drug-free, act as if they were strung out on cocaine.

For years scientists have suspected that genes play a critical role in determining who will become addicted to drugs and who will not. But not until now have they had molecular tools powerful enough to go after the prime suspects. Caron's mice are just the most recent example. By knocking out a single gene—the so-called dopamine-transporter gene—Caron and his colleagues may have created a strain of mice so sated with dopamine that they are oblivious to the allure of cocaine, and possibly alcohol and heroin as well. "What's exciting about our mice," says Caron, "is that they should allow us to test the hypothesis that all these drugs funnel through the dopamine system."

Several dopamine genes have already been tentatively, and controversially, linked to alcoholism and drug abuse. Inherited variations in these genes modify the efficiency

COKE'S HIGH IS DIRECTLY TIED TO DOPAMINE LEVELS

A.A.'S PATH TO RECOVERY STILL SEEMS THE BEST

with which nerve cells process dopamine, or so the speculation goes. Thus, some scientists conjecture, a dopamine-transporter gene that is superefficient, clearing dopamine from the synapses too rapidly, could predispose some people to a form of alcoholism characterized by violent and impulsive behavior. In essence, they would be mirror images of Caron's mice. Instead of being drenched in dopamine, their synapses would be dopamine-poor.

The dopamine genes known as D2 and D4 might also play a role in drug abuse, for similar reasons. Both these genes, it turns out, contain the blueprints for assembling what scientists call a receptor, a minuscule bump on the surface of cells to which biologically active molecules are attracted. And just as a finger lights up a room by merely flicking a switch, so dopamine triggers a sequence of chemical reactions each time it binds to one of its five known receptors. Genetic differences that reduce the sensitivity of these receptors or decrease their number could diminish the sensation of pleasure.

The problem is, studies that have purported to find a basis for addiction in variations of the D2 and D4 genes have not held up under scrutiny. Indeed, most scientists think addiction probably involves an intricate dance between environmental influences and multiple genes, some of which may influence dopamine activity only indirectly. This has not stopped some researchers from promoting the provocative theory that many people who become alcoholics and drug addicts suffer from an inherited condition dubbed the reward-deficiency syndrome. Low dopamine levels caused by a particular version of the D2 gene, they say, may link a breathtaking array of aberrant behaviors. Among them: severe alcoholism, pathological gambling, binge eating and attention-deficit hyperactivity disorder.

The more science unmasks the powerful biology that underlies addiction, the brighter the prospects for treatment become. For instance, the discovery by Fowler and her team that a chemical that inhibits the mopping-up enzyme MAO B may play a role in cigarette addiction has already opened new possibilities for therapy. A number of well-tolerated MAO B inhibitor drugs developed to treat Parkinson's disease could find a place in the antismoking arsenal. Equally promising, a Yale University team led by Eric Nestler and David Self has found that another type of compound—one that targets the dopamine receptor known as D1—seems to alleviate, at least in rats, the intense craving that accompanies withdrawal from cocaine. One day, suggests Self, a D1 skin patch might help cocaine abusers kick their habit, just as the nicotine patch attenuates the desire to smoke.

Like methadone, the compound that activates D1 appears to be what is known as a partial agonist. Because such medications stimulate some of the same brain pathways as drugs of abuse, they are often addictive in their own right, though less so. And while treating heroin addicts with methadone may seem like a cop-out to people who have never struggled with a drug habit, clinicians say they desperately need more such agents to tide addicts—particularly cocaine addicts—over the first few months of treatment, when the danger of relapse is highest.

REALISTICALLY, NO ONE BELIEVES better medications alone will solve the drug problem. In fact, one of the most hopeful messages coming out of current research is that the biochemical abnormalities associated with addiction can be reversed through learning. For that reason, all sorts of psychosocial interventions, ranging from psychotherapy to 12-step programs, can and do help. Cognitive therapy, which seeks to supply people with coping skills (exercising after work instead of going to a bar, for instance), appears to hold particular promise. After just 10 weeks of therapy, before-and-after PET scans suggest, some patients suffering from obsessive-compulsive disorder (which has some similarities with addiction) manage to resculpt not only their behavior but also activity patterns in their brain.

In late 20th century America, where drugs of abuse are being used on an unprecedented scale, the mounting evidence that treatment works could not be more welcome. Until now, policymakers have responded to the drug problem as though it were mostly a criminal matter. Only a third of the $15 billion the U.S. earmarks for the war on drugs goes to prevention and treatment. "In my view, we've got things upside down," says Dr. David Lewis, director of the Center for Alcohol and Addiction Studies at Brown University School of Medicine. "By relying so heavily on a criminalized approach, we've only added to the stigma of drug abuse and prevented high-quality medical care."

Ironically, the biggest barrier to making such care available is the perception that efforts to treat addiction are wasted. Yet treatment for drug abuse has a failure rate no different from that for other chronic diseases. Close to half of recovering addicts fail to maintain complete abstinence after a year—about the same proportion of patients with diabetes and hypertension who fail to comply with their diet, exercise and medication regimens. What doctors who treat drug abuse should strive for, says Alan Leshner, director of the National Institute on Drug Abuse, is not necessarily a cure but long-term care that controls the progress of the disease and alleviates its worst symptoms. "The occasional relapse is normal," he says, "and just an indication that more treatment is needed."

Rafael Rios has been luckier than many. He kicked his habit in one lengthy struggle that included four months of in-patient treatment at a residential facility and a year of daily outpatient sessions. During that time, Rios checked into 12-step meetings continually, sometimes attending three a day. As those who deal with alcoholics and drug addicts know, such exertions of will power and courage are more common than most people suspect. They are the best reason yet to start treating addiction as the medical and public health crisis it really is.

—With reporting by Alice Park/New York

The Fear of Heroin Is
Shooting Up

Kids on dope are still rare, but parents are right to be scared

JOHN LELAND

JANE HOWLAND LIKES TO TRY AN EXPERIMENT when she talks to kids about drugs. Howland is a middle-school guidance counselor in Greenwich Conn., one of the wealthiest suburbs in America. The kids are maybe 10 or 11. "I ask them who knows what it means to be a high-risk-taker," she says. Every hand goes up. Then she asks those who consider themselves high-risk-takers to go to one part of the room, low- and middle-riskers to another. Invariably, every boy goes to the high-risk group. "They push each other out of the way to get there first. It's cool." These are just preteens; to them risk means shoplifting, vandalism, marijuana, maybe inhalants. But many of her fifth graders are in the thrall of Kurt Cobain; they think he was "really cool," she says. Howland worries that, by the eighth and ninth grades, the biggest risk-takers might want to follow Cobain's path into heroin.

After a decade in low relief, heroin is now scaring the heck out of people like Howland, in cities and suburbs nationwide. "The bad news," says Gen. Barry McCaffrey, the new drug czar, "is heroin is back." Schools that used to discuss heroin in the late high-school years now teach it in the eighth grade. The Partnership for a Drug-Free America, best known for its "This is your brain on drugs" campaign of the '80s, now worries that heroin will be *the* drug of the '90s. (James E. Burke, chairman of the partnership, sits on the board of The Washington Post Company, NEWSWEEK'S corporate parent.) Earlier this summer the organization rolled out the most expensive publicity campaign ever to target heroin. Spurred by images of junkie celebs, and anecdotes about middle-class heroin use, the press has touted a new epidemic since 1989. Now, says Yale medical historian David Musto, "this is the nearest we've come."

How near are we? The answers are not so clear. There are an estimated 500,000 to 750,000 heroin addicts in this country, a figure that has held steady for decades. But for the past five years, heroin use has been on the rise. Since heroin is illegal, no one knows just how many people use it. But by rough government estimates, U.S. heroin consumption has doubled since the mid-'80s, to about 10 to 15 metric tons per year. Last year 2.3 percent of *eighth graders* said they had tried heroin, nearly double the rate of 1991. (Note: eighth graders always show higher rates than high-schoolers, because heroin users tend to drop out of school.) "Obviously this is not a runaway epidemic among teens," says Lloyd Johnston of the University of Michigan, who monitors adolescent drug use. "But it should give rise to some caution."

Most heroin users today are still old-timers, battered by decades of addiction, arrest and rehab. As crack use has stabilized, many crack smokers have also turned to heroin to ease their cocaine jitters. Dealers, increasingly, are "double breasting," or selling both—bringing crack's widespread availability to heroin. But in many cities, a new class of user is emerging. Drug ethnographers Ansley Hamid and Ric Curtis of John Jay College of Criminal Justice note that as residents of black and Latino communities turned away from heroin in the early '90s, white people started to show up, "infatuated with it," says Curtis. The numbers of new, more affluent users are especially elusive. Because they have resources, they tend not to show up in jail or public treatment centers. "Heroin may be flying *above* the radar," says Mark A. R. Kleiman, a drug-policy analyst at UCLA.

WHY HEROIN AND WHY NOW? If the U.S. auto industry cut the price of its sedans by half and redesigned them to go to 180 mph, no one would wonder why sales hit the roof. In the past five years the heroin industry—a $7 billion-plus retail market in the United States—has wrought a similar revolution, offering a more powerful, cheaper and safer product. In the '80s average $10 bags ran about 2 to 8 percent pure; by 1994 average purity in New York hit 63 percent—pure enough to snort or smoke, without the risk of getting AIDS from dirty needles. This made the drug seem less deadly, more approachable. At the same time, the price has fallen to a historic low. The street price of a milligram in New York fell from $1.81 in 1988 to just 37 cents in 1994. Globally, heroin production has doubled in the past decade, flooding the United States from Burma, Afghanistan, Laos, Pakistan, Colombia and Mexico—and ensuring a competitive market with low prices and

From *Newsweek*, August 26, 1996, pp. 55-56. © 1996 by Newsweek, Inc. All rights reserved. Reprinted by permission.

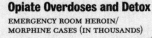

▲SUPPLY IN DEMAND: U.S. heroin consumption has probably doubled since the mid-'80s, and the product sold now (from poppy fields like this one in Pakistan) is much purer

Drug Usage
EIGHTH GRADERS WHO HAVE USED
DRUGS IN THEIR LIFETIME (IN PERCENT)

	1991	1995	PERCENT CHANGE
Crack	1.3	2.7	+108
Heroin	1.2	2.3	+92
Marijuana	10.2	19.9	+95
Cocaine	2.3	4.2	+83
Hallucinogens	3.2	5.2	+63
Stimulants	10.5	13.1	+25
Tranquilizers	3.8	4.5	+18
Cigarettes	44.0	46.4	+5
Been drunk	26.7	25.3	−5

Opiate Overdoses and Detox
EMERGENCY ROOM HEROIN/
MORPHINE CASES (IN THOUSANDS)

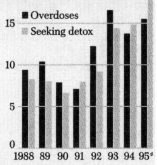

■ Overdoses
▨ Seeking detox

1988 89 90 91 92 93 94 95*

*ESTIMATE BASED ON JAN.–JUNE FIGURES. SOURCES: UNIVERSITY OF MICHIGAN, MONITORING THE FUTURE STUDY; SAMHSA, DRUG ABUSE WARNING NETWORK

high purity. As a recent White House report conceded, "We have yet to substantially influence either the availability or the purity of cocaine and heroin within the United States."

Heroin's rise is also historically predictable. Since 1885 cocaine and opiate waves have succeeded one another, each relieving the chronic maladies of the last. Cocaine epidemics tend to be fast and short, accelerated by binge use. "You can't take cocaine for long periods of time," says Herbert Kleber of the Center on Addiction and Substance Abuse at Columbia University. "It burns you out. People need a sedative to mellow out: sometimes alcohol, sometimes heroin." Heroin booms, by contrast, move slowly. Users take an average of three to 10 years to progress from regular use to treatment or arrest. The heroin-horror stories circulating now suggest a rise in use four or five years ago, and may signal the start of a decline. As Kleber notes, "All drug cycles carry the seed of their own destruction."

New users typically begin by snorting. But many progress to the more efficient method of injecting. According to General McCaffrey, about 50 percent of users seeking treatment last year used needles; this year, the figure has grown to 75 percent. This is doubly dangerous. Injection-drug users now have the highest rates of new HIV infection, nearly twice that of gay men. And wild fluctuations in street purity raise the risk of overdose. Between 3,000 and 4,000 users die of heroin overdoses annually—many using the heroin in lethal combination with alcohol or other drugs. The expanding drug market and the criminal-justice system unwittingly conspire to push this figure higher. As police arrest drug consumers by the thousands, as part of the war on drugs, users are likely to come out of jail with reduced tolerance—and a lower threshold for overdose. Also, says John Jay College's Curtis, some new dealers don't have experience with the substance. He mentions one experienced Brooklyn dealer known as Half, for the way he cuts the dope. "The new guys turn to him to show them how its done." Others, though, "use too much adulterant, or too little," giving people unpredictably strong doses. "I attribute deaths to that instability."

It is too soon to say how high the current heroin wave will rise, or how long it will last. Musto of Yale contends that it "won't be as alarming as the last [in the '70s], because we're much better informed about drugs now. The number of people the 'chic' aspect applies to is very small." But many professionals believe we can't wait around to find out. Already there are too few treatment slots for the addicts on the streets, a woeful shortage of treatment beds in prisons—and no money for more. Wayne Wiebel, an epidemiologist at the University of Illinois at Chicago, offers a chilling scenario. We are unprepared, he says, especially to help the young users just getting hooked. "There are only two pots of money," says Wiebel. "One is for prevention, mostly through schools; and the other is treatment for casualties that have already been fully impacted by the problem. There's virtually nothing in the middle for early intervention." Wiebel has been studying drug trends for more than 15 years. From where he stands, the new wave of heroin use, and our reaction to it, looks horrifyingly familiar. It's going to "unfold like the crack epidemic," he says, "and we're not going to do a hell of a lot about it."

With PETER KATEL *in Miami and* MARY HAGER *in Washington*

Predators: The Disturbing World of the Psychopaths Among Us

Jeffrey Dahmer. Ted Bundy. Hannibal Lechter. These are the psychopaths whose stunning lack of conscience we see in the movies and in tabloids. Yet, as this report makes abundantly clear, these predators, both male *and* female, haunt our everyday lives at work, at home, and in relationships. How to find them before they find you.

Robert Hare, Ph.D.

Robert Hare, Ph.D., a forensic psychologist and psychophysiologist at the University of British Columbia, conducted hundreds of interviews for his book on psychopaths.

She met him in a laundromat in London. He was open and friendly and they hit it off right away. From the start she thought he was hilarious. Of course, she'd been lonely. The weather was grim and sleety and she didn't know a soul east of the Atlantic.

"Ah, traveler's loneliness," Dan crooned sympathetically over dinner. "It's the worst."

After dessert he was embarrassed to discover he'd come without his wallet. She was more than happy to pay for dinner. At the pub, over drinks, he told her he was a translator for the United Nations. He was, for now, between assignments.

They saw each other four times that week, five the week after. It wasn't long before he had all but moved in with Elsa. It was against her nature, but she was having the time of her life.

Still, there were details, unexplained, undiscussed, that she shoved out of her mind. He never invited her to his home; she never met his friends. One night he brought over a carton filled with tape recorders—plastic-wrapped straight from the factory, unopened; a few days later they were gone. Once she came home to find three televisions stacked in the corner. "Storing them for a friend," was all he told her. When she pressed for more he merely shrugged.

Once he stayed away for three days and was lying asleep on the bed when she came in midmorning. "Where have you been?" she cried. "I've been so worried. Where were you?"

He looked sour as he woke up. "Don't ever ask me that," he snapped. "I won't have it."

"What—?"

"Where I go, what I do, who I do it with—it doesn't concern you, Elsa. Don't ask."

He was like a different person. But then he seemed to pull himself together, shook the sleep off, and reach out to her. "I know it hurts you," he said in his old gentle way, "but think of jealousy as a flu, and wait to get over it. And you will, baby, you will." Like a mother cat licking her kitten, he groomed her back into trusting him.

One night she asked him lightly if he felt like stepping out to the corner and bringing her an ice cream. He didn't reply, and when she glanced up she found him glaring at her furiously. "Always got everything you wanted, didn't you?" he asked in a strange, snide way. "Any little thing little Elsa wanted, somebody always jumped up and ran out and bought it for her, didn't they?"

"Are you kidding? I'm not like that. What are you talking about?"

He got up from the chair and walked out. She never saw him again.

There is a class of individuals who have been around forever and who are found in every race, culture, society, and walk of life. Everybody has met these people, been deceived and manipulated by them, and forced to live with or repair the damage they have wrought. These often charming—but always deadly—individuals have a clinical name: *psychopaths.* Their hallmark is a stunning lack of conscience; their game is self-gratification at the other person's expense. Many spend time in prison, but many do not. All take far more than they give.

The most obvious expressions of psychopathy—but not the only ones—involve the flagrant violation of society's rules. Not surprisingly, many psychopaths are criminals, but many others manage to remain out of prison, using their charm and chameleonlike coloration to cut a wide swathe through society and leaving a wake of ruined lives behind them.

A major part of my own quarter-century search for answers to this enigma has been a concerted effort to develop an accurate means of detecting the psychopaths among us. Measurement and categorization are of course fundamental to any scientific endeavor, but the implications of being able to identify psychopaths are as much practical as academic. To put it simply, if we can't spot them we are doomed to be their victims, both as individuals and as a society.

My role in the search for psychopaths began in the 1960s at the psychology department of the University of British Columbia. There, my growing interest in

From *Psychology Today*, January/February 1994, pp. 54-56, 58, 60-63. Excerpted from *Without Conscience: The Disturbing World of the Psychopaths among Us* by Robert Hare. © 1993 by Robert Hare. Reprinted by permission of Pocket Books, a division of Simon & Schuster.

psychopathy merged with my experience working with psychopaths in prison to form what was my life work.

I assembled a team of clinicians who would identify psychopaths in the prison population by means of long, detailed interviews and close study of file information. From this eventually developed a highly reliable diagnostic tool that any clinician or researcher could use and that yielded a richly detailed profile of the personality disorder called psychopathy. We named this instrument the *Psychopathy Checklist* (Multi-Health Systems; 1991). The checklist is now used worldwide and provides clinicians and researchers with a way of distinguishing with reasonable certainty true psychopaths from those who merely break the rules.

What follows is a general summary of the key traits and behaviors of a psychopath. *Do not use these symptoms to diagnose yourself or others.* A diagnosis requires explicit training and access to the formal scoring manual. If you suspect that someone you know conforms to the profile described here, and if it is important for you to have an expert opinion, you should obtain the services of a qualified (registered) forensic psychologist or psychiatrist.

Also, be aware that people who are *not* psychopaths may have *some* of the symptoms described here. Many people are impulsive, or glib, or cold and unfeeling, but this does not mean that they are psychopaths. Psychopathy is a *syndrome*—a cluster of related symptoms.

Key Symptoms of Psychopathy
Emotional/Interpersonal:
—Glib and superficial
—Egocentric and grandiose
—Lack of remorse or guilt
—Lack of empathy
—Deceitful and manipulative
—Shallow emotions
Social Deviance:
—Impulsive
—Poor behavior controls
—Need for excitement
—Lack of responsibility
—Early behavior problems
—Adult antisocial behavior

GLIB AND SUPERFICIAL
Psychopaths are often voluble and verbally facile. They can be amusing and entertaining conversationalists, ready with a clever comeback, and are able to tell unlikely but convincing stories that cast themselves in a good light. They can be very effective in presenting themselves well and are often very likable and charming.

One of my raters described an interview she did with a prisoner: "I sat down and took out my clipboard," she said, "and the first thing this guy told me was what beautiful eyes I had. He managed to work quite a few compliments on my appearance into the interview, so by the time I wrapped things up, I was feeling unusually . . . well, pretty. I'm a wary person especially on the job, and can usually spot a phony. When I got back outside, I couldn't believe I'd fallen for a line like that."

EGOCENTRIC AND GRANDIOSE
Psychopaths have a narcissistic and grossly inflated view of their own self-worth and importance, a truly astounding egocentricity and sense of entitlement, and see themselves as the center of the universe, justified in living according to their own rules. "It's not that I don't follow the law," said one subject. "I follow my own laws. I never violate my own rules." She then proceeded to describe these rules in terms of "looking out for number one."

Psychopaths often claim to have specific goals but show little appreciation regarding the qualifications required—they have no idea of how to achieve them and little or no chance of attaining these goals, given their track record and lack of sustained interest in formal education. The psychopathic inmate might outline vague plans to become a lawyer for the poor or a property tycoon. One inmate, not particularly literate, managed to copyright the title of a book he was planning to write about himself, already counting the fortune his best-selling book would bring.

LACK OF REMORSE OR GUILT
Psychopaths show a stunning lack of concern for the effects their actions have on others, no matter how devastating these might be. They may appear completely forthright about the matter, calmly stating that they have no sense of guilt, are not sorry for the ensuing pain, and that there is no reason now to be concerned.

When asked if he had any regrets about stabbing a robbery victim who subsequently spent time in the hospital as a result of his wounds, one of our subjects replied, "Get real! He spends a few months in the hospital and I rot here. If I wanted to kill him I would have slit his throat. That's the kind of guy I am; I gave him a break."

Their lack of remorse or guilt is associated with a remarkable ability to rationalize their behavior, to shrug off personal responsibility for actions that cause family, friends, and others to reel with shock and disappointment. They usually have handy excuses for their behavior, and in some cases deny that it happened at all.

LACK OF EMPATHY
Many of the characteristics displayed by psychopaths are closely associated with a profound lack of empathy and inability to construct a mental and emotional "facsimile" of another person. They seem completely unable to "get into the skin" of others, except in a purely intellectual sense.

They are completely indifferent to the rights and suffering of family and strangers alike. If they do maintain ties, it is only because they see family members as possessions. One of our subjects allowed her boyfriend to sexually molest her five-year-old daughter because "he wore me out. I wasn't ready for more sex that night." The woman found it hard to understand why the authorities took her child into care.

DECEITFUL AND MANIPULATIVE
With their powers of imagination in gear and beamed on themselves, psychopaths appear amazingly unfazed by the possibility—or even by the certainty—of being found out. When caught in a lie or challenged with the truth, they seldom appear perplexed or embarrassed—they simply change their stories or attempt to rework the facts so they appear to be consistent with the lie. The result is a series of contradictory statements and a thoroughly confused listener.

And psychopaths seem proud of their ability to lie. When asked if she lied easily, one woman laughed and replied, "I'm the best. I think it's because I sometimes admit to something bad about myself. They think, well, if she's admitting to that she must be telling the truth about the rest."

SHALLOW EMOTIONS
Psychopaths seem to suffer a kind of emotional poverty that limits the range and depth of their feelings. At times they appear to be cold and unemotional while nevertheless being prone to dramatic, shallow, and short-lived displays of feeling. Careful observers are left with the impression they are play-acting and little is going on below the surface.

A psychopath in our research said that he didn't really understand what others meant by fear. "When I rob a bank," he said, "I notice that the teller shakes. One barfed all over the money. She must have been pretty messed up inside, but I don't know why. If someone pointed a gun at me I guess I'd be afraid, but I wouldn't throw up." When asked if he ever felt his heart pound or his stomach churn, he replied, "Of course! I'm not a robot. I really get pumped up when I have sex or when I get into a fight."

IMPULSIVE

Psychopaths are unlikely to spend much time weighing the pros and cons of a course of action or considering the possible consequences. "I did it because I felt like it," is a common response. These impulsive acts often result from an aim that plays a central role in most of the psychopath's behavior: to achieve immediate satisfaction, pleasure, or relief.

So family members, relatives, employers, and coworkers typically find themselves standing around asking themselves what happened—jobs are quit, relationships broken off, plans changed, houses ransacked, people hurt, often for what appears as little more than a whim. As the husband of a psychopath I studied put it: "She got up and left the table, and that was the last I saw of her for two months."

POOR BEHAVIOR CONTROLS

Besides being impulsive, psychopaths are highly reactive to perceived insults or slights. Most of us have powerful inhibitory controls over our behavior; even if we would like to respond aggressively we are usually able to "keep the lid on." In psychopaths, these inhibitory controls are weak, and the slightest provocation is sufficient to overcome them.

As a result, psychopaths are short-tempered or hotheaded and tend to respond to frustration, failure, discipline, and criticism with sudden violence, threats or verbal abuse. But their outbursts, extreme as they may be, are often short-lived, and they quickly act as if nothing out of the ordinary has happened.

For example, an inmate in line for dinner was accidentally bumped by another inmate, whom he proceeded to beat senseless. The attacker then stepped back into line as if nothing had happened. Despite the fact that he faced solitary confinement as punishment for the infraction, his only comment when asked to explain himself was, "I was pissed off. He stepped into my space. I did what I had to do."

Although psychopaths have a "hair trigger," their aggressive displays are "cold"; they lack the intense arousal experienced when other individuals lose their temper.

A Survival Guide

Although no one is completely immune to the devious machinations of the psychopath, there are some things you can do to reduce your vulnerability.

• *Know what you are dealing with.* This sounds easy but in fact can be very difficult. All the reading in the world cannot immunize you from the devastating effects of psychopaths. Everyone, including the experts, can be taken in, conned, and left bewildered by them. A good psychopath can play a concerto on *anyone's* heart strings.

• *Try not to be influenced by "props."* It is not easy to get beyond the winning smile, the captivating body language, the fast talk of the typical psychopath, all of which blind us to his or her real intentions. Many people find it difficult to deal with the intense, "predatory stare" of the psychopath. The fixated stare is more a prelude to self-gratification and the exercise of power rather than simple interest or empathic caring.

• *Don't wear blinders.* Enter new relationships with your eyes wide open. Like the rest of us, most psychopathic con-artists and "love-thieves" initially hide their dark side by putting their "best foot forward." Cracks may soon begin to appear in the mask they wear, but once trapped in their web, it will be difficult to escape financially and emotionally unscathed.

• *Keep your guard up in high-risk situations.* Some situations are tailor-made for psychopaths: singles bars, ship cruises, foreign airports, etc. In each case, the potential victim is lonely, looking for a good time, excitement, or companionship, and there will usually be someone willing to oblige, for a hidden price.

• *Know yourself.* Psychopaths are skilled at detecting and ruthlessly exploiting your weak spots. Your best defense is to understand what these spots are, and to be extremely wary of anyone who zeroes in on them.

Unfortunately, even the most careful precautions are no guarantee that you will be safe from a determined psychopath. In such cases, all you can do is try to exert some sort of damage control. This is not easy but some suggestions may be of help:

• *Obtain professional advice.* Make sure the clinician you consult is familiar with the literature on psychopathy and has had experience in dealing with psychopaths.

• *Don't blame yourself.* Whatever the reasons for being involved with a psychopath, it is important that you not accept blame for his or her attitudes and behavior. Psychopaths play by the same rules—their rules—with everyone.

• *Be aware of who the victim is.* Psychopaths often give the impression that it is *they* who are suffering and that the victims are to blame for their misery. Don't waste your sympathy on them.

• *Recognize that you are not alone.* Most psychopaths have lots of victims. It is certain that a psychopath who is causing you grief is also causing grief to others.

• *Be careful about power struggles.* Keep in mind that psychopaths have a strong need for psychological and physical control over others. This doesn't mean that you shouldn't stand up for your rights, but it will probably be difficult to do so without risking serious emotional or physical trauma.

• *Set firm ground rules.* Although power struggles with a psychopath are risky, you may be able to set up some clear rules—both for yourself and for the psychopath—to make your life easier and begin the difficult transition from victim to a person looking out for yourself.

• *Don't expect dramatic changes.* To a large extent, the personality of psychopaths is "carved in stone." There is little likelihood that anything you do will produce fundamental, sustained changes in how they see themselves or others.

• *Cut your losses.* Most victims of psychopaths end up feeling confused and hopeless, and convinced that they are largely to blame for the problem. The more you give in the more you will be taken advantage of by the psychopath's insatiable appetite for power and control.

• *Use support groups.* By the time your suspicions have led you to seek a diagnosis, you already know that you're in for a very long and bumpy ride. Make sure you have all the emotional support you can muster.

A NEED FOR EXCITEMENT

Psychopaths have an ongoing and excessive need for excitement—they long to live in the fast lane or "on the edge," where the action is. In many cases the action involves the breaking of rules.

Many psychopaths describe "doing crime" for excitement or thrills. When asked if she ever did dangerous things just for fun, one of our female psychopaths replied, "Yeah, lots of things. But what I find most exciting is walking though airports with drugs. Christ! What a high!"

The flip side of this yen for excitement is an inability to tolerate routine or monotony. Psychopaths are easily bored and are not likely to engage in activities that are dull, repetitive, or require intense concentration over long periods.

LACK OF RESPONSIBILITY

Obligations and commitments mean nothing to psychopaths. Their good intentions—"I'll never cheat on you again"—are promises written on the wind.

Horrendous credit histories, for example, reveal the lightly taken debt, the loan shrugged off, the empty pledge to contribute to a child's support. Their performance on the job is erratic, with frequent absences, misuse of company resources, violations of company policy, and general untrustworthiness. They do not honor formal or implied commitments to people, organizations, or principles.

Psychopaths are not deterred by the possibility that their actions mean hardship or risk for others. A 25-year-old inmate in our studies has received more than 20 convictions for dangerous driving, driving while impaired, leaving the scene of an accident, driving without a license, and criminal negligence causing death. When asked if he would continue to drive after his release from prison, he replied, "Why not? Sure, I drive fast, but I'm good at it. It takes two to have an accident."

EARLY BEHAVIOR PROBLEMS

Most psychopaths begin to exhibit serious behavioral problems at an early age. These might include persistent lying, cheating, theft, arson, truancy, substance abuse, vandalism, and/or precocious sexuality. Because many children exhibit some of these behaviors at one time or another—especially children raised in violent neighborhoods or in disrupted or abusive families—it is important to emphasize that the psychopath's history of such behaviors is more extensive and serious than most, even when compared with that of siblings and friends raised in similar settings.

One subject, serving time for fraud, told us that as a child he would put a noose around the neck of a cat, tie the other end of the string to the top of a pole, and bat the cat around the pole with a tennis racket. Although not all adult psychopaths exhibited this degree of cruelty when in their youth, virtually all routinely got themselves into a wide range of difficulties.

ADULT ANTISOCIAL BEHAVIOR

Psychopaths see the rules and expectations of society as inconvenient and unreasonable impediments. to their own behavioral expression. They make their own rules, both as children and as adults.

Many of the antisocial acts of psychopaths lead to criminal charges and convictions. Even within the criminal population, psychopaths stand out, largely because the antisocial and illegal activities of psychopaths are *more varied and frequent* than are those of other criminals. Psychopaths tend to have no particular affinity, or "specialty," for one particular type of crime but tend to try everything.

But not all psychopaths end up in jail. Many of the things they do escape detection or prosecution, or are on "the shady side of the law." For them, antisocial behavior may consist of phony stock promotions, questionable business practices, spouse or child abuse, and so forth. Many others do things that, though not necessarily illegal, are nevertheless unethical, immoral, or harmful to others: philandering or cheating on a spouse to name a few.

ORIGINS

Thinking about psychopathy leads us very quickly to a single fundamental question: Why are some people like this?

Unfortunately, the forces that produce a psychopath are still obscure, an admission those looking for clear answers will find unsatisfying. Nevertheless, there are several rudimentary theories about the cause of psychopathy worth considering. At one end of the spectrum are theories that view psychopathy as largely the product of genetic or biological factors (nature), whereas theories at the other end posit that psychopathy results entirely from a faulty early social environment (nurture).

The position that I favor is that psychopathy emerges from a complex—and poorly understood—interplay between biological factors and social forces. It is based on evidence that genetic factors contribute to the biological bases of brain function and to basic personality structure, which in turn influence the way an individual responds to, and interacts with, life experiences and the social environment. In effect, the core elements needed for the development of psychopathy—including a profound inability to experience empathy and the complete range of emotions, including fear—are in part provided by nature and possibly by some unknown biological influences on the developing fetus and neonate. As a result, the capacity for developing internal controls and conscience and for making emotional "connections" with others is greatly reduced.

CAN ANYTHING BE DONE?

In their desperate search for solutions people trapped in a destructive and seemingly hopeless relationship with a psychopath frequently are told: Quit indulging him and send him for therapy. A basic assumption of psychotherapy is that the patient needs and wants help for distressing or painful psychological and emotional problems. Successful therapy also requires that the patient actively participate, along with the therapist, in the search for relief of his or her symptoms. In short, the patient must recognize there is a problem and must want to do something about it.

But here is the crux: Psychopaths don't feel they have psychological or emotional problems, and they see no reason to change their behavior to conform with societal standards they do not agree with.

Thus, in spite of more than a century of clinical study and decades of research, the mystery of the psychopathy still remains. Recent developments have provided us with new insights into the nature of this disturbing disorder, and its borders are becoming more defined. But compared with other major clinical disorders, little research has been devoted to psychopathy, even though it is responsible for more social distress and disruption than all other psychiatric disorders combined.

So, rather than trying to pick up the pieces after the damage has been done, it would make far greater sense to increase our efforts to understand this perplexing disorder and to search for effective early interventions. The alternatives are to continue devoting massive resources to the prosecution, incarceration, and supervision of psychopaths after they have committed offenses against society, and to continue to ignore the welfare and plight of their victims. We have to learn how to socialize them, not resocialize them. And this will require serious efforts at research and early intervention. It is imperative that we continue the search for clues.

Dissociative Disorders and Memory

Who are you? What do you do for a living? What are your most pleasant memories? What are your most unpleasant memories? Answers to questions such as these reveal the importance of memory as a connection of our present to our past. Memory is also a crucial component of the self. This process is central to a number of mental disorders as well as the focus of a major controversy involving mental health professionals and the legal system. The significance of this controversy is evident in the fact that the American Psychological Association and the British Psychological Association have asked groups of experts to study the issue and write policy statements. The key question concerns the validity of reports about recently recovered memories of sexual abuse that occurred many years in the past, usually during childhood.

No one doubts that childhood sexual abuse exists, although its actual incidence is difficult to determine. Decades ago, Sigmund Freud thought that sexual abuse might be the cause of the symptoms he observed in many of his patients. However, he eventually decided that the sexual activity reported by his patients had not actually occurred; he believed that they were reporting their fantasies. In an example of history repeating itself, similar issues concerning memories of childhood sexual abuse are being raised today.

The typical situation that leads to recovered memories occurs when an individual seeks therapy for any of a number of problems. Many therapists, encouraged by books and the media, believe that childhood sexual abuse is associated with a range of problems. In an attempt to reach what they believe is the root cause of these problems, some therapists encourage their clients to retrieve long-buried memories of childhood sexual abuse by parents, teachers, baby-sitters, neighbors, and friends. During the first session, some therapists have asked about the existence of sexual abuse, and they have even insisted that the abuse occurred, despite the client's denials. They argue that the inability to retrieve the memory is due to the powerful effects of repression.

An alternative explanation is that the therapists may actually encourage repressed sexual abuse reports. Some therapeutic methods such as hypnosis are known to be capable of inducing false memories. This issue has become so controversial that an organization called the False Memory Syndrome Foundation is tracking examples of false reports of abuse. In one case of a recovered memory not associated with therapy, a California man was found guilty of murdering his daughter's friend. The conviction was based on his daughter's recovered memory about 20 years after the murder. (The conviction has been reversed by a higher court.) Many individuals who have recovered memories of abuse are encouraged to stop all contact with family members, and some have sued for damages. A number of states have extended the statute of limitations to enable individuals who retrieve memories of sexual abuse to sue alleged perpetrators many years after the alleged abuse took place.

This controversy pits the experiences of therapists against the results reported by laboratory researchers. In the first unit article, Elizabeth Loftus has offered strong evidence that imagination and suggestion may play key roles in false memories. The debate is also evident in the articles by David Holmes and Mardi Horowitz. From a therapeutic standpoint, there are many examples that support the possibility of repressing memories. Forgetting anxiety-arousing events is a rather common experience. Laboratory researchers, however, report that there is no convincing evidence for repressed memories. Clinicians wonder if research on college students is relevant to the real-life traumas that their clients bring to therapy. Researchers counter that it is necessary to study this phenomenon under careful and controlled conditions in order

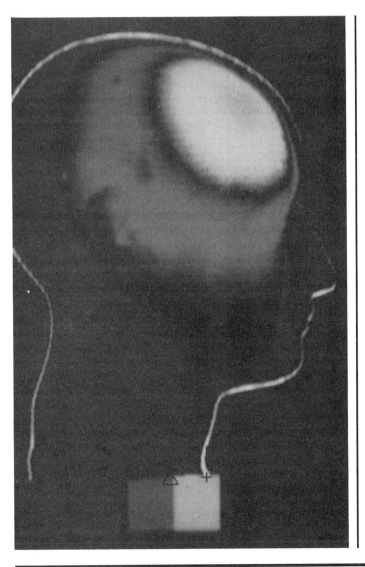

to understand it. Some experts are concerned that this debate will make society so skeptical of reports of sexual abuse that genuine cases will not be believed.

Over the last few decades, the reported incidence of multiple personality has increased substantially from a handful to thousands of cases. Sexual trauma early in life is the most frequently cited cause of this disorder. Thus, it too is a matter of controversy, as researchers search to explain its increased incidence. Is multiple personality disorder caused by severe childhood trauma? Are some therapists subtly suggesting the existence of alternative personalities to their clients?

At the most basic level, the brain is involved in what we process, record, and eventually recall. This point is most evident in situations in which changes in the brain have dramatic effects on memory, as in Alzheimer's disease. The death of brain cells in this disease leads to a number of symptoms; the most fundamental signs of the disease involve memory and language.

Looking Ahead: Challenge Questions

Discuss whether or not we can differentiate true memories from memories of events that never happened.

How might therapists encourage clients to recall past events that may not have occurred? What safeguards could be put in place to reduce the chances that this would happen?

How should jurors view sexual abuse evidence that is based on recovered memories?

What is the connection between the symptoms of post-traumatic stress disorder and those found in cases related to recovered memories of sexual abuse?

What does the recent increase in diagnoses of multiple personality tell us about various influences on diagnostic processes and procedures?

Creating False Memories

Researchers are showing how suggestion and imagination can create "memories" of events that did not actually occur

by Elizabeth F. Loftus

In 1986 Nadean Cool, a nurse's aide in Wisconsin, sought therapy from a psychiatrist to help her cope with her reaction to a traumatic event experienced by her daughter. During therapy, the psychiatrist used hypnosis and other suggestive techniques to dig out buried memories of abuse that Cool herself had allegedly experienced. In the process, Cool became convinced that she had repressed memories of having been in a satanic cult, of eating babies, of being raped, of having sex with animals and of being forced to watch the murder of her eight-year-old friend. She came to believe that she had more than 120 personalities—children, adults, angels and even a duck—all because, Cool was told, she had experienced severe childhood sexual and physical abuse. The psychiatrist also performed exorcisms on her, one of which lasted for five hours and included the sprinkling of holy water and screams for Satan to leave Cool's body.

When Cool finally realized that false memories had been planted, she sued the psychiatrist for malpractice. In March 1997, after five weeks of trial, her case was settled out of court for $2.4 million.

Nadean Cool is not the only patient to develop false memories as a result of questionable therapy. In Missouri in 1992 a church counselor helped Beth Rutherford to remember during therapy that her father, a clergyman, had regularly raped her between the ages of seven and 14 and that her mother sometimes helped him by holding her down. Under her therapist's guidance, Rutherford developed memories of her father twice impregnating her and forcing her to abort the fetus herself with a coat hanger. The father had to resign from his post as a clergyman when the allegations were made public. Later medical examination of the daughter revealed, however, that she was still a virgin at 22 and had never been pregnant. The daughter sued the therapist and received a $1-million settlement in 1996.

About a year earlier two juries returned verdicts against a Minnesota psychiatrist accused of planting false memories by former patients Vynnette Hamanne and Elizabeth Carlson, who under hypnosis and sodium amytal, and after being fed misinformation about the workings of memory, had come to remember horrific abuse by family members. The juries awarded Hammane $2.67 million and Carlson $2.5 million for their ordeals.

In all four cases, the women developed memories about childhood abuse in therapy and then later denied their authenticity. How can we determine if memories of childhood abuse are true or false? Without corroboration, it is very difficult to differentiate between false memories and true ones. Also, in these cases, some memories were contrary to physical evidence, such as explicit and detailed recollections of rape and abortion when medical examination confirmed virginity. How is it possible for people to acquire elaborate and confident false memories? A growing number of investigations demonstrate that under the right circumstances false memories can be instilled rather easily in some people.

My own research into memory distortion goes back to the early 1970s, when I began studies of the "misinformation effect." These studies show that when people who witness an event are later exposed to new and misleading information about it, their recollections often become distorted. In one example, participants viewed a simulated automobile accident at an intersection with a stop sign. After the viewing, half the participants received a suggestion that the traffic sign was a yield sign. When asked later what traffic sign they remembered seeing at the intersection, those who had been given the suggestion tended to claim that they had seen a yield sign. Those who had not received the phony information were much more accurate in their recollection of the traffic sign.

My students and I have now conducted more than 200 experiments involving over 20,000 individuals that document how exposure to misinformation induces memory distortion. In these studies, people "recalled" a conspicuous barn in a bucolic scene that contained no buildings at all, broken glass and tape recorders that were not in the scenes they viewed, a white instead of a blue vehicle in a crime scene, and Minnie Mouse when they actually saw Mickey Mouse. Taken together, these studies show that misinformation can change an individual's recollection in predictable and sometimes very powerful ways.

Misinformation has the potential for invading our memories when we talk to other people, when we are suggestively interrogated or when we read or view media coverage about some event that we may have experienced ourselves. After more than two decades of exploring the power of misinformation, research-

 Reprinted with permission from *Scientific American*, September 1997, pp. 70-75. © 1997 by Scientific American, Inc. All rights reserved.

ers have learned a great deal about the conditions that make people susceptible to memory modification. Memories are more easily modified, for instance, when the passage of time allows the original memory to fade.

False Childhood Memories

It is one thing to change a detail or two in an otherwise intact memory but quite another to plant a false memory of an event that never happened. To study false memory, my students and I first had to find a way to plant a pseudomemory that would not cause our subjects undue emotional stress, either in the process of creating the false memory or when we revealed that they had been intentionally deceived. Yet we wanted to try to plant a memory that would be at least mildly traumatic, had the experience actually happened.

My research associate, Jacqueline E. Pickrell, and I settled on trying to plant a specific memory of being lost in a shopping mall or large department store at about the age of five. Here's how we did it. We asked our subjects, 24 individuals ranging in age from 18 to 53, to try to remember childhood events that had been recounted to us by a parent, an older sibling or another close relative. We prepared a booklet for each participant containing one-paragraph stories about three events that had actually happened to him or her and one that had not. We constructed the false event using information about a plausible shopping trip provided by a relative, who also verified that the participant had not in fact been lost at about the age of five. The lost-in-the-mall scenario included the following elements: lost for an extended period, crying, aid and comfort by an elderly woman and, finally, reunion with the family.

After reading each story in the booklet, the participants wrote what they remembered about the event. If they did not remember it, they were instructed to write, "I do not remember this." In two follow-up interviews, we told the participants that we were interested in examining how much detail they could remember and how their memories compared with those of their relative. The event paragraphs were not read to them verbatim, but rather parts were provided as retrieval cues. The participants recalled something about 49 of the 72 true events (68 per-

cent) immediately after the initial reading of the booklet and also in each of the two follow-up interviews. After reading the booklet, seven of the 24 participants (29 percent) remembered either partially or fully the false event constructed for them, and in the two follow-up interviews six participants (25 percent) continued to claim that they remembered the fictitious event. Statistically, there were some differences between the true memories and the false ones: participants used more words to describe the true memories, and they rated the true memories as being somewhat more clear. But if an onlooker were to observe many of our participants describe an event, it would be difficult indeed to tell whether the account was of a true or a false memory.

Of course, being lost, however frightening, is not the same as being abused. But the lost-in-the-mall study is not about real experiences of being lost; it is about planting false memories of being lost. The paradigm shows a way of instilling false memories and takes a step toward allowing us to understand how this might happen in real-world settings. Moreover, the study provides evidence that people can be led to remember their past in different ways, and they can even be coaxed into "remembering" entire events that never happened.

Studies in other laboratories using a similar experimental procedure have produced similar results. For instance, Ira Hyman, Troy H. Husband and F. James Billing of Western Washington University asked college students to recall childhood experiences that had been recounted by their parents. The researchers told the students that the study was about how people remember shared experiences differently. In addition to actual events reported by parents, each participant was given one false event—either an overnight hospitalization for a high fever and a possible ear infection, or a birthday party with pizza and a clown—that supposedly happened at about the age of five. The parents confirmed that neither of these events actually took place.

Hyman found that students fully or partially recalled 84 percent of the true events in the first interview and 88 percent in the second interview. None of the participants recalled the false event during the first interview, but 20 percent said they remembered something

about the false event in the second interview. One participant who had been exposed to the emergency hospitalization story later remembered a male doctor, a female nurse and a friend from church who came to visit at the hospital.

In another study, along with true events Hyman presented different false events, such as accidentally spilling a bowl of punch on the parents of the bride at a wedding reception or having to evacuate a grocery store when the overhead sprinkler systems erroneously activated. Again, none of the participants recalled the false event during the first interview, but 18 percent remembered something about it in the second interview and 25 percent in the third interview. For example, during the first interview, one participant, when asked about the fictitious wedding event, stated, "I have no clue. I have never heard that one before." In the second interview, the participant said, "It was an outdoor wedding, and I think we were running around and knocked something over like the punch bowl or something and made a big mess and of course got yelled at for it."

Imagination Inflation

The finding that an external suggestion can lead to the construction of false childhood memories helps us understand the process by which false memories arise. It is natural to wonder whether this research is applicable in real situations such as being interrogated by law officers or in psychotherapy. Although strong suggestion may not routinely occur in police questioning or therapy, suggestion in the form of an imagination exercise sometimes does. For instance, when trying to obtain a confession, law officers may ask a suspect to imagine having participated in a criminal act. Some mental health professionals encourage patients to imagine childhood events as a way of recovering supposedly hidden memories.

Surveys of clinical psychologists reveal that 11 percent instruct their clients to "let the imagination run wild," and 22 percent tell their clients to "give free rein to the imagination." Therapist Wendy Maltz, author of a popular book on childhood sexual abuse, advocates telling the patient: "Spend time imagining that you were sexually abused, without worrying about accuracy, proving anything, or having your ideas make sense.... Ask yourself...these questions: What time of day is it? Where are you? Indoors or outdoors? What kind of things are happening? Is there one or more person with you?" Maltz further recommends that therapists continue to ask questions such as "Who would have been likely perpetrators? When were you most vulnerable to sexual abuse in your life?"

The increasing use of such imagination exercises led me and several colleagues to wonder about their consequences. What happens when people imagine childhood experiences that did not happen to them? Does imagining a childhood event increase confidence that it occurred? To explore this, we designed a three-stage procedure. We first asked individuals to indicate the likelihood that certain events happened to them during their childhood. The list contains 40 events, each rated on a scale ranging from "definitely did not happen" to "definitely did happen." Two weeks later we asked the participants to imagine that they had experienced some of these events. Different subjects were asked to imagine different events. Sometime later the participants again were asked to respond to the original list of 40 childhood events, indicating how likely it was that these events actually happened to them.

Consider one of the imagination exercises. Participants are told to imagine playing inside at home after school, hearing a strange noise outside, running toward the window, tripping, falling, reaching out and breaking the window with their hand. In addition, we asked participants questions such as "What did you trip on? How did you feel?"

In one study 24 percent of the participants who imagined the broken-window scenario later reported an increase in confidence that the event had occurred, whereas only 12 percent of those who were not asked to imagine the incident reported an increase in the likelihood that it had taken place. We found this "imagination inflation" effect in each of the eight events that participants were asked to imagine. A number of possible explanations come to mind. An obvious one is that an act of imagination simply makes the event seem more familiar and that familiarity is mistakenly related to childhood memories rather than to the act of imagination. Such source confusion—when a person does not remember the source of informa-

tion—can be especially acute for the distant experiences of childhood.

Studies by Lyn Goff and Henry L. Roediger III of Washington University of recent rather than childhood experiences more directly connect imagined actions to the construction of false memory. During the initial session, the researchers instructed participants to perform the stated action, imagine doing it or just listen to the statement and do nothing else. The actions were simple ones: knock on the table, lift the stapler, break the toothpick, cross your fingers, roll your eyes. During the second session, the participants were asked to imagine some of the actions that they had not previously performed. During the final session, they answered questions about what actions they actually performed during the initial session. The investigators found that the more times participants imagined an unperformed action, the more likely they were to remember having performed it.

Impossible Memories

It is highly unlikely that an adult can recall genuine episodic memories from the first year of life, in part because the hippocampus, which plays a key role in the creation of memories, has not matured enough to form and store long-lasting memories that can be retrieved in adulthood. A procedure for planting "impossible" memories about experiences that occur shortly after birth has been developed by the late Nicholas Spanos and his collaborators at Carleton University. Individuals are led to believe that they have well-coordinated eye movements and visual exploration skills probably because they were born in hospitals that hung swinging, colored mobiles over infant cribs. To confirm whether they had such an experience, half the participants are hypnotized, age-regressed to the day after birth and asked what they remembered. The other half of the group participates in a "guided mnemonic restructuring" procedure that uses age regression as well as active encouragement to re-create the infant experiences by imagining them.

Spanos and his co-workers found that the vast majority of their subjects were susceptible to these memory-planting procedures. Both the hypnotic and guided participants reported infant memories. Surprisingly, the guided group did so somewhat more (95 versus 70 per-

cent). Both groups remembered the colored mobile at a relatively high rate (56 percent of the guided group and 46 percent of the hypnotic subjects). Many participants who did not remember the mobile did recall other things, such as doctors, nurses, bright lights, cribs and masks. Also, in both groups, of those who reported memories of infancy, 49 percent felt that they were real memories, as opposed to 16 percent who claimed that they were merely fantasies. These findings confirm earlier studies that many individuals can be led to construct complex, vivid and detailed false memories via a rather simple procedure. Hypnosis clearly is not necessary.

How False Memories Form

In the lost-in-the-mall study, implantation of false memory occurred when another person, usually a family member, claimed that the incident happened. Corroboration of an event by another person can be a powerful technique for instilling a false memory. In fact, merely claiming to have seen a person do something can lead that person to make a false confession of wrongdoing.

This effect was demonstrated in a study by Saul M. Kassin and his colleagues at Williams College, who investigated the reactions of individuals falsely accused of damaging a computer by pressing the wrong key. The innocent participants initially denied the charge, but when a confederate said that she had seen them perform the action, many participants signed a confession, internalized guilt for the act and went on to confabulate details that were consistent with that belief. These findings show that false incriminating evidence can induce people to accept guilt for a crime they did not commit and even to develop memories to support their guilty feelings.

Research is beginning to give us an understanding of how false memories of complete, emotional and self-participatory experiences are created in adults. First, there are social demands on individuals to remember; for instance, researchers exert some pressure on participants in a study to come up with memories. Second, memory construction by imagining events can be explicitly encouraged when people are having trouble remembering. And, finally, individuals can be encouraged not to think about whether their constructions are real or not. Creation of false memories is most likely to occur when these external factors are present, whether in an experimental setting, in a therapeutic setting or during everyday activities.

False memories are constructed by combining actual memories with the content of suggestions received from others. During the process, individuals may forget the source of the information. This is a classic example of source confusion, in which the content and the source become dissociated.

Of course, because we can implant false childhood memories in some individuals in no way implies that all memories that arise after suggestion are necessarily false. Put another way, although experimental work on the creation of false memories may raise doubt about the validity of long-buried memories, such as repeated trauma, it in no way disproves them. Without corroboration, there is little that can be done to help even the most experienced evaluator to differentiate true memories from ones that were suggestively planted.

The precise mechanisms by which such false memories are constructed await further research. We still have much to learn about the degree of confidence and the characteristics of false memories created in these ways, and we need to discover what types of individuals are particularly susceptible to these forms of suggestion and who is resistant.

As we continue this work, it is important to heed the cautionary tale in the data we have already obtained: mental health professionals and others must be aware of how greatly they can influence the recollection of events and of the urgent need for maintaining restraint in situations in which imagination is used as an aid in recovering presumably lost memories.

The Author

ELIZABETH F. LOFTUS is professor of psychology and adjunct professor of law at the University of Washington. She received her Ph.D. in psychology from Stanford University in 1970. Her research has focused on human memory, eyewitness testimony and courtroom procedure. Loftus has published 18 books and more than 250 scientific articles and has served as an expert witness or consultant in hundreds of trials, including the McMartin preschool molestation case. Her book *Eyewitness Testimony* won a National Media Award from the American Psychological Foundation. She has received honorary doctorates from Miami University, Leiden University and John Jay College of Criminal Justice. Loftus was recently elected president of the American Psychological Society.

Further Reading

THE MYTH OF REPRESSED MEMORY. Elizabeth F. Loftus and Katherine Ketcham. St. Martin's Press, 1994.
THE SOCIAL PSYCHOLOGY OF FALSE CONFESSIONS: COMPLIANCE, INTERNALIZATION, AND CONFABULATION. Saul M. Kassin and Katherine L. Kiechel in *Psychological Science*, Vol. 7, No. 3, pages 125–128; May 1996.
IMAGINATION INFLATION: IMAGINING A CHILDHOOD EVENT INFLATES CONFIDENCE THAT IT OCCURRED. Maryanne Garry, Charles G. Manning, Elizabeth F. Loftus and Steven J. Sherman in *Psychonomic Bulletin and Review*, Vol. 3, No. 2, pages 208–214; June 1996.
REMEMBERING OUR PAST: STUDIES IN AUTOBIOGRAPHICAL MEMORY. Edited by David C. Rubin. Cambridge University Press, 1996.
SEARCHING FOR MEMORY: THE BRAIN, THE MIND, AND THE PAST. Daniel L. Schacter. BasicBooks, 1996.

Is There Evidence for Repression? Doubtful

David S. Holmes

David S. Holmes, Ph.D., is Professor of Psychology at the University of Kansas. He is the author of more than 120 articles in professional journals and a widely used text on psychopathology.

This is the first part of a debate [between David S. Holmes, Ph.D., and] Mardi J. Horowitz, M.D. [See the next *Annual Editions* article for Horowitz's reply.]

Sigmund Freud, who introduced the concept of repression into psychological theory, used it differently at various times, but it is now usually defined as the involuntary selective removal from consciousness of anxiety-provoking memories. These memories are said to be stored in the unconscious but capable of returning to consciousness if the anxiety associated with them is eliminated. The concept of repression is central to many theories of personality and psychopathology. For Freud it was a major defense mechanism of the ego and a cornerstone of psychoanalytic theory. Yet, despite a 70-year search, investigators have not been able to find objective evidence that the process actually occurs.

The earliest research concentrated on whether people recalled pleasant experiences more readily than unpleasant ones, which are presumably more likely to be repressed. Subjects kept diaries and were later tested for their recall of pleasant and unpleasant experiences. The main finding was that more emotionally intense experiences, both pleasant and unpleasant, were recalled more easily than less intense ones. Subjects also recalled pleasant experiences somewhat better than unpleasant ones, but only because intense feelings associated with unpleasant experiences dissipated faster. The feelings dissipated because subjects re-evaluated their experiences when consequences they anticipated did not come about.

These early findings did not provide direct evidence against repression, because the experiences involved, although unpleasant, were not necessarily threatening or anxiety-provoking. Investigators later took a different approach. In a typical experiment they would have a group of people learn a list of words, and then expose half of the group to stress by telling them they had failed a test or revealed personality defects. The other half were told they had passed the test or were given neutral comments on their personalities. All were then asked to recall the word list. The people exposed to stress recalled fewer words, and it seemed plausible at first that they were repressing memories associated with the stress. This conclusion was apparently strengthened when they were tested again after being told that they had passed a difficult test or that the earlier information about personality was false. Now they remembered the words as well as the control group. It looked as though stress had induced repression and removal of the stress had lifted it.

But when researchers inquired more closely, they found that many of the people exposed to stress in this way had been concentrating on the experience instead of shutting it out; they recalled the words poorly because of distraction rather than repression. Preoccupied with their own recent "failures," they were less capable of paying attention to a routine memorization task. Further research confirmed this interpretation: information that enhanced self-esteem was equally distracting and had similar effects on memorization.

It still seemed possible that even if most people did not use repression as a defense against stress, certain personality types did. But when investigators looked

From *The Harvard Mental Health Newsletter*, June 1994, pp. 4-6. © 1994 by the President and Fellows of Harvard College. Reprinted by permission.

at the links between personality, stress, and recall, they did not find what they expected. For example, people with high achievement motivation, whom they expected to be more distressed by failure on a test, recalled the failure better than people who were less strongly motivated to succeed. Furthermore, hysteria, ego strength, and other traits considered important in psychoanalytic theory were unrelated to the recall of stressful experiences. Other research has shown that socially conforming people with little anxiety are less likely to admit that they have undergone distressing or unpleasant experiences. But there are good reasons to believe that these people are simply unwilling to report the events; they are consciously suppressing rather repressing them.

Clinicians often dismiss the laboratory research on repression as artificial, superficial, or irrelevant. They argue that the real evidence is to be found only in the behavior of patients during psychotherapy. Unfortunately, what a patient does and says in psychotherapy is difficult for an outsider to judge. At a recent conference attended by some of the world's leading experts on repression, a group of investigators decided to overcome that difficulty by showing videotapes of therapy sessions. The conferees would be allowed to look into the consulting room and observe repression as it was taking place. Alas, the experts at the meeting could not even agree on when or whether a patient seen on the videotape was using repression.

In the absence of good laboratory or clinical evidence for repression, proponents of the concept have begun to emphasize dissociation instead. But that is simply another name for repression; if one dissociates oneself from an event (is no longer aware of it), one has repressed it. Dissociative amnesia is supposed to occur after certain traumatic experiences. Yet alleged cases of this phenomenon are very rare, although many people undergo overwhelming stress (wars, airplane crashes, devastating earthquakes, and so on). If the truly terrifying disasters that afflict millions of persons rarely result in dissociative amnesia, it seems unlikely that the relatively mild emotional conflicts and upsetting situations described by clinicians could possibly cause repression. In other words, even if the existence of dissociative amnesia were admitted, it would not prove that repression was common.

Dissociative amnesia was originally observed in soldiers who lost their memory of terrifying battles in which they had just fought, and later seemed to recover the experiences through hypnosis and drugs.

There are two reasons why these cases are not evidence for repression. First, the amnesia might have been the result of physical trauma; injuries as minor as whiplash can cause amnesia. Second, when hypnosis and drugs are used in this way, possibilities for suggestion and influence are almost unlimited. Investigators inducing their patients to reenact battle scenes while drugged are concocting an ideal recipe for false memories.

The most striking and hotly disputed evidence for recovery of forgotten traumatic events comes from patients who remember alleged childhood sexual abuse after many years of amnesia. In the most recent research on this subject, investigators interviewed a group of women who had been treated in a hospital emergency department as children after reported sexual abuse. Thirty-eight percent of the women did not mention the abuse, and researchers therefore concluded that they had repressed the memory of it. But the women were never directly asked about the documented abuse, and another investigation using the same procedures indicated that they had simply chosen not to report it. In the second study, 38% of the women again failed to mention the abuse at the first interview, but all reported it when asked. These findings clearly provide no evidence for the repression of childhood sexual abuse.

Memory is undoubtedly selective. Mood, cognitive set, and associative links influence what we perceive, store, and recall. The concept of repression could be rescued if we simply used the word to describe these well-attested mental processes. That might win the approval of the famous Wonderland theorist H. Dumpty, who declared, "When I use a word, it means just what I choose it to mean — neither more nor less." But the workings of cognitive set, associations, and mood at the time of recall bear no resemblance to repression as it is traditionally conceived; for example, these processes are not defenses against anxiety and do not imply the existence of the unconscious. Any such Humpty-Dumptyish redefinition would eliminate what makes the idea of repression unique and gives it interest.

Some readers, surprised to learn how weak the evidence for repression is, may conclude that the topic has not been adequately studied. Surely evidence will appear as soon as more investigators turn their attention to the issue. But the present negative conclusion has withstood refutation for at least 20 years. The many elegant theoretical explanations of repression may seem convincing, but they are meaningless because its existence has never been demonstrated. Although it is impossible to prove that repression does not exist, we are no more justified in using the concept to explain a patient's behavior than we are in expecting the patient to ride home on a unicorn. Given the current trend toward full disclosure and truth in packaging, it may be appropriate for psychotherapists who insist on the significance of repression to issue the following warning: since there is no objective evidence for this concept, use of it may be hazardous to your treatment.

Does Repression Exist? Yes

Mardi J. Horowitz

Mardi J. Horowitz, M.D., is Professor of Psychiatry at the University of California at San Francisco and Director of the Program on Conscious and Unconscious Mental Processes of the John D. and Catherine T. MacArthur Foundation. He is the author of several books including Person Schemas and Maladaptive Interpersonal Patterns *(University of Chicago Press: 1991).*

In the [previous *Annual Editions* article,] *David S. Holmes, Ph.D., argued that there was no good evidence for the existence of repression. Dr. Horowitz replies below.*

People often have experiences in which they do not remember something important despite conscious willed effort; for example, a grieving person may be unable to form a mental image of the face of a loved one who has recently died. But the information is recorded in the mind and may be recalled in a later phase of mourning. The fact that repressive phenomena exist is indicated by such experiences in which conscious thinking about stored mental information is omitted and later recovered.

David Holmes concludes that there is no objective evidence for repression after 70 years of research. In my disagreement I have the support of the clinicians who compile the diagnostic manual of the American Psychiatric Association. Among the clinical signs and symptoms of posttraumatic stress disorder they have included avoidance and numbing, which are repressive phenomena. Furthermore, a new diagnosis based on posttraumatic dissociative experiences will be included in the next edition of the manual.

Nevertheless, difficulties arise when we try to define and describe repression. The term is used both to describe a mental process, such as a defense mechanism, and to define a set of outcomes or phenomena: conscious experiences in which people should and could be paying attention to certain information but instead are unaware of it. The word "omission" is often appropriate to describe such episodes. In many of these experiences there is no distinct cleavage between what is consciously represented, what is preconsciously processed, and what is non-consciously stored.

Freud believed that most mental activity was conscious. Memories, fantasies, motivations, and conceptions of the self and others became unconscious only in defense against anxiety that would be provoked by conscious awareness of them. Freud called the material warded off in this way "the repressed," and the process of warding it off "repressing." Today we have a more complex view of mental activity. There are many kinds of unconscious mental processes, and much of our knowledge is unconscious. Although Freud could speak only of "repressing," we now know many different ways in which information processing is regulated in order to control emotional experiences. The mechanisms of warding off are ways of inhibiting that processing, and the results are omissions. Broadly, then, repression refers to omissions rooted in unconscious defensive motives and mediated by inhibitory controls over mental information processing. We need not define the term as Freud did a century ago. When repression is seen this way, all of Holmes's arguments can be refuted.

Holmes summarizes studies pairing stress with recollection of word lists and concludes that people usually concentrate on rather than repress stressful experiences. His interpretation is correct for average results in a group of normal college students, but clinicians are concerned with experiences that are out of the ordinary. In the experiments described by Holmes, the rare student who was too anxious to recall what he or she felt during the memory test would be showing evidence of omissions of the type also called repression.

In fact, the increased focus on the stressful event found in these experiments may be a mild variant of the kind of intrusive experience recognized as a symptom of posttraumatic stress. Intrusions alternate with involuntary avoidance and omission in

From *The Harvard Mental Health Newsletter*, July 1994, pp. 4-6. © 1994 by the President and Fellows of Harvard College. Reprinted by permission.

many stress response syndromes. I and others have demonstrated the empirical reliability and validity of this cycle in laboratory experiments with stress-provoking films, field studies of populations exposed to stress, and clinical studies of patients with posttraumatic symptoms. There is strong evidence that during the avoidant phase people try to remove certain topics from contemplation. This repression is not permanent, since the very topics that are warded off in one phase may become intrusive in another state of mind. Mental contents avoided in phases of denial are apparently held unconsciously in active storage for eventual processing. During the treatment, intrusions become less insistent and the patient becomes capable of both remembering the traumatic events and putting them out of mind at will — a sign that unconscious information processing of the stressful experience has been more or less completed. The American Psychiatric Association has accepted the diagnosis of posttraumatic stress disorder partly on the basis of such research.

Some patients in psychotherapy sessions alternate in a shorter cycle between heightened intrusiveness and defensive avoidance. An unbidden image with precursors stored in active memory may interrupt and disrupt the patient's focus of attention. When observed on video recordings, patients try to avoid such intrusions in a way that suggests non-conscious motivation.

Holmes describes a conference at which, according to him, no one could determine from tapes of therapy sessions whether or not a patient was using repression. He is referring to videotapes that I presented in order to show that the classic psychoanalytical terminology of defense mechanisms is inadequate to describe the on-the-spot formation of psychiatric signs and symptoms. The theory can now be reformulated usefully in the language of information processing. My colleagues and I expected disagreement on what was observed and how it could be explained: argument about evidence was the point of the scientific workshop. We believe that the presence of repression can be judged by many different signs of defensive control processes affecting expression. We have published new classifications of these processes as well as data on the reliability of independent observers in identifying signs of defensiveness.

Although omissions may result in amnesia, they are far more likely to involve simply an absence of conscious thinking about the implications of an event. Sometimes complete forgetting occurs because of defensive avoidance, but more often the patient's attention touches some aspects of a theme while other aspects are unrecognized. At the beginning of psychotherapy, patients may avoid certain aspects of an emotional dilemma, especially those lying at the heart of an emotional conflict. When thoughts and feelings about the issue emerge, the themes embodied in them may at first take the form of involuntary repressed memories or flashbacks. For a while, then, the patient may feel as if the mind is acting simply as a camera flashing back to a memory. But in many cases the same themes are later examined in a less and less passive way, until the patient feels himself or herself to be deliberately thinking by both remembering and imagining. The mind constructs rather than photographs, and apparent memories shift in different states of mind.

Failure to translate meanings across mental systems is another type of omission that deserves the name of repression. It too is best explained as the result of many processes of control over different mental activities. Visual images may not be "known" in words; gestures leak emotional information that is not "known" in conscious verbal representation or mental images. Omissions also take the form of conspicuous and purposive inattention to emotionally relevant aspects of the environment or the self.

As I have mentioned, experiences of omission often occur during mourning and after traumatic events. In the early stages of a stress response syndrome, a person may be unable to address certain topics related to the events, although other topics can be contemplated. Inability to imagine or recall the voice or face of someone who has died is one example of such conceptual denial and emotional numbing. These experiences may even evoke a fear of forgetting the person who has died. Later, for reasons beyond the mourner's conscious knowledge, he or she may once again see the face, hear the voice, and recall memories of the deceased at will.

Holmes doubts the authenticity of such experiences. He also doubts the authenticity of experiences that involve the return of the long repressed in the form of adult recovered memories of childhood trauma. He believes that these memories have been implanted by suggestion. It is true that amnesia and the recovery of memories are often overdramatized. The process is less spectacular and the work of mastery is harder and slower than one would guess from watching a film like Hitchcock's "Spellbound." But recovery of forgotten traumatic events does occur, and these phenomena can be called repressive because they involve information that is absent from central conscious attention but attains conscious representation in another state of mind. Comparing discoveries that emerge in therapy with home movies made decades earlier, Herman Serota has reported that memories returning after decades of omission can be validated by evidence. These memories are not always accurate, but they are often strikingly detailed and illuminating.

As for the issue of suggestion, modern integrated psychodynamic and cognitive theories of the mind regard all thinking as constructive. No one can be sure that a subjective experience is real, and no one hearing a report of the experience can tell for sure whether it is a memory, a fantasy, or a construction with elements of both. Suggestion can be powerful, and there are false memory syndromes, but there are also false fantasy syndromes in which real events are recalled as daydreams, dreams, or hallucinations.

Psychotherapists often encounter less dramatic forms of long-term repression in patients with personality disorders who habitually avoid conscious awareness of certain desires and fears. They may ignore certain aspects of their emotional relationships but repeat the maladaptive pattern and resist understanding it. In psychotherapy the pattern becomes known, but not in a progressive series of blazing insights. There are stages of learning and forgetting, staggering forward and back. The backward shifts may appear purposive, but the underlying defensive aims and control processes are partly beyond conscious awareness.

In treating personality disorders, psychotherapists often encounter a type of omission that has been called "unconscious fantasy." The term refers to motivated scenarios in which the same maladaptive roles and relationships involving the self and others are repeatedly re-enacted. For example, some people allow themselves to be exploited, not because they are masochistic (receive erotic pleasure from suffering), but because they have unconscious fantasy scripts in which suffering to meet the demands of another person is a role they must play in order to be granted a desired role later on. They expect loving attention after being exploited but often have no awareness of this unrealistic expectation — only a dim recognition that their behavior is bringing no satisfaction.

Conscious representation of the expected sequence of relationship transactions may help these patients to exercise conscious control over enactments of unconscious fantasy at the beginning of a new repetition. Conscious overriding of unconscious tendencies can help patients plan and try out alternative patterns of behavior that may then lead to more realistic ways of viewing themselves and others. As a result, they may form new schemas that can organize more adaptive behavior in a more automatic, less consciously controlled manner.

The inhibition of specific associations is thus not enough to explain all episodes of omission. My colleagues and I have developed a model we call person schemas theory, which integrates psychoanalytic object relations theory, self-psychology, and the theory of cognitive schemas. We have concluded that different information is available to consciousness in different states of mind partly because these states of mind are associated with different ways of controlling self-concepts and different models of the relationship between self and others. Role relationship models and other schemas, by affecting patterns of association, serve to organize even memories, fantasies, and thoughts about specific stressful events and thus determine the states of mind in which they will be omitted, intrusive, or contemplated in a well-modulated way.

To sum up, repression cannot be fully explained by theoretical models advanced decades ago, but the omissions to which the term refers are genuine. What feels like a memory may not represent a real event. What feels like a fantasy may have elements of past reality. What feels like "forgetting forever" may be a transitory state. We must examine such unusual conscious episodes to understand how conscious and unconscious mental processes transform meanings and emotions. And when we hold these episodes up to the light, we should not dismiss certain aspects of the resulting picture just because we do not completely understand them. Repressive phenomena are genuine, and we must continue to develop theories to explain them.

Multiple Personality Disorder

Paul R. McHugh

Paul R. McHugh, M.D. is Henry Phipps Professor of Psychiatry and Director of the Department of Psychiatry and Behavioral Science at the Johns Hopkins Medical Institutions, Baltimore, MD.

This article is the first part of a debate. [See *The Harvard Mental Health Newsletter*, October 1993 issue for a reply by Richard P. Kluft, M.D.]

Prompted by the unexpected flourishing of this extraordinary diagnosis, students often ask me whether multiple personality disorder (MPD) really exists. I usually reply that the symptoms attributed to it are as genuine as hysterical paralysis and seizures and teach us lessons already learned by psychiatrists more than a hundred years ago.

Consider the dramatic events that occurred at the Salpêtrière Hospital in Paris in the 1880s. For a time the chief physician, Jean-Martin Charcot, thought he had discovered a new disease he called "hystero-epilepsy," a disorder of mind and brain combining features of hysteria and epilepsy. The patients displayed a variety of symptoms, including convulsions, contortions, fainting, and transient impairment of consciousness. Charcot, the acknowledged master of Parisian neurologists, demonstrated the condition by presenting patients to his staff during teaching rounds in the hospital auditorium.

A skeptical student, Joseph Babinski, decided that Charcot had invented rather than discovered hystero-epilepsy. The patients had come to the hospital with vague complaints of distress and demoralization. Charcot had persuaded them that they were victims of hystero-epilepsy and should join the others under his care. Charcot's interest in their problems, the encouragement of attendants, and the example of others on the same ward prompted patients to accept Charcot's view of them and eventually to display the expected symptoms.

These symptoms resembled epilepsy, Babinski believed, because of a municipal decision to house epileptic and hysterical patients together (both having "episodic" conditions). The hysterical patients, already vulnerable to suggestion and persuasion, were continually subjected to life on the ward and to Charcot's neuropsychiatric examina-

tions. They began to imitate the epileptic attacks they repeatedly witnessed.

Babinski eventually won the argument. In fact, he persuaded Charcot that doctors can induce a variety of physical and mental disorders, especially in young, inexperienced, emotionally troubled women. There was no "hystero-epilepsy." These patients were afflicted not by a disease but by an idea.

With this understanding, Charcot and Babinski devised a two-stage treatment consisting of isolation and countersuggestion. First, "hystero-epileptic" patients were transferred to the general wards of the hospital and kept apart from one another. Thus they were separated from everyone else who was behaving in the same way, and also from staff members who had been induced by sympathy or investigatory zeal to show great interest in the symptoms. The success of this first step was remarkable. Babinski and Charcot were reminded of the rare but impressive epidemics of fainting, convulsions, and wild screaming in convents and boarding schools that ended when the group of afflicted persons was broken up and scattered.

The second step, countersuggestion, was designed to give the patients a view of themselves that would persuade them to abandon their symptoms. Dramatic countersuggestions, such as electrical stimulation of "paralyzed" muscles, proved to be unreliable. The most effective technique was simply ignoring the hysterical behavior and concentrating on the present circumstances of these patients. They were suffering from many forms of stress, including sexual feelings and traumas, economic fears, religious conflicts, and a conviction (perhaps correct) that they were being exploited or neglected by their families. In some cases their distress had been provoked by a mental or physical illness. The hysterical symptoms obscured the underlying emotional conflicts and traumas. How trivial a sexual fear seemed to a patient in whom convulsive attacks produced paralysis and temporary blindness every day!

From *The Harvard Mental Health Newsletter*, September 1993, pp. 4-6. © 1993 by the President and Fellows of Harvard College. Reprinted by permission.

Staff members expressed their withdrawal of interest in hysterical behavior subtly, in such words as, "You're in recovery now and we will give you some physiotherapy, but let us concentrate on the home situation that may have brought this on." These face-saving countersuggestions reduced a patient's need to go on producing hystero-epileptic symptoms in order to certify that her problems were real. The symptoms then gradually withered from lack of nourishing attention. Patients began to take a more coherent and disciplined approach to their problems and found a resolution more appropriate than hysterical displays.

The rules discovered by Babinski and Charcot, now embedded in psychiatric textbooks and confirmed by decades of research in social psychology, are being overlooked in the midst of a nationwide epidemic of alleged MPD that is wreaking havoc on both patients and therapists. MPD is an iatrogenic behavioral syndrome, promoted by suggestion and maintained by clinical attention, social consequences, and group loyalties. It rests on ideas about the self that obscure reality, and it responds to standard treatments.

To begin with the first point: MPD, like hystero-epilepsy, is created by therapists. This formerly rare and disputed diagnosis became popular after the appearance of several best-selling books and movies. It is often based on the crudest form of suggestion. Here, for example, is some advice on how to elicit alternative personalities (alters, as they have come to be called), from an introduction to MPD by Stephen E. Buie, M.D., who is director of the Dissociative Disorders Treatment Program at a North Carolina hospital:

> It may happen that an alter personality will reveal itself to you during this [assessment] process, but more likely it will not. So you may have to elicit an alter . . . You can begin by indirect [sic] questioning such as, "Have you ever felt like another part of you does things that you can't control?" If she gives positive or ambiguous responses ask for specific examples. You are trying to develop a picture of what the alter personality is like . . . At this point you may ask the host personality, "Does this set of feelings have a name?" . . . Often the host personality will not know. You can then focus upon a particular event or set of behaviors. "Can I talk to the part of you that is taking those long drives in the country?"

Once patients have permitted a psychiatrist to "talk to the part . . . that is taking these long drives," they are committed to the idea that they have MPD and must act in ways consistent with this self-image. The patient may be placed on a hospital service (often called the dissociative service) with others who have given the same compliant responses. The emergence of the first alter breaches the barrier of reality, and fantasy is allowed free rein. The patient and staff now begin a search for further alters surrounding the so-called host personality. The original two or three personalities proliferate into 90 or 100. A lore evolves. At least one alter must be of the opposite sex (Patricia may have Penny but also must have Patrick). Sometimes it is even suggested that one alter is an animal. A dog, cat, or cow must be found and made to speak! Individual alters are followed in special notes for the hospital record. Every time an alter emerges, the hospital staff shows great interest. The search for fresh symptoms sustains the original commitment while cultivating and embellishing the suggestion. It becomes harder and harder for a patient to say to the psychiatrist or to anyone else, "Oh, let's stop this. It's just me taking those long drives in the country."

The cause of MPD is supposed to be a childhood sexual trauma so horrible that it has to be split off (dissociated) from the host consciousness and lodged in the alters. Patient and therapist begin a search for alters who remember the trauma and can identify the abuser. Thus commitment to the diagnosis of MPD is enhanced by the sense that a crime is being exposed and justice is being done. The patient now has such a powerful vested interest in sustaining the MPD enterprise that it almost becomes an end in itself.

Certainly these patients, like Charcot's, have many emotional conflicts and have often suffered traumatic experiences. But everyone is distracted from the patient's main problems by a preoccupation with dramatic symptoms, and perhaps by a commitment to a single kind of psychological trauma. Furthermore, given that treatment may become interminable when therapists concentrate on fascinating symptoms, it is no wonder that MPD is regarded as a chronic disorder that often requires long stretches of time on dissociative units.

Charcot removed his patients from the special wards when he realized what he had been inventing. We can do the same. These patients should be treated by the same methods Charcot used — isolation and countersuggestion. Close the dissociation services and disperse the patients to general psychiatric units. Ignore the alters. Stop talking to them, taking notes on them, and discussing them in staff conferences. Pay attention to real present problems and conflicts rather than fantasy. If these simple, familiar rules are followed, multiple personalities will soon wither away and psychotherapy can begin.

IS IT NORMAL AGING—OR ALZHEIMER'S?

Forgetfulness usually doesn't signal senility—and there are ways to bolster a failing memory.

You draw a blank trying to recall an acquaintance's name. You can't recall where you set down the television remote. You misplace your keys—again. Could this be the start of Alzheimer's?

Last November, former President Ronald Reagan's disclosure that he was suffering from Alzheimer's drew national attention to this devastating disease. Then, in May, a large study of elderly people in East Boston, Mass., suggested that Alzheimer's is more common than previously believed, striking nearly one in five people who live to age 80. Of course, that also means that four out of five people who reach the age of 80 do *not* have Alzheimer's disease. At age 70, the researchers figured, only 1 in 20 people will have the disease.

So while memory lapses do tend to become more common with age, they're usually not a sign of Alzheimer's disease. In fact, worrying about whether you're "going senile" is itself a good sign that you're not (see box, Alzheimer's: Tarnishing the Golden Years). In some cases, severe memory loss may be due to an underlying condition that can be remedied. Most of the time, however, occasional forgetfulness is nothing to worry about. And there are a variety of simple strategies that anyone can use to bolster a weak memory.

The aging brain

The overall mental decline that accompanies aging is not as dramatic as many people think. After all, young people forget names and misplace things, too; they just don't suspect Alzheimer's when they do. Forgetfulness in a 30-year-old is considered "spacey," not "senile."

While the average 80-year-old is not as quick-minded as a 30-year-old, the differences are not great. "An elderly person might be able to press a lever in response to a signal just as fast as a younger person can," explains Paul Coleman, Ph.D., director of the Alzheimer's Center at the University of Rochester. "But if the test involves pressing one lever when a *green* light goes on and another lever when a *red* light goes on, an elderly person will respond at a slightly more sluggish pace."

As a practical matter, an older person's experience or perceptiveness can offset that touch of mental sluggishness. In one study, for instance, older typists typed just as fast as younger typists, despite slower reaction times. Puzzled, the researchers investigated and found that the seniors were compensating for their handicap by taking in more words with each glance at the written page.

Age-related memory deficits seem to involve a diminished ability to store *new* information. The ability to retrieve old information tends to remain intact, as anyone knows who has listened to a grandparent recount days of old. In recent studies, for example, scientists from the National Institute on Aging and the National Institute of Mental Health found that older people (aged 64 to 76) had a harder time memorizing new faces than did younger people (aged 23 to 27). Brain scans revealed less activity in the hippocampal region—an area thought to be important in memory storage—among the older volunteers. However, they were just as good as their younger counterparts on perception tests that involved matching identical faces.

Part of the reason that older people tend to do worse than younger people on memory tests may also be that they're tested at the wrong time of day. Duke University researchers have found that older people perform better on tests given in the morning than in the afternoon. So the age-related declines in mental acuity seen in some studies may have been exaggerated.

All told, a debilitating decline in mental powers just doesn't seem to be an inevitable consequence of aging. Ordinarily, the changes that do occur cause

IS POOR MEMORY A PROBLEM?

Follow the flowchart below to see if a perceived memory problem is really anything to be concerned about. Medical evaluation may be in order if depression appears to be a factor or if memory is seriously impaired (see memory test, next page).

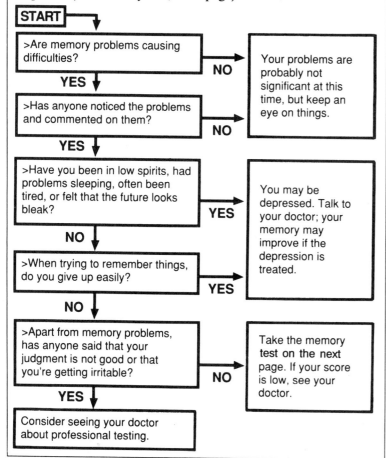

START

>Are memory problems causing difficulties? — NO → Your problems are probably not significant at this time, but keep an eye on things.

YES ↓

>Has anyone noticed the problems and commented on them? — NO →

YES ↓

>Have you been in low spirits, had problems sleeping, often been tired, or felt that the future looks bleak? — YES → You may be depressed. Talk to your doctor; your memory may improve if the depression is treated.

NO ↓

>When trying to remember things, do you give up easily? — YES →

NO ↓

>Apart from memory problems, has anyone said that your judgment is not good or that you're getting irritable? — NO → Take the memory test on the next page. If your score is low, see your doctor.

YES ↓

Consider seeing your doctor about professional testing.

Reprinted with permission from *Consumer Reports on Health*, October 1995, pp. 114-116. © 1995 by Consumers Union of U.S., Inc., Yonkers, NY 10703-1057.

only minor problems, if any. When problems with memory or learning skills are severe, they may be the result of an underlying condition other than Alzheimer's. Those include alcohol abuse, depression, severe nutrient deficiencies, sleep disorders, stroke, and thyroid imbalance—all of which can usually be prevented or treated. Mental cloudiness may also be a side effect of medications. Older people, of course, are more likely to be taking medication—often, more than one.

Finally, what appears to be poor memory may reflect poor hearing or failing eyesight, rather than actual memory loss. Those age-related declines can interfere with the ability to receive information—to hear a person's name when introduced, or to see the television remote sitting on the sofa.

Preserve your memories

As we reported in May, regular exercise, a nutritious diet, and other healthy habits may help older people preserve their mental faculties. A study of some 5000 Seattle residents found that those who stayed physically healthy were more likely to remain mentally sharp in their 70s and 80s. One possible explanation is that chronic illnesses such as hypertension, coronary heart disease, and lung disease may reduce the brain's oxygen supply or even cause tiny, unnoticed strokes. Or it may also be that people who feel sick avoid mentally challenging activity. Research suggests that such mental exercise may help preserve the mind, just as physical exercise preserves the body.

It's never too late to become mentally active—learn a language, study a new subject, play chess. Indeed, some studies suggest that becoming mentally active may help older people reverse any decline in memory and other mental abilities. (For more detail, see [Consumer Reports'] May report on healthy habits.)

Clearing the cobwebs

If forgetfulness causes problems in your life, there are ways to give your natural powers an assist, regardless of your age. The most fundamental step is to focus your attention, since memory often fails due to sensory overload—too many things going on at once. Try to limit yourself to one task at a time. Beyond that, studies have found that various mnemonic techniques—tricks for remembering things—do work. Here are some of the most effective techniques for different situations.

To remember names:

■ Pause after an introduction and use the person's name. Say "Glad to meet you, Mr. Feltman." Recite the name to yourself. Don't hesitate to ask a new acquaintance to repeat his or her name.

■ Try to associate a new name with something distinctive about that person. John Feltman, for example, may have hair like felt. Liz Jones may have eyes like Liz Taylor.

■ Before a social gathering, think about who might be there and practice linking names and faces.

A HOME TEST OF FAILING MEMORY

The following test is designed to provide a rough measure of the severity of memory problems. Lower-than-normal scores on this test don't necessarily signal Alzheimer's disease or other forms of dementia. Low scoring can occur for a number of reasons—but medical evaluation may be warranted.

THE PERSON WHO IS GOING TO TAKE THIS TEST SHOULD STOP READING HERE. A close friend or family member can read on to administer the test. Complete all items in turn and add up points at the end. The maximum possible score is 35 points.

20 to 35 points: Normal. No serious memory problem.

15 to 19 points: Borderline. Repeat the test in a few months; if worse, consult a doctor for evaluation.

Below 15 points: Low. Consult a doctor for evaluation.

STOP

1 Examiner: "I'm going to tell you a short story. Remember all you can about it. After the story, I'll ask you to repeat it to me. At the end of this test, I'll ask you to repeat the story again. 'An airplane with 203 people on board left New York for Washington. The experienced pilot became ill but the confident young co-pilot landed the plane safely.'"

Score one point for each of these seven details recalled immediately after story: • 203 people on board • Airplane • From New York • Washington • Pilot ill • Confident co-pilot • Safe landing

2 Examiner: "I'm going to say three words. I want you to repeat them right after I'm done. I'll ask you the words again in a few minutes, 'CAT, BOOK, PEN.'"

Score one point for each word.

3 Examiner: "I'll now tell you a word and I would like you to spell it backward. The word is 'WORLD.'"

Score one point for each letter in the correct place.

4 Examiner: "Could you now remember the three words that I told you earlier?"

Score one point for each word.

5 Examiner: "Please subtract 7 from 100." (If the answer given is incorrect, go on to question 6. If the answer is correct, ask the subject to continue subtracting 7 from each successive answer until he or she reaches 30 or has given 10 answers. The correct sequence is 93, 86, 79, 72, 65, 58, 51, 44, 37, 30.)

Score one point for each correct answer.

6 Examiner: "Tell me about the story we started with, giving as much detail as you can."

Score one point for each of the seven details listed in question 1. (This is the most important part of the test. Normal recall at this point is four to seven details. But more significant is how many details have been lost since the start of the test; there should be no more than one fewer detail recalled now than had been recalled initially. A person with dementia may recall a total of only one or two details by now.)

Memory test and flowchart courtesy of "Which? Way to Health," a magazine published by Consumers Union's sister organization, Consumers' Association, London, England.

And don't set out to learn the name of every new face you meet; instead, concentrate on remembering just the ones that might matter most to you.

Summing up

The decline in memory that accompanies aging is usually mild—annoying, not debilitating. Severe memory loss can signal Alzheimer's disease, but it may also be due to medication, depression, or some other underlying condition that can be remedied.

What to do

- If you're concerned about memory loss, follow the flowchart and take the home test to gauge the severity of memory problems and to help determine the need for professional evaluation.
- To shore up a sagging memory, practice the mnemonic techniques for help remembering names, things, actions, and lists and processes.
- Stay physically fit and mentally active to preserve your mind along with your body.

To remember actions:

■ Jot everything down. Record appointments in a pocket calendar. Use adhesive notes, such as *Post-its*. Keep a notebook or even a tape recorder handy.

■ Set a watch alarm to help remember appointments. Use a watch or a cooking timer to remind you to follow through on necessary tasks—like turning off the stove when the potatoes are done.

To remember things:

■ Set fixed locations for the things you tend to misplace—keys, wallet, television remote. Always return each item to its assigned spot.

■ Designate a place near the front door for anything you'll want to take with you. Put each item there as soon as you decide you'll need it.

■ Set standard places to put your belongings when you're away from home—such as the front seat of your car, or the left side of your chair in a restaurant.

To remember lists and processes:

■ String items together according to their similarities, importance, location, or whatever method fits. For example, if you've got several errands to run, remember them by the route you'll be taking.

■ Visualize yourself going through the steps of a new process. Once you've deciphered the instructions on a new VCR, for example, imagine yourself performing all the operations.

■ Invent an acronym. For example, FILM (Fred, Irene, Louise, Mark) would help you recall the names of a relative's children. Telephone numbers work especially well as acronyms, using the letters on the push buttons. Even if you can't devise a good word, the attempt itself may fix the items in your mind.

■ Do regular chores at the same time every day. Feed the goldfish, for example, right after you've had your breakfast.

■ Take medications at the same times every day. Keep pills on your dresser, on the breakfast table, or near anything else you use routinely. To keep track of whether you've taken your pills, fill out a calendar with "P's" for each time you're supposed to take them. Then circle a "P" whenever you do. Or use a multi-compartment pill box, sold in drugstores.

■ Focus your attention as you complete tasks that you might wonder about later. Say to yourself, for example, "I'm locking the door now." To help remember you did it *today*, not yesterday, note the weather or what you're wearing as you lock the door.

ALZHEIMER'S: TARNISHING THE GOLDEN YEARS

If memory lapses have you worried about Alzheimer's disease, you can probably relax. Fretting and complaining about such lapses and seeking reassurance that they're not a sign of impending senility are normal responses to normal, age-related memory impairment. Experts say that a person with true brain disease is more likely to exhibit signs of denial or to try to hide the deficit.

It takes a battery of physical, neurological, and psychological tests to diagnose Alzheimer's with 80 to 90 percent accuracy. A sure diagnosis can be made only on autopsy. Still, the following signs suggest a serious problem that might indicate Alzheimer's:

■ **Severe memory loss.** Anyone can misplace keys. A person with Alzheimer's might not *recognize* keys.

■ **Extreme disorientation.** It's easy to get lost when you're away from home; Alzheimer's victims can get lost in their own backyard.

■ **Changes in mood or personality.** A person with Alzheimer's may move suddenly from laughter to tears, or may become suspicious for no reason.

■ **Speech problems.** An Alzheimer's victim often has trouble finding the right words for things, or mixes up words in a sentence.

■ **Loss of reasoning.** This deficit can show up as the inability to generalize from or interpret simple proverbs.

■ **Inappropriate behavior.** Anyone might forget to wear gloves in cold weather. Someone with Alzheimer's can forget a coat or even pants.

There's clearly a genetic component to Alzheimer's disease; this summer, researchers reported several breakthroughs in the discovery of genes that appear to play a key role in the development of the disease in some people. Aluminum, long suspected of promoting Alzheimer's, apparently doesn't, judging by reviews of dozens of studies covering every kind of exposure to aluminum. Now zinc has come under suspicion. But there are as yet no solid data to justify avoiding that important nutrient.

Recent studies have hinted that the risk of developing Alzheimer's disease may be lower in women on estrogen replacement therapy and in people who regularly use nonsteroidal anti-inflammatory drugs, typically prescribed for arthritis. Those findings have provided researchers with interesting leads to pursue, but the evidence is far too preliminary to suggest preventive regimens.

The only drug specifically approved for Alzheimer's disease is tacrine (*Cognex*), which can improve brain function somewhat in anywhere from 5 to 40 percent of patients, though it won't halt the disease. Several other drugs are being tested. For details on clinical trials, or for more information on Alzheimer's, including a referral to services in your area, call the Alzheimer's Association at 800-272-3900. Or contact your county or state department of health.

Physical Symptoms

Although we may tend to associate only psychological symptoms with mental disorders, a significant number of symptoms of these disorders are physical in nature. For example, although we know about the emotional and cognitive symptoms of depression, this disorder is frequently diagnosed when individuals seek help from a family physician for the physical symptoms associated with their depression. A growing body of research is explicating the intricate connections between the mind and the body. This connection is apparent in research that describes how stress affects the body in a number of ways, including its effects on the immune system.

Everyone is familiar with the word stress; it is part of the vocabulary of our times. Moreover, most people view modern society as filled with stress. We see ourselves as victims of a long and growing list of stressors. The majority of visits to physicians are related to the effects of stress. Hans Selye's general adaptation syndrome describes the bodily changes that occur when we are stressed. Nowadays, there is growing recognition that we must add an important element to the stress equation: how individuals perceive potential stressors is a significant factor in understanding stress reactions. There is a growing awareness that people are stressed not by things but by their interpretation of things. In arriving at this conclusion, we have returned to an understanding that was first enunciated by a Greek orator centuries ago. Researchers also suggest that psychological factors such as stress and depression may play roles in the development of physical disorders such as heart disease. Moreover, these findings suggest that behavioral medicine and health psychology interventions can reduce the costs of delivering medical care. Evidence for this cost reduction strengthens a belief in the close association between physical and psychological health.

One of the most devastating disorders that affects young people, especially females, is anorexia nervosa. This disorder occurs primarily in Western cultures such as the United States, so, naturally, one wonders what it is about our culture that leads to the disorder. In "Dying to Win," the tragic story of a world-class gymnast who died of anorexia nervosa, focuses attention on the disorder and its possible causes. Anorexia nervosa involves the interaction of biological, social, and cultural factors. Moreover, it has a high rate of comorbidity—the tendency for other disorders to exist simultaneously.

Not all of the disorders we may encounter are outlined in the *Diagnostic and Statistical Manual of Mental Disorders* (*DSM-IV*) published by the American Psychiatric Association. For example, the *DSM* does not use the term *Mun-*

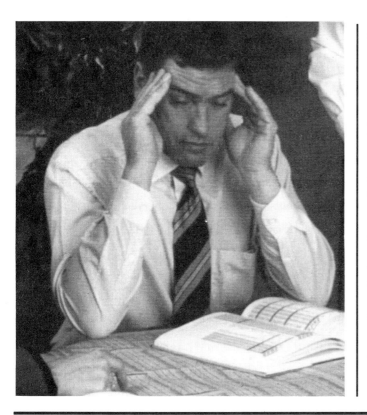

chausen by proxy, which is a tragic and bizarre disorder. Patients exhibiting Munchausen syndrome produce physical symptoms in themselves. It is named for a German baron who was well known for telling embellished, but basically true stories. In trying to understand this disorder, we must recognize that physical symptoms often lead to attention and sympathy, which can be powerful motivators. In another version of this disorder, Munchausen by proxy, an adult produces physical symptoms in another person (usually the adult's child). Mental health practitioners are just beginning to investigate and treat this very dangerous disorder.

Looking Ahead: Challenge Questions

How have the stressors that affect people changed over the last century? How do you anticipate that they will change over the next century?

What is the role of psychology in the delivery of health services to the public? How can psychologists make health delivery more effective and efficient?

How could we reduce the incidence of anorexia nervosa, especially among groups such as female athletes?

What safeguards should be put in place in order to recognize potential cases of Munchausen by proxy?

Hearts and Minds — Part I

In the constant search for ways to thwart heart disease, physicians and scientists have repeatedly examined the effects of mental states. Anything that might throw light on the causes or treatment of myocardial infarction (heart attacks) and coronary artery disease would be of enormous medical significance. Researchers are especially interested in learning whether psychotherapy may be useful, either to prolong life and maintain health in patients with these disorders or to prevent the disorders from developing in the first place. The main subjects under investigation have been depression and anxiety, personality, anger, stress, loneliness, and the suppression or repression of feelings. The findings present many problems of interpretation because the relationships are so complex and difficult to unravel. Both credulity and incredulity must be avoided in considering claims about the influence of our emotions on the chief killer in the industrial world.

The role of depression

In the United States, 2% of the population is depressed at any given time, but in patients with heart disease the number is closer to 20%. One in six people in the general population but (according to some estimates) nearly 50% of heart patients have suffered an episode of major depression. In a recent large survey, the Center for Health Statistics found that even moderate depression was associated with a 60% greater likelihood of high blood pressure. In another study, depression raised the rate of ischemic heart disease (caused by obstructed coronary arteries) by 60% and the rate of heart attacks by 50% after adjustment for smoking, drinking, poor nutrition, and lack of exercise. In another survey of 3,000 subjects, the National Health and Nutrition Examination Epidemiological Follow-up Study, researchers recently found that after adjustment for age, sex, weight, diabetes, and stroke, depression and anxiety significantly raised the risk that high blood pressure would develop within 7 to 16 years.

In 1996, researchers in Baltimore presented the results of a 10-year study with 1,500 participants. They found that after statistical correction for age, sex, high blood pressure, and other health risks, people with a history of depression were four times more likely to have a heart attack. The flaws in this study were a high dropout rate and reliance for evidence of past depression on the subjects' memories, which might have been biased by present poor health.

A 1992 study of 1,200 middle-age Finnish men indicated that although mild to moderate depression alone was not directly associated with arteriosclerosis, men who smoked were three and a half times more likely to suffer from arteriosclerosis if they suffered from depression as well. The depressed men also had twice the average level of low density lipoprotein (LDL, the dangerous kind), even when they had no symptoms of heart disease. In a 1988 report, members of the Harvard classes of 1939 to 1944 were evaluated as pessimistic or optimistic on the basis of essays they had written in college. The more pessimistic they had been, the greater the chance that they would develop atherosclerosis and other chronic diseases by age 45.

A 27-year study of more than 700 Danish men and women suggests that depressive symptoms, even in the absence of clinical depression, can play a role in a person's first heart attack or first symptoms of heart disease. The risk of a heart attack rose steadily with ratings for depression on the Minnesota Multiphasic Personality Inventory (MMPI), a personality questionnaire. People whose scores stood in the top 15% were 71% more likely to have a heart attack and 59% more likely to die than those in the lowest 15%. The association persisted even after statistical correction for physical symptoms (loss of appetite, insomnia, backaches, headaches, chronic fatigue) that might have resulted from either depression or a heart condition. As further evidence that the symptoms were not just signs of incipient heart disease, the researchers found that the sub-

From *Harvard Mental Health Letter,* July 1997, pp. 1-4. © 1997 by the President and Fellows of Harvard College. Reprinted by permission.

jects had no heart attacks in the first year after the original evaluation.

Depression also seems to affect the chance of survival after a heart attack. Researchers in St. Louis found that patients with recently diagnosed heart disease who had symptoms of major depression in the hospital were more likely to suffer a "cardiac event" (heart attack, surgery, or death) in the next year. In fact, major depression was more highly associated with cardiac events than age, high cholesterol, smoking, high blood pressure, or diabetes.

Canadian researchers studying 200 patients who had recently had heart attacks came to similar conclusions. After six months, 12 had died, and 6 of them were among the 35 who had been seriously depressed at the original interview. At 18 months, the death rate in the most depressed was 20%, as compared with an average of 6%. Depression predicted death as well as previous heart attacks or poor heart functioning did. Of patients with a previous history of depression who were also depressed after their heart attack, 50% died within 18 months, compared with 10% of patients who became depressed in the hospital for the first time in their lives. Pessimism at the time of the heart attack was also an accurate predictor of death — in fact, better than artery blockage, high blood pressure, cholesterol, and damage to the heart muscle. Eight years after their heart attack, 21 of the 25 most pessimistic and only 6 of the 25 most optimistic patients had died.

Anxiety and panic disorder

Anxiety has also been associated with heart disease and death from heart attacks. In a long-term study of the population of Framingham, Massachusetts, men with high levels of anxiety early in life — as indicated by their own reports of tension, tightness, restlessness, headaches, and other symptoms — had twice the average rate of high blood pressure 20 years later. None of the standard dietary and health risk factors predicted the development of high blood pressure. In the same study, researchers found that high anxiety more than tripled the risk of a fatal heart attack over a 32-year period. But highly anxious men did not have a higher rate of angina (chest pain caused by obstructed coronary arteries) or nonfatal heart disease, and neither anxiety nor any other psychological state in youth was associated with later high blood pressure in women.

Panic disorder is another condition sometimes associated with heart disease. A British study of 1,500 middle-age men found that those with symptoms of panic, although otherwise healthy, had an increased risk of dying from heart disease. In a two-year Harvard study of 34,000 men, those with a high rating for phobic symptoms were more likely to die from heart attacks (although not more likely to have heart attacks). Overlapping symptoms present a problem here, since chest pain, shortness of breath, and dizzy spells can be warning signs of a heart problem as well as symptoms of a panic attack.

Type A personality

Much research and analysis has been devoted to the subject of heart disease and the Type A personality. A 1964 study found that middle-age people considered Type A — ambitious, competitive, workaholic, sometimes irritable and impatient — had a much greater risk of heart disease than calmer, more passive or even-tempered personalities, even after correction for standard medical risk factors. But results since then have been inconclusive and mostly negative. In a recent 22-year study of 750 subjects, men described as "pressured" and "socially dominant" had a higher death rate from heart disease than those who were more placid. But other studies have found no relationship, and a 1995 meta-analysis (compilation and statistical re-analysis) of nearly 300 studies including 25,000 subjects suggests that Type A personality is not associated with high blood pressure.

One problem is that the traits described as Type A may have different meanings in different circumstances; for example, the personality style is less distinctive in a culture that values and promotes individualism and achievement. There may be class differences as well. In the Framingham Heart Study, the risk of heart disease was high for Type A personalities not among blue-collar men but only among middle-class. The concept of Type A itself has been challenged as obscuring more than it explains. It is not a personality disorder or even a term ordinarily used by psychiatrists to describe a personality type. Critics believe the label has been applied to a mixture of traits and symptoms that are better analyzed separately. For example, Type A personality is sometimes associated with emotional distress, neurosis, and anger, but these are not necessary correlates of drive and ambition or even of a tendency toward impatience.

High levels of hostility alone may better indicate both the danger of developing heart disease and the chance that a person with a heart condition will suffer sudden death. In a seven-year study of men over 60, those who showed the highest level of anger on the MMPI had three times the average risk of a heart attack and fatal heart disease. In a study of 800 subjects, Yale researchers found that students who scored high in hostility on a personality test as freshmen had higher levels of cholesterol and were more likely to be smokers 20 years later. A study of 1,300 men in Boston revealed that those with high scores for anger on a questionnaire (with such statements as "At times I feel like picking a fistfight" and "I have been so angry that I felt as if I would explode") were three times more likely than low scorers to develop heart disease in the next seven years (after correction for the usual medical risk factors).

In the long-term Finnish study of 1,200 middle-age men, those who admitted to being argumentative, irritable, or easily angered were considerably more likely to die if they had both high blood pressure and ischemic heart disease (the result of narrowed and inflexible arteries). Angina was almost three times more common in the 5% with the highest level of hostility than in the 35% with the lowest level. The overall death rate of the most hostile was three times higher, and their death rate from heart disease 2.4 times higher. Among men with high blood pressure and heart disease, those with the highest hostility levels had 13 times the death rate of men with more placid temperaments.

Anger and heart disease

Anger can also be dangerous once heart disease sets in. When people with heart disease are asked to recall an incident that made them angry, their blood pressure rises and the amount of blood pumped by the heart at each beat (the ventricular ejection fraction) falls significantly. In a Harvard study of 1,600 men and women who had had a heart attack, 2% said they had been enraged, with such symptoms as clenched fists and table pounding, at some time in the two hours before the attack. The researchers estimated that the risk of a heart attack was doubled in the two hours following one of these episodes.

The findings on this subject are not entirely consistent. In the Framingham Heart Study, a high level of anger at the original interview was not associated with high blood pressure 20 years later. In a 20-year study at the Mayo Clinic, researchers found that high hostility (believing others to be dishonest or immoral) raised the risk of heart disease and death, but the correlations vanished after corrections for age, sex, and weight. The weaknesses of this study included a high dropout rate and a lack of information on smoking and cholesterol.

Suppressing anger may also be risky. A Belgian study found that heart attack survivors with a strong tendency to suppress their feelings were 27% more likely to die within ten years (after correction for the usual medical risk factors). In another study, women who indicated at age 18 that they often suppressed anger were three times more likely to have died than

women who either expressed their anger or rarely became angry. In this study, competitiveness and work addiction alone were not dangerous to the heart.

Chronic resentment, grudge carrying, cynicism, and mistrust are difficult to judge and measure and are not necessarily correlated with overt rage. Another possibly related condition is alexithymia (the Greek means "no words for emotions"), or an inability to identify and describe one's feelings, even after an outburst of anger or tears (see *Mental Health Letter*, June 1989). Alexithymic persons are often said to be unimaginative, boring, and lacking in empathy; some studies suggest that individuals with this personality type have an increased susceptibility to heart disease and other illnesses. The 1996 meta-analysis of 300 studies revealed an association between high blood pressure and what the reviewers interpreted as defensiveness (presumably unfelt or denied anger), but no association with conscious anger, either expressed or suppressed.

Stress takes a toll

The cardiac effects of stress have been studied apart from specific feelings and personality traits. Acute stress raises blood pressure and can be especially dangerous for people with heart conditions. In an experiment at Duke University, researchers induced mental stress in patients with coronary artery disease by asking them to perform arithmetic calculations, draw from a reflected image, and make a public speech. After adjustment for age and prior heart condition, patients who developed angina during the experiment had three times the average rate of heart attacks, surgery, or death from heart disease in the next five years. That was higher than the rate of cardiac events among patients who developed angina during a bicycle exercise test. In another experiment, 63 patients with atherosclerosis were asked to wear devices that recorded the heart's activity for a day or two while they made notes on their physical activities and emotional states. Recordings indicating ischemia (an insufficient supply of blood to the heart muscle, sometimes resulting in chest tension or angina) were just as closely associated with intense anger or anxiety as with strenuous physical activities like climbing stairs.

Chronic stress, like chronic hostility and resentment, is more difficult to identify and measure. A study of more than 2,400 Danish bus drivers found a high risk of heart disease among those with more traffic congestion on their routes. In another study, the risk for Italian railway workers was found to rise with greater job responsibility as well as less physical activity. In contrast, Swedish researchers found a higher rate of heart disease in men who lacked decision-making power and discretion in their work than in those who had some control and independence (independence and discretion were judged by the job description). But work that was mentally strenuous or performed under time pressure did not raise the risk of heart disease.

Most researchers have not found a strong relationship between death from chronic physical illness and "objectively" stress-provoking events — those that most people would regard as disturbing, disappointing, or demoralizing. One exception is a study in which Swedish researchers followed the lives of 750 50-year-old men for seven years, during which 41 died — 13 from heart disease, 18 from cancer, and 11 from alcohol-related illnesses. The chance of dying was not affected by a man's cholesterol level, weight, or blood pressure at 50, nor by his stated belief that he was under stress. Men were more likely to die if their marriages had broken up or they had financial troubles or had lost a job in the previous year.

Part 2 can be found in the August 1997 issue of *The Harvard Mental Health Letter.*

FOR FURTHER READING

George C. Chrousos and Philip W. Gold. The concepts of stress and stress system disorders: Overview of physical and behavioral homeostasis. *Journal of the American Medical Association 267: 1244–1252 (March 4, 1992).*

Catherine Frank and Stephen Smith. Stress and the heart: Biobehavioral aspects of sudden cardiac death. *Psychosomatics 31: 255–264 (1990).*

Randall S. Jorgensen, Blair T. Johnson, Monika E. Kolodziej, and George E. Schreer. Elevated blood pressure and personality: A meta-analytic review. *Psychological Bulletin 120: 293–320 (1996).*

W. Linden, C. Stossel, and J. Maurice. Psychosocial intervention for patients with coronary artery disease: A meta-analysis. *Archives of Internal Medicine 156: 745–752 (April 8, 1996).*

Bert N. Uchino, John T. Cacioppo, and Janice K. Kiecolt-Glaser. The relationship between social support and physiological processes: A review with emphasis on underlying mechanisms and implications for health. *Psychological Bulletin 119: 488–531 (1996).*

Behavioral Medicine, Clinical Health Psychology, and Cost Offset

Richard Friedman
State University of New York at Stony Brook
and Deaconess Hospital, Harvard Medical School

David Sobel
Kaiser Permanente Medical Care Program,
Northern California Region

Patricia Myers
State University of New York at Stony Brook

Margaret Caudill and Herbert Benson
Deaconess Hospital, Harvard Medical School

The use of medical services is a function of several interacting psychological and social variables as well as a function of physical malfunction. The clinical significance of addressing patients' psychosocial issues has only occasionally been considered. However, the shift in health care economics toward health care maintenance is responsible for the increased interest in interventions in the domain of behavioral medicine and health psychology. Evidence is reviewed for 6 mechanistic pathways by which behavioral interventions can maximize clinical care and result in significant economic benefits. The rationale for further integration of behavioral and biomedicine interventions is also reviewed.

Key words: cost offset, behavioral medicine

The current health care reform agenda represents both a threat and an opportunity for mental health providers and behavioral scientists. The health care system is reeling under the impact of escalating costs, limited access, and the prospect of an aging population with multiple chronic illnesses that will increase demand for health care. Traditionally, the primary focus of most mental health providers has been on the diagnosis and treatment of mental illness—an important and challenging undertaking in itself. However, the current health care debate challenges health care providers to look beyond diagnostic categories and disciplinary boundaries, beyond the dysfunctional distinction between mind and body, and beyond traditional psychotherapeutic interventions. The challenge is to most effectively address the true needs that people bring into the health care system and to do so with maximum efficiency.

Increasingly, the focus of health care reform is controlling costs, and the secondary focus is on improving health and quality outcomes. Although studies have shown that providing psychological services can reduce health care costs (Pallak, Cummings, Dorken, & Henke, 1995), the national health care reform agenda, driven by a concern for cost containment, ensures that medical services in general and mental health services in particular will be examined in great detail. There is

Richard Friedman, Department of Psychiatry and Behavioral Science, State University of New York at Stony Brook, and Mind/Body Medical Institute, Deaconess Hospital, Harvard Medical School; David Sobel, Regional Health Education Department, Kaiser Permanente Medical Care Program, Northern California Region; Patricia Myers, Department of Psychiatry and Behavioral Science, State University of New York at Stony Brook; Margaret Caudill and Herbert Benson, Mind/Body Medical Institute, Deaconess Hospital, Harvard Medical School.

Correspondence concerning this article should be addressed to Richard Friedman, Department of Psychiatry and Behavioral Science, State University of New York at Stony Brook, Putnam Hall, South Campus, Stony Brook, New York 11794-8790.

reason for optimism, however, partly on the basis of the evidence summarized below and elsewhere that psychosocial interventions can improve both health and cost outcomes (Sobel, 1995).

Most recommendations offered to reduce health care costs involve "supply-side" strategies such as altering access to health care, improving the efficiency of services, examining more closely the utilization and capitated payments, decreasing practice variation, and limiting technology. Seldom is the "demand side" of the health care equation given equal consideration. What determines the demand and need for medical service? Patients are more likely to seek care when they have symptoms, but the presence or severity of symptoms or conditions account for a surprisingly small portion of the variability in health care use. Studies have found that only 12–25% of health care use can be predicted by objective disability or morbidity alone (Berkanovic, Telesky, & Reeder, 1981). It appears that health care seeking is a complex behavior that is influenced strongly by psychosocial factors such as individual attitudes, perceptions, cultural norms, and levels of psychosocial distress. Lynch (1993) has conceptualized the demand for health care as having four components: morbidity (the presence or absence of illness), perceived need (individuals' perceptions of the severity of a given problem), patient preference (patients differ in the treatment options they choose on the basis of their knowledge and beliefs about risks and benefits), and nonhealth motives (patients may manipulate the system just for benefits such as time off from work).

Clearly, behavioral and psychosocial variables significantly influence the need and demand for health services (Fries et al., 1993). Unhealthy behaviors, from smoking to diet and drug use to a sedentary lifestyle, are the major contributors to morbidity. In addition to behavior patterns contributing to illness, psychosocial variables have increasingly been implicated in health care utilization. For example, Kroenke and Mangelsdorff (1989) reviewed the records of over 1,000 patients in

From *Health Psychology*, Vol. 14, No. 6, 1995, pp. 509-518. © 1995 by the American Psychological Association. Reprinted by permission.

an internal medicine clinic over a 3-year period. In less than 16% of cases was the origin of the most common somatic complaints identified as being organic. The authors concluded that in 74% of the cases with unknown etiology "it was probable that many of the symptoms ... were related to psychosocial factors" (p. 265).

Evidence that attending to the psychological needs of medical patients was advantageous both clinically and economically was provided by Cummings and Follette (1968). They found that for patients at a large health maintenance organization (HMO) more than 60% of all visits were made by the "worried well" with no diagnosable disorder. Not only did psychotherapy help these patients but the direct costs of providing treatment was "offset" by reductions in subsequent general medical use.

Understanding that the demand for medical services is motivated not solely on the basis of the physical components of disease is crucial to improving medical care and reducing medical costs. Managing demand to control costs can be done by developing interventions to address the "pathways" by which psychosocial factors influence the need and decision to seek medical care. For description purposes we have identified six pathways by which psychosocial factors drive medical utilization and costs. We also provide examples of the evidence that addressing the psychological and behavioral aspects of illness can decrease medical utilization and costs. The savings from reduced medical utilization can also more than offset the cost of providing the behavioral interventions, resulting in total cost savings. The pathway categories clearly overlap and interact. Patients often present with a combination of psychosocial factors that motivate their medical utilization. Similarly, most of the cost-effective behavioral interventions that we use as examples cross over to impact multiple pathways to utilization.

Information and Decision-Support Pathway

The medical community has traditionally placed patients in a very passive role. Patients frequently feel that their only responsibility is the selection of a competent health care provider who will then diagnose and prescribe. This dependency on health professionals undermines patients' self-confidence and ability to distinguish symptoms and problems that can be safely self-managed and those that would benefit from professional attention. Many unnecessary and costly visits to professionals are occasioned by a lack of information and confidence in appropriate self-management and use of the health care system. Patients are not just consumers of health care. With over 80% of all illness episodes self-diagnosed and self-treated without professional consultation, patients are, in fact, the true primary health care providers in the health care system (Demers, Altamore, Mustin, Kleinman, & Leonardi, 1980; White, Williams, & Greenberg, 1961).

With both acute and chronic conditions, maximal clinical efficacy and economic efficiency require a far more active participation on the part of patients. Teaching patients how to effectively distinguish those symptoms and circumstances that require professional attention from those that can be self-treated is becoming increasingly important. For a variety of illnesses, patients can be taught specific intervention strategies that can be safely and effectively applied to remediate symptoms. In many cases, the clinician can assume the role of

teacher who will naturally want to maintain a sufficiently good relationship with the patient so that the patient feels comfortable turning to the clinician should the circumstances dictate.

Empowering patients in appropriate self-care can be enhanced through print and audiovisual materials, professional teaching one-on-one or in groups, as well as the emergence of peer-led support groups. Such interventions are paying remarkable dividends in terms of improved quality of care, reduced symptoms, enhanced satisfaction, and reduced costs (Kemper, Lorig, & Mettler, 1993).

Evidence of Cost Offset

Parents of children sick with a fever are naturally fearful, confused, and concerned. These feelings often result in a visit to the pediatrician for reassurance. In nearly 25% of all acute pediatric visits, fever is a chief complaint. A randomized clinical study was conducted at Kaiser Permanente in southern California to evaluate the cost effectiveness of an office health education program designed to improve knowledge, skills, and sense of confidence about fever in children. At follow-up the group receiving the health intervention evidenced decreased medical visits for fever and for other acute illnesses (Robinson, Schwartz, Magwene, Krengel, & Tamburello, 1989).

In a controlled study, patients were offered a self-care book, a telephone information service, and individual counseling by a trained nurse. The self-care guide contained information on nearly 100 common symptoms and advice about home treatment and when to call a physician. In patients exposed to the intervention, visits for minor illnesses were reduced by 35% as a result of the program, and the total use of ambulatory care services was reduced by 17%. For every $1 that was spent on self-care education in the program, $2.50 was saved in medical costs (Vickery et al., 1983).

Teaching self-management skills is particularly critical for patients with chronic illness. Providing patients with social support, skill building, and accurate information regarding the nature and treatment of disease stimulates and engenders feelings of self-control, empowerment, and self-efficacy, which further enhance clinical outcome. The clinical and economic importance of self-efficacy was examined in a series of studies conducted at the Stanford Arthritis Center (Lorig et al., 1989; Lorig, Mazonson, & Holman, 1993). Patients and their families participated in an arthritis self-management course conducted by lay leaders who themselves often had arthritis. Results showed that it was not the patients who learned more about arthritis that did better but rather those who evidenced a greater sense of self-efficacy, or a conviction in their ability to manage their arthritis. At 4-year follow-up, in addition to participants experiencing a marked increase in self-efficacy and a 20% reduction in pain, they also reported a 43% decrease in physician visits as compared with pretreatment levels. On the basis of the reduced physician visit rates, adjusted 4-year health care savings were $648 per person with rheumatoid arthritis and $189 per person with osteoarthritis. Given these figures, if only 1% of the patients in the United States with moderate-to-severe osteoarthritis of the hand (103,000) and only 1% of the patients with classical or definite rheumatoid arthritis (21,000) participated in the arthritis self-management program, total discounted savings over 4 years would equal $19.5 million for osteoarthritis and $13.6 million for rheumatoid arthritis.

Psychophysiological Pathway

Psychological stress itself can generate profound effects on the body by stimulating what has been termed the fight-or-flight response (Cannon, 1941). The fight-or-flight response is a heightened state of sympathetic nervous system arousal that prepares the body for vigorous muscular activity. Repeated exposure to everyday annoyances or prolonged stress can trigger the fight-or-flight response, which in turn effects the skeletal muscular system, the autonomic nervous system, and the neuroendocrine system. The importance of stress in the etiology and exacerbation of a wide variety of illnesses is documented in an extensive experimental literature and a growing clinical literature (Gatchel & Blanchard, 1993).

The physiological opposite of the fight-or-flight response is the relaxation response. Whereas the fight-or-flight response involves central and peripheral nervous system changes that prepare the organism for action, the relaxation response involves central and peripheral nervous system changes that prepare the organism for calmness and behavioral inactivity. The same physiological relaxation response pattern (Benson & Stuart, 1992) can be achieved in numerous ways, including progressive muscle relaxation, focused attention, yoga, meditation, prayer (Benson, Beary, & Carol, 1974), or even repetitive exercise (Benson, Dryer, & Hartley, 1978). There is a substantial literature that documents the significance of the control of stress in the treatment of many diseases such as arthritis (Lorig et al., 1993) as well as hypertension, cardiac arrhythmias, insomnia, premenstrual syndrome, infertility, and the nausea and vomiting associated with chemotherapy (Benson & Stuart, 1992). There is a growing literature suggesting the efficacy of stress management in the treatment of cancer (Fawzy et al., 1993; Spiegel, Bloom, Kraemer, & Gottheil, 1989). To the extent that stress plays a role in either etiology or exacerbation of disease and to the extent that increased disease is costly to society, it is economically reasonable to include stress management in comprehensive treatment.

Evidence of Cost Offset

The impact of modifying and controlling autonomic reactivity through biofeedback and relaxation albeit considerable can only be estimated. As Schneider (1987) has pointed out in her review, there are no studies that examine the cost effectiveness of biofeedback alone because biofeedback is generally administered as part of a clinical package. Several studies have attempted to estimate cost effectiveness by examining reductions in physician visits and medication use.

A study of medicated and nonmedicated patients with hypertension conducted at the Menninger Clinic (Fahrion, Norris, Green, Green, & Schnar, 1987) reported decreased medication use as well as lowered blood pressure readings following a multi-modal biobehavioral treatment that included biofeedback-assisted training to regulate the vasodilation in patients' hands and feet. Over half of the medicated patients were able to eliminate hypertensive medication and reduce their blood pressure after treatment. Of the unmedicated patients in the sample, 22% showed clinically significant reductions in blood pressure readings. Fahrion et al. estimated that the cost savings for medication over a 5-year period would be $738. This savings was assuming that the group treatment cost was $600 per patient and that the average 5-year medication cost was $1,338 per patient.

Shellenberger, Turner, Green, and Cooney (1986) reported that physician visits were significantly reduced among a group of individuals who participated in a biofeedback and stress management program. Participants received a stress profile and 10 weeks of biofeedback-assisted relaxation training. Control participants received only a stress profile. At 2-year follow-up, the stress management group reported a 70% reduction in visits to physicians, whereas the control group reported a 26% increase.

Numerous studies have attempted to reduce the acute stress of hospitalization and surgery. The effects of psychoeducational interventions on postsurgical outcome was examined through a meta-analysis on 191 studies conducted between 1963 and 1989 (Devine, 1992). Seventy-nine percent to 84% of the studies indicated that there were beneficial effects from interventions, such as providing health care information, skill building, and psychosocial support. Length of hospital stay following surgery for patients given such interventions was decreased by an average of 1.5 days. Using a conservative estimate of $200 in savings from hospital expenses and $20 in educational costs, $10 would have been saved for every $1 invested in patient education.

Behavior Change Pathway

There is little doubt that overt behavior patterns have a great impact on disease. How a patient eats, drinks, smokes, takes prescribed or illegal drugs, and exercises has profound implications for health. Those with higher health risks do tend to have higher medical costs. To the extent that diet, smoking, and exercise patterns could be positively modified, rates of our most widespread illnesses, heart disease and cancer, would be reduced (Ornish et al., 1990). Formal behavior modification programs make sense both clinically and economically because systematic efforts at changing behavior have been shown to be more successful than informal unsystematic efforts (Black & Bruce, 1989).

Along with efforts to change behavior patterns such as smoking, drinking alcohol, and overeating, it is also important both clinically and economically to establish ways to maintain healthy habits and reduce relapse rates. For many patients stressful events can increase the likelihood that they will reengage in anxiety-reducing behaviors that they have used in the past, such as smoking and eating high-fat foods (Heatherton & Renn, 1995). This common pattern has been termed the stress-disinhibition effect (Marlatt, 1985). Coping with stress and anxiety has a "psychic cost" that takes the form of lowered self-regulatory capacity (e.g., Glass, Singer, & Friedman, 1969). Relaxation training has been demonstrated to be a very effective acute coping strategy for anxiety reduction (American Psychiatric Association, 1989) and for maintaining abstinence among ex-smokers (Wynd, 1992). Health care utilization rates can thus be reduced by incorporating strategies that assist patients to stop engaging in unhealthy behaviors and can be further reduced by integrating strategies that help patients maintain their healthy habits.

Attempts to fully integrate systematic behavior modification programs into medical care have been hampered to a significant degree by the reimbursement policies and health plan contracts of insurers and providers. However, it is clear that such behavioral interventions would pay economic dividends to the extent that they obviate the need for more expensive interventions.

Evidence of Cost Offset

Ornish and his colleagues (1990) provided a good example of how an intensive lifestyle change program consisting of maintaining a low-fat diet, exercise, yoga, meditation, and group support can reverse the effects of heart disease and potentially save money. It was widely publicized that Mutual of Omaha would reimburse patients who chose to participate in the program, and it was the first time that such a costly, nonpharmacologic intervention program for heart disease reversal had received such coverage. On the one hand, the motivation on the part of the insurance company to cover the costs of the program, about $3,500 per year, could have been based on the clinical results reported by Ornish and his colleagues that program participants showed reductions in the narrowing of coronary arteries. On the other hand, given the average cost of coronary bypass surgery, about $35,000, the motivation for covering the costs may have made good economic sense as well. If by virtue of participation in behavioral medicine intervention programs only a few bypass operations could be prevented, such programs become cost effective.

Less intensive, low-cost programs to support positive lifestyle and behavior change also appear to have favorable effects on the bottom line. For example, Fries et al. (1993) conducted a study with 4,712 senior citizens in which information was mailed to participants about ways to improve health habits, increase feelings of personal self-efficacy, and increase the appropriate use of health care services. Participants in the experimental group received books and newsletters on health care, a health habits questionnaire, a computer-based personal health risk report every 6 months, and individualized recommendation letters from a physician. Results showed that compared with controls who received only mailed questionnaires, those who received the intervention had overall health risk scores 20% lower than baseline. Improvements were seen in blood pressure, body weight, seat belt use, dietary intake of salt and fat, alcohol use, exercise, smoking, cholesterol levels, and stress levels. Health care expenditures were reduced by 10–20%. The cost of the program was approximately $30 per person per year and reduced health care expenditures by an average of $164 in the 1st year alone. In the control groups, average costs increased $15.

Behavioral medicine interventions can be quite nonintrusive and not labor intensive. They need also not be restricted to the clinic environment. Several studies have demonstrated that behavior modification and stress management programs provided directly at the work site reduce clinical symptoms in targeted populations and reduce use of health services (Pelletier, 1993). These work site studies also afford the opportunity to suggest additional economic advantages of providing behavioral medicine services. The interventions tend to generally increase health and result in positive psychological changes. Most studies have also reported increases in worker productivity and decreases in absenteeism. These effects further increase the economic viability of behavioral medicine above those ascribed to decreased clinic utilization.

Social Support Pathway

Many patients feel isolated and confront perceived or real medical problems without social support. These patients frequently enter the health care system to obtain social support as well as traditional diagnostic and therapeutic services. Even patients who have high levels of social support under ordinary circumstances may develop feelings of isolation when they experience chronic illness. There is evidence that providing social support not only results in increased psychological benefits but may reduce physical symptoms as well. Most studies on social support have not focused on reduced costs as an outcome measure. However, some studies allow economic conclusions to be drawn.

Evidence of Cost Offset

A good example of a positive impact of social support in medical settings was reported by Frasure-Smith (1991). Male patients with myocardial infarction ($n = 461$) were examined over a 5-year period. Participants completed a 20-item General Health Questionnaire (GHQ) a few days before hospital discharge, and those assigned to an experimental group completed the GHQ on a monthly basis through telephone interviews. Participants assigned to a control group received routine medical care. Experimental group patients were supported by nurses' visits when they reported high GHQ stress scores. Patients receiving routine care exhibited an increased risk of cardiac events relative to those receiving the support visits. Although this study demonstrates the important clinical impact of providing social support, it did not directly address economic outcomes. However, by reducing the frequency of nonfatal myocardial infarctions some cost savings may be inferred.

Emotional support during labor and delivery also appears to have a positive effect on health and cost outcomes. Cesarean section (C-section) is the most common surgical procedure performed in the United States, affecting about one in every five deliveries. Delivery by C-section extends the hospital stay of mother and child and increases the risk of maternal infection and other complications.

Five studies have confirmed that the continuous presence of a supportive woman during labor and delivery can reduce the need for C-section, shorten labor and delivery, and reduce perinatal problems (Kennell, Klaus, McGrath, Robertson, & Hinkley, 1991; Klaus, Kennell, Berkowitz, & Klaus, 1992). The intervention was a *doula*—a trained lay person who provided emotional support consisting of praise, reassurance, physical contact (such as rubbing the mother's back or holding her), explanations of what was happening, and a continuous presence. In one study of the 204 patients in the control group, 18% had C-sections, and of the 212 in the group supported by doulas only 8% had C-sections—a reduction of 56%. The presence of a doula also reduced rates of epidural anesthesia by 85%, labor was an average of 2 hr shorter, and only half as many babies required more than 48 hr of hospitalization because of neonatal problems. The cost savings from reduced surgical and anesthesia procedures alone would greatly exceed the $200 cost of providing continuous emotional support from a doula.

Undiagnosed Psychiatric Problem Pathway

In many cases, patients present with somatic symptoms but have undiagnosed psychiatric illnesses. The problems that are increasing medical utilization in this case are not related entirely to physical symptoms but rather to problems such as depression (Jacobs, Kopans, & Reizes, 1995) and generalized anxiety disorder (GAD; Carter & Maddock, 1992). Failure to appropriately diagnose these conditions can have profound clinical and economic implications.

A recent study examining acute chest pain typifies the problem. Patients with acute chest pain ($n = 334$) were prospectively evaluated for panic disorder and depression over an 8-week period. Panic disorder was identified in 17.5% of the cases, and depression was identified in 23.1% of the cases. Importantly, the likelihood of an emergency room visit for chest pain in the previous year was significantly higher for those patients identified as panic disordered and depressed than for those patients without psychiatric disorder. This suggests that psychiatric variables may identify frequent utilizers of emergency room services for chest pain (Yingling, Wulsin, Arnold, & Rouan, 1993). The authors postulated that a third of all patients with chest pain making emergency visits have a current psychiatric disorder. Because the prevalence of psychiatric disturbance is so high, and because it is so clearly a contributor to the unnecessarily high utilization of medical services, careful assessment of psychiatric disorders is required in patients with coronary artery disease (Wulsin & Yingling, 1991). These examples regarding anxiety, depression, and chest pain are indicative of a widespread but poorly defined set of relationships between medical symptom reports and underlying but underdiagnosed psychiatric conditions. Because most physicians are not trained in diagnosing and treating these widespread conditions, an expanded role for experts in psychological and behavioral issues may result in better diagnosis and treatment and also save money.

Although the importance of diagnosing psychiatric problems within the medical population is recognized, standardized psychological screening inventories and interviews are often lengthy and thus impractical for clinical use. Recently, however, Spitzer et al. (1994) developed the Primary Care Evaluation of Mental Disorders (PRIME-MD), a 30-item self-report inventory that assesses four groups of mental disorders (mood, anxiety, somatoform, and alcohol) commonly seen in the clinical settings. The inventory was tested among 1,000 adult patients, and on average it took approximately 8 min for clinicians to complete an evaluation. Spitzer et al. found that 48% of the patients who, through the use of the PRIME-MD, were diagnosed as having a disorder and who had been fairly well-known by their physicians had not had the disorder detected by the physician prior to the assessment. Of more relevance to the current discussion, it was also found that compared with patients without PRIME-MD diagnoses, those diagnosed with disorders had significantly ($p < .005$) lower functioning, more disability days, and higher health care utilization rates.

Evidence of Cost Offset

A particularly good example of how the treatment of psychiatric disorders can reduce health care costs was reported by Strain et al. (1991), who studied a group of elderly patients with hip fractures who had been admitted to the hospital for surgical repair. Strain and his colleagues had noted that relatively few such patients were screened for psychiatric problems before surgery. To determine the degree to which

depression and other psychiatric disorders occurred in this population, 452 consecutive patients who were admitted to the hospital received a psychiatric screening consultation. Sixty percent of the patients met diagnostic criteria and received treatment. The control group in this case consisted of a cohort of patients admitted to the hospital under normal circumstances. For this cohort, the average length of the postsurgical hospital stay was reduced by 2.2 days. However, the experimental cohort, consisting of the 452 screened patients, had a reduction in mean postsurgical stay of 1.7 days. This reduction in postsurgical hospitalization translated into a significant net savings for the hospital of nearly $1,300 per patient. This study provides a good example of the need to look at total reduction in cost. Although the cost for psychiatric and psychological services in this study was $40,000, medical expenses were reduced by $270,000. Thus, the intervention was cost effective from an institutional perspective.

Another example was reported by Carter and Maddock (1992), who studied the relationship between chest pain and GAD. They found that among 50 patients with GAD 48% had a history of chest pain. Sixteen of the GAD patients associated episodes of excess worry with their chest pain. Seven of the patients also reported having had panic attacks. However, of these 7 patients, 4 reported that their pain was not associated with their panic attacks. The Yingling et al. (1993) study described previously is also relevant. The results do not directly address the issue of cost offset. However, they do indicate a need for evaluating and treating anxiety disorders among patients with chest pain. In an environment that readily provides access to medical services but restricts access to psychological services, such patients are more likely to receive expensive electrocardiographic evaluations than psychological evaluations.

Somatization Pathway

Patients presenting with somatic complaints may have an organic disease, a psychiatric disorder, or significant emotional distress being expressed through somatic symptoms (Barsky, 1981). Although some somatizing patients qualify for a formal psychiatric diagnosis, a far greater number are expressing psychosocial distress in bodily terms. In either case, the medical system is overused by some patients who complain of physical symptoms to their physicians but who are primarily in need of relief from emotional distress (Smith, Monson, & Ray, 1986). Physicians trained primarily to diagnose and treat somatic complaints will typically respond with tests and interventions that may fail to produce symptom relief. This may in turn magnify symptom reporting, initiate a round of more exotic and more expensive tests to find "the problem," or trigger a round of doctor shopping, all which increase costs. A recent review by Ross, Hamilton, and Smith (1995) has suggested that a simple screening procedure, which involves counting the number of symptoms presented, may help physicians detect this disorder. With early diagnosis and recognition regarding attention to the emotional needs of the patient the primary care clinician can alter their treatment accordingly. Although referral to a mental health professional may be appropriate in many cases, Ross et al. suggested that physicians can forestall excessive medical utilization and reduce costs by providing services directly appropriate to the emotional problems at the root of the patient's complaint.

Evidence of Cost Offset

Some patients are particularly sensitive to changes in physical sensations and are quick to seek medical attention. Organic causes for physical symptoms are generally not discovered for these patients, and for the majority of this group emotional distress appears to aggravate their sensitivity. Psychological interventions before or in conjunction with treatment have been found to reduce medical utilization.

Smith et al. (1986) studied 38 patients who had been diagnosed with somatization disorder prospectively for 18 months. Patients in the treatment group received a psychiatric consultation, and treatment recommendations were given to the patients' primary physicians. The control group received the same intervention after 9 months. Results showed that the quarterly health care charges in the treatment group declined by 53% ($p < .05$), and the control group showed no overall change. However, after the control group was crossed over and received treatment, their quarterly charges declined by 49% ($p < .05$). The authors concluded that psychiatric consultation reduced medical costs significantly in patients with somatization disorder.

More recently Smith, Rost, and Kashner (1995) reported the results of a randomized intervention for somatizing patients who had a history of seeking help for 6 to 12 lifetime unexplained physical symptoms but who did not meet the formal diagnostic criteria for somatization disorder. Physicians in the intervention group received a consultation letter recommending specific behavioral strategies for managing their somatizing patients. Patients of physicians who received the consultation letter reported significant increases in physical functioning and had reduced annual medical charges of $289, which equated to a 33% reduction in the annual median cost of their medical care.

The largest study to date of the cost-offset effect of mental health treatment involved an examination of a group of high utilizers of Medicaid services. This study found that 80% of medical costs were distributed in 15% of the Medicaid population (Pallak et al., 1995). Although no specific attempt was made to determine the degree to which the utilization patterns of this high-use group were due to somatization, the results of previous studies suggested that it was likely that a significant percentage of medical visits were prompted by psychological distress.

On the basis of this presumption, an intervention study was initiated. Two thirds of the high-use group were offered and received brief psychological intervention, and one third were assigned to a control group and did not receive therapy. Those patients who received brief psychotherapy showed significant reductions in medical costs. Differences were found depending on the length of time patients had been enrolled for Medicaid services. For those enrolled 6 months, medical costs declined by 20–23%. For those enrolled 12 months, costs declined by 36–25%.

Access to appropriate, focused mental health treatment clearly reduces medical care costs. Addressing the emotional distress of patients, whether because of psychological problems or medical illness, decreases the utilization of costly medical services. It makes health and economic sense to offer high medical utilizers the benefits of focused mental health services through referral and outreach. Health care systems that make use of appropriate expertise directed at both medical and emotional distress can provide superior patient care and medical cost reductions.

Psychosocial interventions do not always have to consist of individual counseling. A study at the Harvard Community Health Plan investigated the effectiveness of two group behavioral interventions among high-utilizing primary care patients who experienced physical symptoms (e.g., palpitations, shortness of breath, gastrointestinal complaints, headaches, sleeplessness, musculoskeletal complaints, malaise, etc.) with significant psychosocial components (Hellman, Budd, Borysenko, McClelland, & Benson, 1990). Both interventions offered patients educational materials, relaxation–response training, and awareness training, and both included cognitive restructuring. These groups were compared with a randomized control group that received only information about stress management. The behavioral medicine intervention groups met for 90-min sessions once a week for 6 weeks. The information-only group met for just two 90-min sessions. Six months after treatment, only patients in the behavioral medicine groups reported less physical and psychological discomfort and averaged nearly two fewer visits to the health plan than the patients in the control group. The estimated net savings to the HMO above the cost of the intervention for the 46 behavioral medicine patients was $85 per participant in the first 6 months.

The implications of these representative studies are clear. For many patients who are heavy utilizers of the medical system, psychological interventions pay economic dividends. In the Smith et al. (1986) study, the patients were identified on the basis of a psychiatric diagnosis. In the Medicaid (Pallak et al., 1995) study, patients were identified on the basis of utilization patterns. The former strategy is more effective for smaller studies, whereas the latter strategy is more effective for larger studies. It is also worth emphasizing that the cost offset associated with these studies is realized immediately. Furthermore, these cost savings are real and not a function of cost shifting from one clinical service to another.

Chronic Pain Management: An Example of a Cost-Effective Intervention

The arbitrary distinction between mind and body undermines clinical efficacy and economic savings. Psychiatric, psychological, behavioral, and biomedical evaluations and interventions should be integrated. Although such combination makes it more difficult from a research point of view to tease out the active ingredients, more often than not effective clinical care of patients will involve a multidisciplinary approach. Multidimensional back pain centers are a good example of successful integration of behavioral medicine interventions with biomedical treatment. Such centers generally treat patients who have been unsuccessful with the use of usual medical and surgical treatments. Relaxation, cognitive restructuring, exercise, and nutritional counseling are integrated with physical, occupational, and vocational therapy, as well as pharmacological and surgical interventions.

Several studies have now demonstrated that multidimensional pain centers are a cost-effective way to treat patients with chronic back pain. As an example, Simmons, Avant, Demski, and Parisher (1988) compared the medical costs for patients in the year before treatment and the year after treatment in a multidimensional pain center. In the year before treatment at the pain center, medical costs averaged

$13,284 per patient and in the year after averaged $5,596. For the 16 patients sampled, this represented a total savings of $123,000 in medical costs. Turk and Stacey (in press) extrapolated the savings reported by Simmons et al. to a much larger sample. Specifically, they estimated the savings that would occur if the 2,318 patients successfully treated in pain centers as reported in a meta-analysis by Flor, Fydrich, and Turk (1992) exhibited reductions similar to those in the Simmons et al. study. With a 3% correction for inflation, Turk and Stacey estimated a cost savings of $20 million in medical expenses in the 1st year following treatment. They further extrapolated the cost savings that would occur if disability payments could be eliminated. The Flor et al. meta-analysis estimated that 50% of patients treated in pain centers receive some form of disability. Turk and Stacey calculated that if 1,544 patients, half the patients in the cohort described by Flor et al., were to stop receiving disability payments, the savings in reduced disability payments would be over $90 million.

Caudill, Schnable, Zuttermeister, Benson, and Friedman (1991) also investigated the effect of a behavioral group intervention on clinic usage in an HMO for patients with chronic pain. One hundred nine patients who had been suffering with chronic pain for an average of 6.5 years participated in the study. The patients attended 90-min group sessions once a week for 10 weeks. The behavioral medicine intervention resulted in decreases in negative psychological symptoms such as anxiety, depression, and hostility. In addition, clinic use decreased by 36% among patients who had received the intervention in the 1st and 2nd year after the program. The program cost $1,000 per group of 10 patients. However, the net savings in clinic visits alone was estimated to average $110 per patient in the 1st year and $210 per patient in the 2nd year after the behavioral intervention. These estimates do not include possible savings from reduced prescription drugs and reassuring diagnostic tests.

Barriers to Integration of Behavioral Medicine and Biomedical Interventions

If the case for integrating behavioral and biomedical interventions from both a clinical and cost viewpoint is so compelling, why has there not been more investment in such integration? One reason is that the data are incomplete. Although we have highlighted some of the evidence supporting the cost-offset effect, the majority of behavioral and psychosocial interventions have never been thoroughly investigated to assess their impact on medical utilization and costs. Along with the message that incorporation of mental health services into routine medical care can save money comes the responsibility to define what mental health services are most cost effective for which patients and under what circumstances. No intervention works for everyone in every case. Admittedly, much more data is required to address the issue of specificity.

It is unlikely that the incorporation of behavioral medicine into the treatment of all chronic disease would have equally profound cost savings. Where there is good data, often providers of medical, and even psychological, services are not aware of it. Even when hard data on cost and health outcomes are reported for soft psychosocial interventions, medical professionals too often dismiss or ignore such studies. For one, over the past century, the medical community has been focused on improving technology and clinical services. The prevailing attitudes toward the origin of disease has emphasized biological explanations.

Patients also may be resistant to psychosocial explanations and behavioral interventions. Somatizing patients, in particular, are often focused on finding a medical explanation and treatment to fix their somatic concerns. Psychosocial interventions, especially those associated with traditional psychiatric diagnoses and treatment, unfortunately still carry with them a stigmatizing shadow.

There continues to be confusion between behavioral medicine and clinical health psychology on the one hand, and psychotherapy on the other (Friedman, Vasile, Gallagher, & Benson, 1994). Patients, third-party insurers, and policy makers still tend to view all behavioral medicine interventions as the equivalent of psychotherapy. The traditional, long-term psychotherapy model consisting of several individual counseling sessions per week that can persist for several years is likely to have quite different outcomes than the more efficient and targeted behavioral approaches described above.

Another practical problem that must be confronted to achieve maximal integration is the issue of cost–benefit accounting and budgeting. The Strain et al. (1991) study of a psychiatric consultation-liaison intervention for postsurgical patients noted previously is a good example of the problem. Although medical costs, or more specifically, hospital costs, were reduced, the "bottom line" for the provision of psychiatry services was increased. An important part of increasing use of psychological, or in this case psychiatric, interventions in medicine is a readjustment of accounting. It is usually the case that profits and losses are independently calculated for each clinical services. Furthermore, it is also frequently the case that insurance coverage for medical problems is handled by one company, whereas coverage for mental health problems is handled by another. Trying to convince the latter to spend money so that the former would save money is problematic at best. Developing mechanisms for addressing these problems is critical if health policy and the delivering of health services is brought into better alignment with the underlying psychosocial and behavioral issues that determine overall medical utilization and cost.

Caveat Emptor: The Limits of Cost Analysis

Many studies of psychosocial interventions have not included utilization or cost impact in their outcome analysis. Often we have to infer or project potential savings. For example, psychosocial interventions that reduce anxiety and depression, boost smoking cessation, or enhance adherence to medical regimens might be assumed to have favorable impact on health and cost outcomes even though use may not have been directly measured. For the purposes of this review, however, we primarily have used examples where cost-related data are available.

The primary purpose of psychosocial interventions should be to improve health outcomes, not just reduce medical costs or utilization. Although on balance, many psychosocial interventions appear to reduce overall health care costs through the cost-offset effect, some may very well increase costs. For example, by extending the life of patients with metastatic breast cancer (Spiegel et al., 1989) by means of a support group, the total lifetime medical costs are likely to increase. In the rush toward cost-effective interventions, we should not lose sight of the true purpose of all health care interventions—to improve the quality and, when appropriate, quantity of life.

Conclusion

The economic pressures prompting more consistent incorporation of cost-effective behavioral medicine into clinical practice come at a propitious moment. The empirical evidence documenting clinical efficacy of behavioral medicine over the past 20 years continues to accumulate. There are patient-specific and disease-specific intervention strategies that can be integrated into clinical care with the same degree of scientific credibility as pharmaceutical or surgical interventions. Although the current economic climate provides a new impetus for integration, practitioners must appreciate the need to incorporate only those interventions that have been scientifically validated.

Fortunately, there is growing evidence that attending to the multiple psychosocial reasons that prompt patients to visit physicians can be both health and cost effective. Interventions can be designed and targeted to address each of six pathways that reflect the psychosocial drivers of medical utilization and medical costs. It is important to emphasize that enhancing self-management skills and self-efficacy, reducing psychophysiological arousal, altering specific behavior patterns while preventing relapse through stress management, and enhancing social support are not independent interventions but rather components of an overall strategy of psychological and behavioral management. When these four strategies are combined with increased sensitivity to psychiatric and somatoform disorders that prompt medical utilization, maximum clinical and economic gains are to be expected. Providing behavioral interventions better suited to patient needs can often offset the demand for costly medical services.

The studies cited above have addressed a variety of clinical problems and used a variety of interventions to eventuate savings. Some of the studies involved mental health interventions that demonstrated cost-offset benefits from individual brief psychotherapy or psychiatric consultations for medical–surgical patients. Other studies involved multi-faceted behavioral medicine interventions that combined medications, cognitive therapy, group support, biofeedback, relaxation, and behavior modification. The incorporation of psychological, psychiatric, and behavioral interventions into routine medical care has always made clinical sense and is grounded in empirical science. The contemporary economic climate now makes such an integration essential.

References

American Psychiatric Association. (1989). *Task report of the American Psychiatric Association: Treatment of psychiatric disorders* (pp. 1856, 2429–2430). Washington, DC: American Psychiatric Association.

Barsky, A. J. (1981). Hidden reasons some patients visit doctors. *Annals of Internal Medicine, 94,* 492–498.

Benson, H., Beary, J. F., & Carol, M. P. (1974). The relaxation response. *Psychiatry, 37,* 37–45.

Benson, H., Dryer, T., & Hartley, L. H. (1978). Decreased oxygen consumption during exercise with elicitation of the relaxation response. *Journal of Human Stress, 4,* 38–42.

Benson, H., & Stuart, E. M. (1992). *The wellness book.* New York: Simon and Shuster.

Berkanovic, E., Telesky, C., & Reeder, S. (1981). Structural and social psychological factors in the decision to seek medical care for symptoms. *Medical Care, 21,* 693–709.

Black, J. L., & Bruce, B. K. (1989). Behavior therapy: A clinical update. *Hospital Community Psychiatry, 40,* 1152.

Cannon, W. B. (1941). The emergency function of the adrenal medulla in pain and the major emotions. *American Journal of Physiology, 33,* 356.

Carter, C. S., & Maddock, R. J. (1992). Chest pain in generalized anxiety disorder. *International Journal of Psychiatry in Medicine, 22,* 291–298.

Caudill, M., Schnable, R., Zuttermeister, P., Benson, H., & Friedman, R. (1991). Decreased clinic use by chronic pain patients: Response to behavioral medicine interventions. *Clinical Journal of Pain, 7,* 305–310.

Cummings, N. A., & Follette, W. T. (1968). Psychiatric services and medical utilization in a prepaid health plan setting: Part II. *Medical Care, 6,* 31–41.

Demers, R. Y., Altamore, R., Mustin, H., Kleinman, A., & Leonardi, D. (1980). An exploration of the dimensions of illness behavior. *Journal of Family Practice, 11,* 1085–1092.

Devine, E. C. (1992). Effects of psychoeducational care for adult surgical patients: A meta-analysis of 191 studies. *Patient Education and Counseling, 19,* 129–142.

Fahrion, S., Norris, P., Green, E., Green, A., & Schnar, R. (1987). Biobehavioral treatment of essential hypertension: A group outcome study. *Biofeedback and Self Regulation, 11,* 257–278.

Fawzy, F. I., Fawzy, N. W., Hyun, C. S., Elashoff, R., Guthrie, D., Fahey, J. L., & Morton, D. L. (1993). Malignant melanoma: Effects of an early structured psychiatric intervention, coping, and affective state on recurrence and survival 6 years later. *Archives of General Psychiatry, 50,* 681–689.

Flor, H., Fydrich, T., & Turk, D. C. (1992). Efficacy of multidisciplinary pain treatment centers: A meta-analytic review. *Pain, 49,* 221–130.

Frasure-Smith, N. (1991). In-hospital symptoms of psychological stress as predictors of long-term outcome after acute myocardial infarction in men. *American Journal of Cardiology, 67,* 121–127.

Friedman, R., Vasile, R., Gallagher, R. M., & Benson, H. (1994). Behavioral medicine and psychiatry. *Directions in Psychiatry, 14,* 1–8.

Fries, J. F., Koop, C. E., Beadle, C. E., Cooper, P. P., England, M. J., Greaves, R. F., Sokolov, J. J., & Wright, D. (1993). Reducing health care costs by reducing the need and demand for medical services. *The New England Journal of Medicine, 329,* 321–325.

Gatchel, R. J., & Blanchard, E. B. (Eds.). (1993). *Psychophysiological disorders: Research and clinical applications.* Washington, DC: American Psychological Association.

Glass, D. C., Singer, J. E., & Friedman, L. N. (1969). Psychic cost of adaption to an environmental stressor. *Journal of Personality and Social Psychology, 12,* 200–210.

Heatherton, T. F., & Renn, R. J. (1995). Stress and the disinhibition of behavior. *Mind/Body Medicine, 1,* 72–81.

Hellman, C. J. C., Budd, M., Borysenko, J., McClelland, D. C., & Benson, H. (1990). A study of the effectiveness of two group behavioral medicine interventions for patients with psychosomatic complaints. *Behavioral Medicine, 16,* 165–173.

Jacobs, D. G., Kopans, B. S., & Reizes, J. M. (1995). Reevaluation of depression: What the general practitioner needs to know. *Mind/Body Medicine, 1,* 17–22.

Kemper, D. W., Lorig, K., & Mettler, M. (1993). The effectiveness of medical self-care interventions: A focus on self-initiated responses to symptoms. *Patient Education and Counseling, 21,* 29–39.

Kennell, J., Klaus, M., McGrath, S., Robertson, S., & Hinkley, C. (1991). Continuous emotional support during labor in a U.S. hospital: A randomized controlled trial. *Journal of the American Medical Association, 265,* 2197–2237.

Klaus, M. K., Kennell, J., Berkowitz, G., & Klaus, P. (1992). Maternal assistance and support in labor: Father, nurse, midwife, or doula? *Clinical Consultations in Obstetrics and Gynecology, 4,* 211–217.

Kroenke, K., & Mangelsdorff, A. D. (1989). Common symptoms in ambulatory care: Incidence, evaluation, therapy, and outcome. *American Journal of Medicine, 86*, 262–266.

Lorig, K., Mazonson, P. D., & Holman, H. R. (1993). Evidence suggesting that health education for self-management in patients with chronic arthritis has sustained health benefits while reducing health care costs. *Arthritis and Rheumatism, 36*, 439–446.

Lorig, K., Seleznick, M., Lubeck, D., Ung, E., Chastian, R. L., & Holman, H. R. (1989). The beneficial outcomes of the arthritis self-management course are not adequately explained by behavior change. *Arthritis and Rheumatism, 32*, 91–95.

Lynch, W. D. (1993). The potential impact of health promotion on health care utilization: An introduction to demand management. *Association for Worksite Health Promotion Practitioners' Forum, 8*, 87–92.

Marlatt, G. A. (1985). Relapse prevention: Theoretical rationale and overview of the model. In G. A. Marlatt & J. R. Gordon (Eds.), *Relapse prevention* (pp. 3–70). New York: Guilford.

Ornish, D., Brown, S. E., Scherwitz, L. W., Billings, J. H., Armstrong, W. T., Ports, T. A., McLanahan, S. M., Kirkeeide, R. L., Brand, R. J., & Gould, K. L. (1990). Can lifestyle changes reverse coronary heart disease? The Lifestyle Heart Trial. *Lancet, 336*, 129–133.

Pallak, M. S., Cummings, N. A., Dorken, H., & Henke, C. J. (1995). Effect of mental health treatment on medical costs. *Mind/Body Medicine, 1*, 7–12.

Pelletier, K. R. (1993). A review and analysis of the health and cost-effective outcome studies of comprehensive health promotion and disease prevention programs at the worksite: 1991–1993 update. *American Journal of Health Promotion, 8*, 50–62.

Robinson, J. S., Schwartz, M. M., Magwene, K. S., Krengel, S. A., & Tamburello, D. (1989). The impact of fever health education on clinic utilization. *American Journal of Diseases of Children, 143*, 698–704.

Ross, R. L., Hamilton, G. E., & Smith, G. R. (1995). Somatization disorder in primary care. *Mind/Body Medicine, 1*, 24–29.

Schneider, C. J. (1987). Cost effectiveness of biofeedback and behavioral medicine treatments: A review of the literature. *Biofeedback and Self Regulation, 12*, 71–92.

Shellenberger, R., Turner, J., Green, J., & Cooney, J. (1986). Health changes in a biofeedback and stress management program. *Clinical Biofeedback and Health, 9*, 23–24.

Simmons, J. W., Avant, W. S., Demski, J., & Parisher, D. (1988). Determining successful pain clinic treatment through validation of cost effectiveness. *Spine, 13*, 34.

Smith, G. R., Monson, R. A., & Ray, D. C. (1986). Psychiatric consultation in somatization disorder. *The New England Journal of Medicine, 314*, 1407–1413.

Smith, G. R., Rost, K., & Kashner, T. M. (1995). A trial of the effect of a standardized psychiatric consultation on health outcomes and costs in somatizing patients. *Archives of General Psychiatry, 52*, 238–243.

Sobel, D. S. (1995). Rethinking medicine: Improving health outcomes with cost-effective psychosocial interventions. *Psychosomatic Medicine, 57*, 234–244.

Spiegel, D., Bloom, J., Kraemer, H. C., & Gottheil, E. (1989). Effect of psychosocial treatment on survival of patients with metastatic breast cancer. *Lancet, 2*, 888–891.

Spitzer, R. L., Williams, J. B. W., Kroenke, K., Linzer, M., deGruy, F. V., III, Hahn, S. R., Brody, D., & Johnson, J. G. (1994). Utility of a new procedure for diagnosing mental disorders in primary care: The PRIME-MD 1000 study. *Journal of the American Medical Association, 272*, 1749–1756.

Strain, J. J., Lyons, J. S., Hammer, J. S., Fahs, M., Lebovits, A., Paddison, P. L., Snyder, S., Strauss, E., Burton, R., & Nuber, G. (1991). Cost offset from a psychiatric consultation-liaison intervention with elderly hip fracture patients. *American Journal of Psychiatry, 148*, 1044–1049.

Turk, D. C., & Stacey, B. R. (in press). Multidisciplinary pain centers in the treatment of chronic back pain. In J. W. Frymoyer, T. B. Ducker, N. M. Hadler, J. P. Kostuik, J. N. Weinstein, & T. S. Whitecloud (Eds.), *The adult spine: Principles and practice* (2nd ed.). New York: Raven Press.

Vickery, D. M., Kalmer, H., Lowry, D., Constantine, M., Wright, E., & Loren, W. (1983). Effect of a self-care education program on medical visits. *Journal of the American Medical Association, 250*, 2952–2956.

White, K. L., Williams, T. F., & Greenberg, B. G. (1961). The ecology of medical care. *The New England Journal of Medicine, 265*, 885–891.

Wulsin, L. R., & Yingling, K. (1991). Psychiatric aspects of chest pain in the emergency department. *Medical Clinics of North America, 75*, 1175–1188.

Wynd, C. A. (1992). Relaxation imagery used for stress reduction in the prevention of smoking relapse. *Journal of Advanced Nursing, 17*, 194–202.

Yingling, K. W., Wulsin, L. R., Arnold, L. M., & Rouan, G. W. (1993). Estimated prevalences of panic disorder and depression among consecutive patients seen in an emergency department with acute chest pain. *Journal of General Internal Medicine, 8*, 2315.

DYING TO WIN

For many women athletes, the toughest foe is anorexia.
Gymnast Christy Henrich lost her battle

Merrell Noden

Christy Henrich's fiancé, Bo Moreno, loved her for her sweet side, but he also knew her demons. That's why, when Henrich's parents were preparing to check her into the Menninger Clinic in Topeka, Kans., two years ago for treatment of her eating disorders, Moreno warned them to inspect her suitcase carefully. "It had a false bottom," he says. "She had lined the entire bottom of the suitcase with laxatives. That was part of her addiction." Henrich weighed 63 pounds at the time.

At another treatment center about a year later, the staff had to confine her to a wheelchair to prevent her from running everywhere in an attempt to lose weight. "Another part of the addiction," says Moreno. "Constant movement. Anything to burn calories."

At the peak of her career as a world-class gymnast, the 4' 10" Henrich weighed 95 pounds. But when she died on July 26, eight days past her 22nd birthday, of multiple organ failure at Research Medical Center in Kansas City, she was down to 61 pounds. And that actually represented improvement. On July 4, the day she was discharged from St. Joseph's (Mo.) Medical Center, she had weighed 47 pounds.

"She was getting intensive supportive care," says Dr. David McKinsey, who treated Henrich during the last week of her life, the final three days of which were spent in a coma. "But a person passes the point of no return, and then, no matter how aggressive the care is, it doesn't work. The major problem is a severe lack of fuel. The person becomes so malnourished that the liver doesn't work, the kidneys don't work, and neither do the muscles. The cells no longer function."

Henrich had been in and out off so many hospitals over the past two years that Moreno lost count of them. Her medical bills ran to more than $100,000. There were occasional periods of hope, when she would gain weight and seem to be making progress. But for the most part, as Henrich herself told Dale Brendel of *The Independence* [Mo.] *Examiner* last year, "my life is a horrifying nightmare. It feels like there's a beast inside me, like a monster. It feels evil."

Henrich's funeral was held last Friday morning at St. Mary's Catholic Church in Independence. Her pink casket sat at the front of the church as several hundred mourners filed in. Some were fellow gymnasts; some were friends and relatives; some were former classmates at Fort Osage High, where Henrich had been a straight-A student. In his eulogy Moreno asked those present to do what most people had always had trouble doing when Henrich was alive: to think of her as more than just a gymnast. "She was a talented artist and an unbelievable cook," he said. "But I must admit, her favorite hobby was shopping, for herself and others."

Moreno closed by reading the lyrics to *I Believe in You,* a song he wrote and recorded for Henrich last summer:

> *America's sweetheart brought to her knees*
> *Willing to do anything to please*
> *A product of our country*
> *Pushed too far*
> *You've got to be Extra-Tough, little lady*
> *Now look this way and grin*
> *Remember to hold your head up high*
> *And hold the pain within*

Eating disorders are easily the gravest health problem facing female athletes, and they affect not just gymnasts but also swimmers, distance runners, tennis and volleyball players, divers and figure skaters. According to the American College of Sports Medicine, as many as 62% of females competing in "appearance" sports (like figure skating and gymnastics) and endurance sports suffer from an eating disorder. Julie Anthony, a touring tennis pro in the

Reprinted courtesy of *Sports Illustrated*, August 8, 1994, pp. 52-56, 58-60. © 1994 by Time Inc. Magazine Company. All rights reserved.

1970s who now runs a sports-fitness clinic in Aspen, Colo., has estimated that 30% of the women on the tennis tour suffer from some type of eating affliction. Peter Farrell, who has been coaching women's track and cross-country at Princeton for 17 years, puts the number of women runners with eating disorders even higher. "My experience is that 70% of my runners have dabbled in it in its many hideous forms."

Eating disorders, however, are by no means limited to athletes. The Association of Anorexia Nervosa and Associated Disorders reported before a U.S. Senate subcommittee hearing earlier this year that 18% of females in the U.S. suffer from eating disorders. The illnesses tend to strike women who, like Henrich, are perfectionists, and they often seize those who seem to be the most successful. In 1983 singer Karen Carpenter died following a long battle with eating disorders, and for years Princess Diana waged a well-publicized fight against bulimia.

Girls or women who suffer from depression or low self-esteem are particularly susceptible to eating disorders, as are victims of sexual abuse. The expectations of society, particularly those regarding beauty, also play a role. Not coincidentally, the ideal of the perfect female body has changed dramatically in the past several decades. Marilyn Monroe, as she sashayed away from Jack Lemmon and Tony Curtis in *Some Like It Hot,* looked like "Jell-O on springs." Lemmon's description was a compliment in 1959. A decade later it would make most women cringe.

Given the importance that sport attaches to weight—and, in the subjectively judged sports, to appearance—it isn't surprising that eating disorders are common among athletes. Nor is it surprising that they exact a far greater toll among women than men. In a 1992 NCAA survey of collegiate athletics, 93% of the programs reporting eating disorders were in women's sports. It is true that some male athletes—wrestlers, for example—use extreme methods of weight loss, but there is an important difference between these and the self-starvation practiced by anorexics. A wrestler's perception of his body is not distorted. When he is not competing, he can return to a healthy weight. That is not the case with anorexics, trapped as they are behind bars they can't see.

A study conducted a few years ago at Penn found that while both men and women tend to be unrealistic about how others perceive their bodies, men's perceptions tend to be distorted positively, while women's are more likely to be negative. "Someone feeling really good about herself isn't going to find her self-worth in her looks alone," says Farrell. "But how many girls between the ages of 16 and 22 [when eating disorders tend to strike] feel really good about themselves?"

"Men grow into what they're supposed to be," says Mary T. Meagher, the world-record holder in the 100- and 200-meter butterfly events. "They're supposed to

be big and muscular. A woman's body naturally produces more fat. We grow away from what we're supposed to be as athletes."

Though laymen tend to lump anorexia and bulimia together—perhaps because experimentation with bulimia often leads to anorexia—the two are markedly different. "In a way bulimia is more dangerous," says Pan Fanaritis, who has coached women's track at Georgetown, Missouri and Villanova and is now the men's and women's coach at Denison. "Anorexia you can see."

What you see is frightening. Anorexia is self-starvation driven by a distorted perception of one's appearance. It is not unusual for an anorexic who is 5' 8" to weigh 100 pounds or less—and still think she's too fat. In the women's distance races at the Penn Relays this April, it was not hard to pick out the anorexics: Their arms were shrunken like the vestigial forelimbs of some dinosaurs. And on some a thin layer of downy fur had begun to form as their bodies struggled to compensate for the layers of fat they had lost.

The long-term consequences of anorexia are catastrophic. Deprived of calcium, the body steals it from the bones, leading to osteoporosis. "I've seen X-rays where the bones look like honeycomb," says Fanaritis. "X-rays of an anorexic of four or five years and those of a 70-year-old are very similar." Anorexics have suffered stress fractures just walking down the street.

Bulimia is a binge-purge syndrome in which huge quantities of food—sometimes totaling as much as 20,000 calories in a day—are consumed in a short period of time and then expelled through self-induced vomiting, excessive exercise, the use of diuretics or laxatives, or some combination of those methods. Stomach acids rot the teeth of bulimics and, if they are sticking their fingers down their throats to induce vomiting, their fingernails. Their throats get swollen and lacerated. Electrolyte imbalances disrupt their heart rates. But since bulimics are usually of normal weight, years may pass before a parent, roommate or spouse learns the terrible secret.

"You can always find an empty bathroom," says one recovering bulimic who was an All-America distance runner at Texas. During her worst period of self-abuse she was visiting bathrooms five or six times a day, vomiting simply by flexing her stomach muscles. "It's like a drug," she says of the syndrome. "It controls you. An overwhelming feeling comes over you, like a fog."

In the 1992 NCAA survey 51% of the women's gymnastics programs that responded reported eating disorders among team members, a far greater percentage than in any other sport. The true number is almost certainly higher. Moreno says he knows of five gymnasts on the national team who have eating disorders. Bob Ito, the former women's gymnastics coach at Washington, has estimated that on some of his teams 40% of the athletes had "outright eating disorders." One world-class gymnast has admitted that while she was at UCLA the entire team would binge and vomit together following meets. It was, she said, a "social thing."

Why might gymnasts be more vulnerable to eating disorders than other athletes? The subjectivity of the judging system can't help; nor can the fact that to reach the top, gymnasts must sacrifice having normal childhoods. Moreno also points to authoritarian coaches.

"A large percentage of coaches tell the girls how to count calories, how to act, what to wear, what to say in public," he says. "It becomes a control issue for the girl. They feel the only thing they control is the food they put in their bodies."

Anorexia offers a convenient antidote to what young gymnasts dread most—the onset of womanhood. Not only do anorexics keep their boyish figures, but many go months or even years without their menstrual periods, a side effect that contributes to osteoporosis. "This is a matter of locked-on adolescence," says Scott Pengelly, a psychologist from Eugene, Ore., who has treated athletes with eating disorders. "Chronologically, they may be adults. But they have a 13-year-old's way of looking at life."

In the Lilliputian world of gymnastics, arrested development seems to be an occupational necessity. Women gymnasts "are the most immature people on a college campus," says Rick Aberman, a psychologist and a consultant to the University of Minnesota's athletic department. "They're treated like little kids. When you have 18- or 19-year-old women trying to deny they've matured, you get problems. If [gymnasts] have hips or breasts, it creates inner turmoil that's so destructive. They're trying to deny something that's natural."

No one knows that better than Cathy Rigby, who 20 years ago was the darling of U.S. gymnastics and paid for it with 12 years of bulimia. "As much as [the news of Henrich's death] makes me sad, it makes me angry," Rigby says. "This sort of thing has been going on for so long in our sport, and there's so much denial."

When Rigby competed, every story celebrated her girlishness, which she worked so hard to maintain that she pinned her pigtails back from her face, fastening them so tightly that she got headaches. And the image of the world-class gymnast as waif has only become more exaggerated in the two decades since. The average size of the women on the U.S. Olympic gymnastics team has shrunk from 5′ 3″, 105 pounds in 1976 to 4′ 9″, 88 pounds in 1992. At last year's world championships the all-around gold medalist, 16-year-old Shannon Miller, was 4′ 10″, 79 pounds.

What chance would Vera Caslavska have had in such company? Caslavska, who won the all-around titles at the 1964 and '68 Olympics, was a geriatric giant by today's standards. In Mexico City the 26-year-old Czech was 5′ 3″, 121 pounds. What's more, she and Ludmila Turischeva of the Soviet Union, who succeeded Caslavska as all-around champion, looked like women. Gold medal or not, Turischeva was upstaged in '68 by 13-year-old Olga Korbut, who was 4′ 11″ and 85 pounds. Gymnastics has not been the same since.

At its highest levels gymnastics has evolved in a direction that is incompatible with a woman's mature body. That was plain when Nadia Comaneci, the darling of the 1976 Olympics, showed up at the world championships two years later having grown four inches and put on 21 pounds. She had become a woman, and as John Goodbody wrote in *The Illustrated History of Gymnastics,* "We learnt that week how perfection in women's gymnastics can be blemished by maturity."

By the 1979 world championships, where she won the combined title, Comaneci was her old svelte self, having lost nearly 40 pounds in two months. Eating disorders originate in the mind, and like any disease of self-deception, they are difficult prisons to escape. That was suggested in 1990, in Barbara Grizzuti Harrison's story on Comaneci in LIFE magazine. "I am fat and ugly," Comaneci, then 28, told the writer, although she was a size 6. When they went to dinner, Grizzuti Harrison wrote, "Her appetite for food is voracious. She eats her own food and [her companion] Constantin's too. After each course, she goes to the bathroom. She is gone for a long time. She comes back, her eyes watery, picks her teeth and eats some more. She eats mountains of raspberries and my crème brûlée. She makes her way to the bathroom again. When she returns, she is wreathed in that rank sweet smell."

Henrich's career followed a pattern not unlike that of thousands of little girls who fall in love with gymnastics the first time they see it on television. Henrich started at the age of four. When she was eight she enrolled at the Great American Gymnastics Express in the neighboring suburb of Blue Springs. Al Fong, a 41-year-old former LSU gymnast, founded Great American in 1979, one year before Henrich joined. Even in a sport dominated by monomaniacal men, Fong's determination to produce champion gymnasts is extraordinary. "I work at this seven days a week," he told a reporter last year, "and I look forward to doing it for the next 25 years. It's an obsession with me."

Fong's elite gymnasts are renowned for the hours they train: one three-hour session at six in the morning and then four more hours at five in the afternoon. On meet days they are in the gym to work out two hours before the meet begins. "He pushed them really hard," says Sandy Henrich, Christy's mother. "He wanted them to train no matter what. He didn't want them to get casts [for fractures] because it took away their muscle tone."

For intensity Fong met his match in Henrich. Her nickname at the club was E.T.—hence the Extra-Tough allusion in Moreno's song—and she more than lived up to it, competing with stress fractures and placing second all around in the U.S. nationals just three months after she broke her neck in 1989. "No one can force someone to train 32 hours a week unless they really want to," Fong said last week. "The sacrifices are too great. Christy worked five times harder than anybody else. She became so good because she worked so hard and had this kind of focus."

Henrich made sensational progress. In 1986, at age 14, she finished fifth at the national junior championships and competed in her first international meet, in Italy. In early 1988, when she finished 10th in the all-around competition at the senior nationals, her dream of making the U.S. team at that year's Olympics seemed attainable.

"What's a [high school] dance compared to the Olympics?" she said when she was 15. "It's what I want to do. I want it so bad. I know I have a chance for the Olympics, and that gets me fired up." But Henrich didn't make the Olympic team in 1988. She missed a berth by 0.118 of a point in a vault in the compulsories.

About the same time, her best friend, Julissa Gomez, saw her Olympic dream vanish forever, in devastating circumstances. Gomez broke her neck while performing a practice vault at a meet in Tokyo in May 1988, then went into a coma when an oxygen hose hooked to her respirator became disconnected after she had been given a tracheotomy. She died three years later without ever regaining consciousness.

"Julissa's death devastated Christy," says Moreno. "Christy's condition went downhill after this. She went to the gym and got a photo of Julissa and hung it in her room. It's still there."

Despite the tragedy that had befallen Gomez, in 1989 Henrich had her best year as a gymnast. She finished second in the all-around at the U.S. championships and fourth in the world championships in the uneven parallel bars. By that time she also had a serious eating disorder.

Its inception can be traced in part to an incident in March 1988, at a meet in Budapest, when a U.S. judge remarked that Henrich would have to lose weight if she wanted to make the Olympic team. Sandy Henrich recalls meeting her daughter at the airport upon her return: "The minute she got off the plane, the first words out of her mouth were that she had to lose weight. A judge had told her she was fat. Christy was absolutely devastated. She had a look of panic on her face. And I had a look of panic on my face. She weighed 90 pounds and was beautiful."

Henrich began eating less and less, an apple a day at first, and then just a slice of apple—this while continuing to work out six, seven hours each day.

In one important respect Henrich was different from many anorexics, who tend to live solitary existences. During her junior year at Fort Osage High she began to date Moreno, a friend of her older brother, Paul, and a wrestler on the Fort Osage team. "She was always very tough on herself," says Moreno, "and I could relate

to that." Indeed, he recalls that Henrich got jealous when she learned that his body fat was 8%, while hers was 9%. "I had to tell her men just have lower body fat," he says. They got engaged in 1990 and were to be married later that year, but the wedding had to be postponed when Henrich fell ill. "She wanted to live in Florida and become a nurse," says Moreno. "We'd even named our children. Jesse Joseph and Maya Maria."

Soon after they began dating, Henrich asked Moreno how wrestlers lost weight. "I told her we'd wear plastic. Run in the shower with the steam on. Take Ex-Lax. And," he recalls with a wince, "every one of the things I told her, she tried. That laid real guilt on me, but I had no idea she'd do it. I had always told her how stupid it was."

Moreno says Fong might have spotted the danger signals of anorexia and bulimia earlier. "I find it hard to believe Al would not notice that every day Christy would work out, run five miles and come back. She truly loved Al and would have done anything for him. He'd say, 'Tuck your stomach in. You look like the Pillsbury Doughboy.'"

Kelly Macy, the 1991 NCAA champion on the uneven bars who trained regularly with Henrich at Fong's gym when both were in their early teens, recalls, "Everything was weight, weight, weight. He'd say, 'You could do this if you weighed less.'"

Fong denies ever harping on Henrich's weight or making the Doughboy comment. "It's just not true," he says. "I've heard those comments. Where in the world does that come from?"

Moreno and Sandy and Paul Henrich agree that the blame for Christy's obsession with weight should not fall only on her coach. "It's the whole system," says Sandy. "No matter what you do, it's never, never enough. The whole system has got to change—parents, coaches, the federation."

Christy lived at home, and a former USA Gymnastics official suggests that her parents might have pushed harder for intervention. As Christy's weight dropped precipitously, "they had to be aware of it," the official says, adding that the federation received no complaints from the family. Some of Henrich's friends question if they, too, should have seen the signs earlier.

"I think Christy had a problem a long time before [the obvious symptoms appeared]," says Macy, who herself suffered from anorexia while competing for Georgia and now travels the country speaking about the dangers of eating disorders. "I just didn't realize it. She was always working out, always doing extra stuff after practice. We'd finish, and she'd jump right on the exercise bike. Even my mother commented on it. She said, 'That Christy Henrich looks like she puts 150,000 percent into everything.'"

Moreno has come to understand Henrich's compulsion. "Christy's also to blame for her perfectionist attitude," he says. "The disease strikes people like that. I can remember Christy telling me, 'There's only one first place. Second place sucks.'"

Gail Vaughn, the director of Reforming Feelings, a counseling service in Liberty, Mo., worked with Henrich for six months last year. "Probably one of the things that worked against her most was that label, E.T.," says Vaughn. "She learned to deny pain. She competed in one of her biggest meets with a stress fracture. So when her body broke down and screamed in pain, she ignored it. Because she had learned to push past the pain."

For women, eating disorders are "like steroids are for men," says Liz Natale, a recovering anorexic who was a member of the Texas team that won the 1986 NCAA cross-country title. "You'll get results, but you'll pay for it."

For a time you do get results. That's part of the seduction. As an athlete's weight falls, his or her aerobic power increases. And psychologically there is no lash like anorexia. "To be a great competitor, you need that tunnel vision that anorexia feeds on," says Farrell. "Anybody who can starve herself can run a 10,000 really well."

But ultimately eating disorders exact a severe psychological toll. Distance runner Mary Wazeter was so tormented by constant thoughts of food that in February 1982, after withdrawing from Georgetown in her freshman year, she jumped from a bridge into the ice-covered Susquehanna River in her hometown of Wilkes-Barre, Pa. Her suicide attempt failed, but she broke her back and will spend the rest of her life in a wheelchair.

It does not take much to trigger an eating disorder. Natale recalls watching the mile run at the 1983 NCAA championships while sitting in the stands with her coach. "I remember her telling me to notice how thin all the women in the final were," says Natale. "I hadn't qualified, and I felt bad because I hadn't. I remember thinking if I wanted to run well, I needed to lose weight."

Many coaches aren't that subtle. Some divide their athletes into Lean Machines and Porkers. Tonya Chaplin, an assistant gymnastics coach at Washington, recalls that her club coach would punish female team members if they went much over their assigned weight by abusing them verbally, withholding meals and confining them to a "fat room." Before she quit the team, Chaplin was vomiting 12 times a day.

Regrettably, too many coaches see only what they want to see. Says Fanaritis: "How about the football coach who has the kid come back from summer vacation and he's gained 60 pounds and his neck has grown two inches, and the kid says, 'I lifted my ass off'? It's the same issue. You're not the one who said, 'Go home and use steroids.' You're not the one who said, 'Get skinny so you can run fast.' But you're in that middle ground."

Spurred by Henrich's case, USA Gymnastics has begun to take measures seeking to help prevent eating disorders. Last year the federation measured the bone density of all 32 national team members and found that three of them had deficiencies. It says it is trying to teach young gymnasts that they can say no if they feel too much is being asked by a coach. But how realistic is it to expect children to stop themselves from doing something they love? Especially when, as famed women's gymnastics coach Bela Karolyi once put it, "The young ones are the greatest little suckers in the world. They will follow you no matter what."

Christy Henrich was buried at St. Mary's Cemetery in Independence last Friday afternoon. A line of cars half a mile long moved slowly through the tombstones, which marked the graves of those who had lived 70, 80, even 90 years. For Henrich the time was tragically short. The inscription on her stone will read: 1972–1994.

Munchausen Syndrome by Proxy
Case Accounts

STEPHEN J. BOROS, M.D.
and
LARRY C. BRUBAKER

Dr. Boros is involved with the Infant Apnea Program at Children's Hospital, St. Paul, Minnesota.

Special Agent Brubaker is assigned to the FBI's Minneapolis Division.

Hieronymous Karl Fredrich von Munchausen was an 18th century German baron and mercenary officer in the Russian cavalry. On his return from the Russo-Turkish wars, the baron entertained friends and neighbors with stories of his many exploits. Over time, his stories grew more and more expansive, and finally, quite outlandish. Munchausen became somewhat famous after a collection of his tales was published.[1]

In 1794, at the age of 74, Munchausen married Bernhardine Brun, then 17 years old. It is said that on their wedding night, the baron retired early, and his bride spent the night dancing with another. In 1795, Bernhardine gave birth to a son. Following the birth of this child, it was whispered that "the life of the Munchausen child will likely be short." The boy, named Polle, died at approximately 1 year of age under suspicious circumstances.[2]

Almost a century later, an unusual behavior pattern among young men gained recognition in the writings of Charcot. In 1877, he described adults, who through self-inflicted injuries or bogus medical documents, attempted to gain hospitalization and treatment. Charcot called this condition "mania operativa passiva."[3]

Seventy-four years later, in 1951, Asher described a similar pattern of self-abuse, where individuals fabricated histories of illness. These fabrications invariably led to complex medical investigations, hospitalizations, and at times, needless surgery. Remembering Baron von Munchausen and his apocryphal tales, Asher named this condition Munchausen's Syndrome.[4]

Today, Munchausen's Syndrome is a recognized psychiatric disorder. The American Psychiatric Association's *Diagnostic and Statistical Manual of Disorders* (DSM III-R) describes it as the "intentional production of physical symptoms."

MUNCHAUSEN SYNDROME BY PROXY

The term "Munchausen Syndrome by Proxy" (MSBP) was coined in a 1976 report describing four children who were so severely abused they were dwarfed.[5] In 1977, Meadow described a somewhat less extreme form of child abuse in which mothers deliberately induced or falsely reported illnesses in their children. He also referred to this behavior as MSBP.[6]

Over the years, alternate terms, such as "Polle's syndrome" and "Meadow's syndrome," have been suggested; however, these terms never gained popularity. In contrast to its adult namesake, the American Psychiatric Association's DSM III-R does not consider Munchausen Syndrome by Proxy a psychiatric disorder.

Tragically, MSBP victims are usually children, and the perpetrators are almost always parents or parent substitutes. If and when victims are hospitalized, they may be subjected to multiple, and at times,

From the *FBI Law Enforcement Bulletin*, June 1992, pp. 16-20. Reprinted by permission of the United States Department of Justice, Federal Bureau of Investigation, Washington, DC.

dangerous diagnostic procedures that invariably produce negative or confounding results. When the victim and abuser are separated, however, the victim's symptoms cease. When confronted, the abuser characteristically denies any knowledge of how the child's illness occurred.

CASE REPORTS

In recent years, medical personnel at Children's Hospital in St. Paul, Minnesota, and local law enforcement agencies encountered several MSBP cases, three of which are outlined here. Two of the cases were presented with apnea, a condition where breathing temporarily stops. The third case was presented with recurrent infections masquerading as an immune deficiency.

Case #1

Victim

MA, a 9-month-old boy, was repeatedly admitted to Children's Hospital because of recurrent life-threatening apnea. At 7 weeks of age, he experienced his first apneic event, and his mother administered mouth-to-mouth ventilation. Spontaneous respiration returned, and MA was hospitalized, treated, and discharged with a home monitor.

During the next 9 months, MA experienced 10 similar events and 7 more hospitalizations. Eight of the events required mouth-to-mouth ventilation. All of these episodes occurred while mother and child were alone, and only MA's mother witnessed the actual events. Two episodes occurred in the hospital.

Unfortunately, despite many tests and surgical procedures, MA's apnea persisted, and his growth slowed. Because of his persistent apnea and failure to thrive, MA received home nursing care. During these home visits, several nurses observed that MA would refuse to eat in his mother's presence. If she left the room, however, he would eat.

In time, both medical and nurs-

ing staffs became increasingly suspicious that Mrs. A was somehow responsible for her child's apnea. To better observe mother-child interaction, MA was moved to a hospital room equipped for covert audio-visual surveillance.[7]

On the sixth day, the video clearly recorded Mrs. A bringing on the apnea by forcing the child into her chest, which caused him to lose consciousness. MA became limp and experienced a falling heart rate. Mrs. A then placed the baby back on the bed, called for help, and began mouth-to-mouth resuscitation.

The hospital immediately informed child protection services and police authorities, who reviewed the recording. Shortly thereafter, a team consisting of a physician, nurse, social worker, and police officer confronted the parents. At first, Mrs. A expressed disbelief at the suggestion that she smothered MA, but when she was informed of the video, she made no comment. She was then arrested.

Family History

Mrs. A was a 36-year-old occupational therapist and the mother of three boys. Late into her pregnancy with MA, she worked in an early intervention program for developmentally delayed children. During many of MA's hospitalizations, she appeared caring and concerned, but emotionally distant. Clearly, Mrs. A was the dominant parent, who made all decisions regarding medical treatment.

Followup

Mrs. A subsequently pled guilty to felonious, third-degree assault. At the time, she stated: "The only time I ever caused MA to stop breathing was in the hospital." She received 3 years' probation during which she was to receive psychotherapy. If she successfully completed psychotherapy, the felony charge would be reduced to a misdemeanor. She also had to live apart from her children and could

only visit them in the presence of two adults.

MA had no further apnea, and at 24 months of age, he appeared vigorous, healthy, and normal. Eventually, the family was reunited.

Case #2

Victim

CB, a 10-month-old girl, was admitted to a hospital because of recurrent life-threatening apnea. CB was born in another State and was sexually assaulted at the age of 3 months by an acquaintance of her father. After the assault, local child protection services closely monitored the family.

At 6 months of age, CB experienced her first apneic episode. Her father shook her vigorously, then administered mouth-to-mouth ventilation. She was subsequently admitted to a local hospital. After examination and treatment, she was discharged with a home monitor. During the next 2 months, CB experienced six apneic events and three hospitalizations. The family then moved to Minnesota.

During her first month in Minnesota, CB experienced four apneic episodes and three more hospitalizations. All required vigorous stimulations to restore spontaneous breathing. Other family members observed the child immediately following the events. However, only CB's father ever witnessed all of the actual events. CB was eventually referred to Children's Hospital.

While in the hospital, CB had no clinical apnea or monitor alarms. And, most of the time, she appeared happy and playful. However, when anyone attempted to touch her face, she became hysterical and combative. Over time, both the medical and nursing staffs began to suspect that CB's parents were responsible for her apnea.

Local police and child protection services were notified, and CB was placed in a room with covert audio-visual surveillance.[8] On the third day of video monitoring, the

Help for Investigators

Investigators assigned to work child abuse cases should investigate cases of MSBP as they do similar cases of abuse. In general, however, when confronted with possible cases of MSBP, investigators should:

- Review the victim's medical records to determine condition and illness
- Determine from contact with medical personnel the reporting parent's concerns and reactions to the child's medical treatment
- Compile a complete history of the family to determine previous involvement with law enforcement agencies, medical facilities, and social and child protection services
- Compile a detailed social history of the family, including deaths, injuries, and illnesses
- Interview family members, neighbors, and babysitters
- Use video surveillance in the hospital in accordance with State law, and
- Use a search warrant for the family's residence when collecting evidence of the assaults.

video recording clearly showed CB's father producing an apneic event by smothering her. Mr. B was viewed picking up the sleeping child, placing her prone on the bed, and forcing her face into the mattress. CB awoke and struggled to escape, wildly kicking her legs. Mr. B continued until CB's struggling stopped and she appeared limp and unconscious. Then, he repositioned her on the bed and called for help. A nurse entered the room, stimulated her, and administered supplemental oxygen.

CB's parents were confronted by a physician, nurse, and police officer. Mr. B adamantly denied smothering CB. He was subsequently arrested and removed from the hospital.

Family History

Mr. B. was a 27-year-old, unemployed, semi-literate laborer in good health. He was actively involved in CB's day-to-day medical care and was clearly the dominant parent. He also became very knowledgeable of the mechanics of the various county and hospital welfare systems. Officials described him as "demanding and manipulative." During CB's hospitalizations, the family lived in a hotel adjacent to the hospital with room, board, and radio pagers provided by the hospital. Throughout CB's hospitalization, Mrs. B was passive and deferred all medical decisions to her husband.

> ❝ ...MSBP victims are usually children, and the perpetrators are almost always parents or parent substitutes. ❞

When they first arrived in Minnesota, the family received emergency financial assistance and was closely monitored by local social service agencies. Four years earlier, Mrs. B was allegedly assaulted and raped. Two months prior to CB's monitored episode, Mrs. B was evaluated at a local emergency room for a "hysterical conversion reaction."

Followup

Following the incident at Children's Hospital, Mr. B was taken to the county jail, and upon viewing the video, he admitted to smothering CB. He also was charged with felonious, third-degree assault. The judge ordered a psychiatric examination. Mr. B also received a 10-month sentence in a local workhouse and 5 years' probation. Also, he is to have no contact with his daughter or unsupervised contact with any child in the future.

Case #3

Victim

JC, a 2 1/2-year-old boy suffered from asthma, severe pneumonia, mysterious infections, and sudden fevers. He was hospitalized 20 times during an 18-month period. Doctors were even concerned that he may have AIDS. However, they soon began to suspect that the mother may have caused the child's problems. Finally, when the boy complained to his mother's friend that his thigh was sore because "Mommy gave me shots," the authorities were called.

Upon searching the residence, investigators seized medical charts and information and hypodermic needles. It was also believed that material also entered the boy through a catheter doctors surgically inserted in the arteries near his heart to give him constant medication.

Family History

JC's mother was a 24-year-old homemaker and part-time fast-food restaurant worker. When the mother was 7 years old, an older sister died of a brain tumor at Children's Hospital. During her sister's prolonged

MSBP Warning Signs

- Unexplained, prolonged illness that is so extraordinary that it prompts medical professionals to remark that they've "Never seen anything like it before."

- Repeat hospitalizations and medical evaluations without definitive diagnosis.

- Inappropriate or incongruous symptoms and/or signs that don't make medical sense.

- Persistent failure of a child to tolerate or respond to medical therapy without clear cause.

- Signs and symptoms that disappear when away from the parent.

- A differential diagnosis consisting of disorders less common than MSBP.

- Mothers who are not as concerned by their child's illness as the medical staff, who are constantly with their ill child in the hospital, who are at ease on the children's ward, and who form unusually close relationships with the medical staff.

- Families in which sudden, unexplained infant deaths have occurred and that have several members alleged to have serious medical disorders.

- Mothers with previous medical experience and who often give a medical history similar to the child's.

- Parent who welcomes medical tests of the child, even if painful.

- Increased parental uneasiness as child "recovers" or approaches discharge.

- Parental attempts to convince the staff that the child is more ill than what is apparent.

illness, JC's mother, by necessity, spent long periods of time at the hospital. Although this occurred long ago, JC's mother remembered the experience vividly.

During JC's many hospitalizations, the mother seemed almost obsessively involved in medical matters and hospital routines. She spent hours in the hospital library reading medical texts. She had few friends outside the hospital, and the medical and nursing staff described her as an isolated person.

JC's father was a 24-year-old church janitor, afflicted with many health problems—the most notable being severe insulin-dependent diabetes. During JC's many hospitalizations, his father appeared distant and only marginally involved. JC's 7-year-old sister was in good health and was named after her mother's deceased sister.

Followup

Since JC was removed from his home, he has been healthy. As in previous cases, only Mrs. C was present when the boy became ill, and until investigators showed evidence linking her to her child's illnesses, she denied any wrongdoing. Assault charges were filed, and Mrs. C's case is pending.

CONCLUSION

Today, the consensus is that MSBP is not rare, is notoriously resistant to parental psychotherapy, and carries a very grim prognosis. Approximately 10 percent of MSBP victims die.

Unfortunately, more police agencies and medical professionals will be confronted with this form of abuse in the future. Hopefully, the information discussed here will alert law enforcement officers, especially those who deal with cases of abuse, to the warning signs of MSBP and will assist them in identifying the perpetrators and helping the victims.

ENDNOTES

[1] J.G. Jones, H.L. Butler, B. Hamilton, J.D. Perdue, H.P. Stern, and R.C. Woody, "Munchausen Syndrome by Proxy," *Child Abuse and Neglect*, October 1986, 33-40.

[2] D. Burman and D. Stevens, "Munchausen Family," *Lancet*, August 27, 1977, 456.

[3] M. Signal, M. Gelkopf, and G. Levertov, "Medical and Legal Aspects of Munchausen Syndrome by Proxy Perpetrator," *Medical Law*, September 1990, 739-749.

[4] R. Asher, "Munchausen's Syndrome," *Lancet*, I, 1951, 339-341.

[5] J. Money, "Munchausen's Syndrome by Proxy: Update," *Journal of Pediatric Psychology*, November 1986, 583-584; J. Money, and J. Werlas, "Folie a Deux in Parents of Psychosocial Dwarfs: Two Cases," *Bulletin of the American Academy of Psychiatry and the Law*, April 1976, 351-362.

[6] R. Meadow, "Munchausen Syndrome by Proxy: The Hinterland of Child Abuse," *Lancet*, II, 1977, 343-345.

[7] R. Fiatal, "Lights, Camera, Action: Video Surveillance and the Fourth Amendment," *FBI Law Enforcement Bulletin*, January 1989, 23-30. See also *Sponick* v. *City of Detroit Police Department*, 211 N.W.2d 674, 690 (Mich. Ct. App. Div. 1, 1973).

[8] Ibid.

Therapy: Psychological Approaches

Ever since Sigmund Freud began studying his patients' verbalizations for betrayals of their unconscious motives, a growing number of psychotherapeutic methods have been developed to treat mental illness. When considering these psychologically based therapies, the most fundamental question is, Do they work? Hans Eysenck's criticism of the effectiveness of psychotherapy in the 1950s served as a wake-up call to psychologists, who began a search for compelling evidence of its effectiveness. Despite the large number of available psychotherapies, a general conclusion has emerged: psychotherapy seems to be effective, although not all clients benefit, and some disorders are very difficult to treat. Research also shows that many patients respond well to even small doses of therapy and that some therapies are more effective than others for particular disorders. A major report published by *Consumer Reports* provides strong evidence for the effectiveness of psychotherapy and offers guidelines for those seeking help.

The quality of the relationship between a therapist and client appears to be a key factor in successful outcomes of psychotherapy. For example, in "A Buyer's Guide to Psychotherapy," Frank Pittman recommends that clients seek a therapist who shares similar values. When a therapist and a client share values, there is an increased likelihood that the therapy will be successful, because therapy is often about the values that one holds. Pittman's advice is good to keep in mind if you are looking for a therapist from the variety of mental health professionals available.

The large number of disorders to be treated have led to a plethora of treatments, some very successful, others not worth the effort. How can clients tell the difference? Clients need to ask pertinent and critical questions about therapy. One common question asked by many people when they seek therapy is: How long will it take for my symptoms to respond to treatment? Researchers have now focused some of their efforts on providing answers to questions like this. For example, they have reported the median number of sessions that it takes for a variety of symptoms to respond to treatment. This type of research may prove beneficial in evaluating various psychotherapies as well as the effectiveness of individual therapists.

Is there any evidence that problematic behavior responds to treatment at all? In his essay "What You Can Change and What You Cannot Change," Martin Seligman, from his extensive review of research literature, offers advice about the likelihood of changing problematic behaviors that include panic, depression, and anger. If you suffer from one of the specific phobias, there is good news: Seligman considers specific phobias to be almost curable. However, if you are overweight, the bad news is that the best you can expect is a temporary change. It is probably better to have this information than to search frantically for a treatment that is not likely to work because the problem is intractable. Among the treatments that has shown great promise for a number of disorders is cognitive behavioral therapy.

Looking Ahead: Challenge Questions

Knowing that many states do not license all mental health therapists, how can an individual determine if a therapist is qualified?

Apart from academic degrees, what qualifications and personal characteristics would you look for when seeking the services of a psychotherapist?

How much and what types of information about a particular form of psychotherapy should therapists be required to present and discuss with potential clients?

How could a clearinghouse of therapeutic approaches help individuals make more informed decisions about what form of therapy to select?

UNIT 7

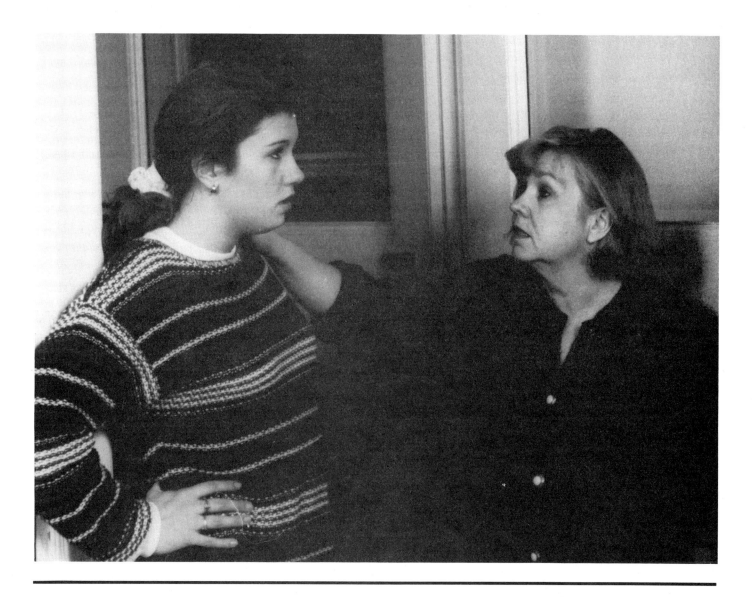

MENTAL HEALTH
DOES THERAPY HELP?

Our ground-breaking survey shows psychotherapy usually works. This report can help you find the best care.

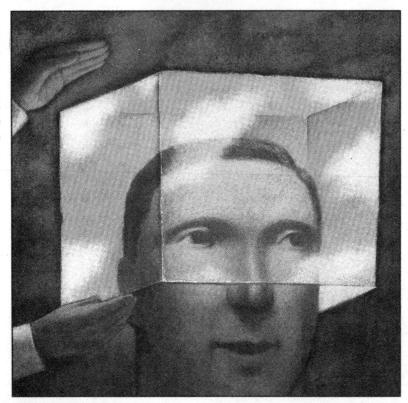

oping with a serious physical illness is hard enough. But if you're suffering from emotional or mental distress, it's particularly difficult to know where to get help. You may have some basic doubts about whether therapy will help at all. And even if you do decide to enter therapy, your health insurance may not cover it—or cover it well.

As a result, millions of Americans who might benefit from psychotherapy never even give it a try. More than 50 million American adults suffer from a mental or addictive disorder at any given time. But a recent Government survey showed that fewer than one-third of them get professional help.

That's a shame. The results of a candid, in-depth survey of CONSUMER REPORTS subscribers—the largest survey ever to query people on mental-health care—provide convincing evidence that therapy can make an important difference. Four thousand of our readers who responded had sought help from a mental-health provider or a family doctor for psychological problems, or had joined a self-help group. The majority were highly satisfied with the care they received. Most had made strides toward resolving the problems that led to treatment, and almost all said life had become more manageable. This was true for all the conditions we asked about, even among the people who had felt the worst at the beginning.

Among our findings

■ People were just as satisfied and reported similar progress whether they saw a social worker, psychologist, or psychiatrist. Those who consulted a marriage counselor, however, were somewhat less likely to feel they'd been helped.

■ Readers who sought help from their family doctor tended to do well. But people who saw a mental-health specialist for more than six months did much better.

■ Psychotherapy alone worked as well as psychotherapy combined with medication, like *Prozac* or *Xanax*. Most people who took drugs like those did feel they were helpful, but many people reported side effects.

■ The longer people stayed in therapy, the more they improved. This suggests that limited mental-health insurance coverage, and the new trend in health plans—emphasizing short-term therapy—may be misguided.

■ Most people who went to a self-help group were very satisfied with the experience and said they got better. People were especially grateful to Alcoholics Anonymous, and very loyal to that organization.

Our survey adds an important dimension to existing research in mental health. Most studies have started with people who have very specific, well-defined problems, who have been randomly assigned to a treatment or control group, and who have received carefully scripted therapy. Such studies have shown which techniques can help which problems (see "What Works Best?"), but they aren't a realistic reflection of most patients' experiences.

Our survey, in contrast, is a unique look at what happens in real life, where problems are diverse and less well-defined, and where some therapists try one technique after another until something works. The success of therapy under these real-life conditions has never before been well studied, says Martin Seligman, former director of clinical training in psychology at the University of Pennsylvania and past president of the American Psychological Association's division of clinical psychology.

Seligman, a consultant to our project, believes our readers' experiences send "a message of hope" for other people dealing with emotional problems.

Like other surveys, ours has several built-in limitations. Few of the people responding had a chronic, disabling condition such as schizophrenia or manic depression. We asked readers about their past experiences, which can be less reliable than asking about the present. We may have sampled an unusually large number of people in long-term treatment. Finally, our data comes from the readers' own perceptions, rather than from a clinician's assessment. However, other studies have shown that such self-reports fre-

Reprinted with permission from *Consumer Reports*, November 1995, pp. 734-739. © 1995 by Consumers Union of U.S., Inc., Yonkers, NY 10703-1057.

quently agree with professionals' clinical judgments.

Who went for help

In our 1994 Annual Questionnaire, we asked readers about their experiences with emotional problems and their encounters with health-care providers and groups during the years 1991 to 1994. Like the average American outpatient client, the 4000 readers who said they had sought professional help were mostly well educated. Their median age was 46, and about half were women. However, they may be more amenable to therapy than most.

Many who went to a mental-health specialist were in considerable pain at the time they entered treatment. Forty-three percent said their emotional state was either very poor ("I barely managed to deal with things") or fairly poor ("Life was usually pretty tough").

Their reasons for seeking therapy included several classic emotional illnesses: depression, anxiety, panic, and phobias. Among the other reasons our readers sought therapy: marital or sexual problems, frequent low moods, problems with children, problems with jobs, grief, stress-related ailments, and alcohol or drug problems.

The results: Therapy works

Our survey showed that therapy for mental-health problems can have a substantial effect. Forty-four percent of people whose emotional state was "very poor" at the start of treatment said they now feel good. Another 43 percent who started out "fairly poor" also improved significantly, though somewhat less. Of course, some people probably would have gotten better without treatment, but the vast majority specifically said that therapy helped.

Most people reported they were helped with the specific problems that brought them to therapy, even when those problems were quite severe. Of those who started out "very poor," 54 percent said treatment "made things a lot better," while another one-third said it helped their problems to some extent. The same pattern of improvement held for just about every condition.

Overall, almost everyone who sought help experienced some relief —improvements that made them less troubled and their lives more pleasant. People who started out feeling the worst reported the most progress. Among people no longer in

MENTAL-HEALTH INSURANCE

WHO PAYS—AND HOW MUCH?

Private insurers have always covered mental disorders and substance abuse more grudgingly than medical illness, either by building in limits or by interposing a case manager between you and your benefit. And very few plans deal well with the lifelong needs of people with chronic, severe mental illness. On the whole, says Kathleen Kelso, executive director of the Mental Health Association of Minnesota, "insurers would just as soon cover us from the neck down."

Almost all traditional fee-for-service plans pay 80 percent or more of the fee when you visit the doctor with a medical problem. But for outpatient therapy, the majority pay just 50 percent, and frequently that's after "capping" bills at well below the therapists' actual fees —which range on average from $80 to $120 according to Psychotherapy Finances, an industry newsletter. Most insurance plans also impose one or more other limits on mental-health coverage, such as the number of outpatient visits and hospital days they will pay for. In addition, many plans have annual or lifetime dollar maximums; for outpatient care, it can be as low as $1000 and $10,000, respectively. In recent years consumer advocates have lobbied for state laws that would equalize coverage for psychiatric and other illnesses. So far, just six states—Maine, Maryland, Minnesota, New Hampshire, Rhode Island, and Texas—have passed so-called "parity" laws. Consumers Union supports such laws, and has actively worked for their passage.

Health maintenance organizations (HMOs) also limit access to psychiatric services, typically providing a maximum of 20 outpatient visits and 30 hospital days a year. Patients usually have to go through their family physician or another gatekeeper to gain access to those benefits, and may get less than the maximum.

In our survey of mental-health care, respondents whose coverage limited the length and frequency of therapy, and the type of therapist, reported poorer outcomes. (However, we found no clear difference in outcome between people with fee-for-service coverage and those in HMOs and preferred provider plans.) Paying for therapy on their own was clearly a hardship for many: Twenty-one percent cited the cost of therapy as a reason for quitting.

To hold down spending, increasing numbers of employers, HMOs, and fee-for-service plans are turning to specialized managed-care companies to run their mental-health benefit. These specialty firms refer patients to a network of clinicians who must adhere to strict treatment guidelines. And they *have* reined in spending, saving some employers as much as 30 percent in the cost of mental-health care.

But many patients—and their therapists— feel they're being shortchanged. Psychiatrists complain about the difficulty of extending a hospital stay for patients considered too sick to leave and the challenge of getting approval for more than brief outpatient care.

Although many plans run by managed-care firms nominally have generous benefits, reality may fall somewhat short. All services must be authorized by a case manager. To get approval for additional sessions, therapists must provide details about a patient's problems and the course of treatment.

With scores of managed-care companies nationwide, there's great variability in how they tend to the needs of their subscribers. Even critics acknowledge that some plans are quite accommodating, and that some overly stringent practices have been curbed. But concern about heavy-handed practices has prompted several states to enact laws regulating managed-care services.

How to choose a plan

If you're picking a health-care plan and are concerned about mental-health coverage, you should ask some pointed questions:

■ **What are the stated benefits?** Pay close attention to the benefit limits, including co-payments, limits on the number of hospital days and outpatient sessions, and annual or lifetime dollar maximums. A typical plan with limits covers 30 days of inpatient care and 50 or fewer outpatient visits. But the cap it sets on covered charges may be low, and the copayments high.

■ **If the benefits cover only "medically necessary" treatment, who makes that determination?** It's best if that decision is left to you and your therapist. But in many managed-care plans it's a case manager who decides whether you need therapy or hospitalization, and how long it should last.

■ **What are your rights of appeal if coverage is denied or cut short?** In many plans the grievance process consists of a single appeal.

■ **In a managed-care plan, how large is the provider panel?** The more therapists in your area, the more likely you'll find one whose personality and expertise are a good match for you.

■ **Will the plan add new providers to its panel?** This can be important if you're already seeing a therapist who's not part of the plan but is willing to join.

■ **Which facilities are approved by the plan?** Be sure there's a hospital that's convenient and that offers a broad spectrum of mental-health and substance-abuse services. Also look for transitional and intermediate-care programs, such as mental-health day centers.

treatment, two-thirds said they'd left because their problems had been resolved or were easier to deal with.

Whom should you see?

In the vast field of mental health, psychiatrists, psychologists, and clinical social workers have long fought for turf. Only psychiatrists, who are medical doctors, can prescribe drugs and have the training to detect medical problems that can affect a person's mental state. Otherwise, each of these professionals is trained to understand human behavior, to recognize problems, and to provide therapy.

Historically, social workers have been the underdogs and have had to fight for state laws requiring insurance companies to cover their services. But many of today's budget-minded insurers *favor* social workers —and psychiatric nurses—because they offer relatively low-cost services.

In our survey, almost three-quarters of those seeking professional help went to a mental-health specialist. Their experiences suggest that any of these therapists can be very helpful. Psychiatrists, psychologists, and social workers received equally high marks and were praised for being supportive, insightful, and easy to confide in. That remained true even when we statistically con-

trolled for the seriousness and type of the problem and the length of treatment.

Those who went to marriage counselors didn't do quite as well, and gave their counselors lower grades for competence. One reason may be that working with a fractured couple is difficult. Also, almost anyone can hang out a shingle as a marriage counselor. In some states the title "marriage and family therapist" is restricted to those with appropriate training. But anyone can use other words to say they *do* marriage therapy, and in most places the title "marriage counselor" is up for grabs.

What about doctors?

Many people are more comfortable taking their problems to their family doctor than to a psychologist or psychiatrist. That may work well for some people, but our data suggest that many would be better off with a psychotherapist.

Readers who exclusively saw their family doctor for emotional problems—about 14 percent of

The worse people felt at the start of therapy, the greater their gains.

those in our survey —had a very different experience from those who consulted a mental-health specialist. Treatment tended to be shorter; more than half of those whose care was complete had been treated for less than two months. People who went to family doctors were much more likely to get psychiatric drugs—83 percent of them did, compared with 20 percent of those who went to mental-health specialists. And almost half the people whose doctors gave them drugs received medication without the benefit of much counseling.

The people who relied on their family doctors for help were less distraught at the outset than those who saw mental-health providers; people with severe emotional problems apparently get themselves to a specialist. Even so, only half were highly satisfied with their family doctor's treatment (compared with 62 percent who were highly satisfied with their mental-health provider). A significant minority felt their doctor had neither the time nor temperament to address emotional issues. In general, family doctors did help people get back on their feet—but longer treatment with a specialist was more effective.

However, if you begin treatment with your family doctor, that's where you're likely to stay. Family doctors referred their patients to a mental-health specialist in only one out of four cases, even when psychotherapy might have made a big difference. Only half of those who were severely distressed were sent on, and 60 percent of patients with panic disorder or phobias were never referred, even though specific therapies are known to work for those problems.

Other research has shown that many family doctors have a poor track record when it comes to mental health. They fail to diagnose some 50 to 80 percent of psychological problems, and sometimes prescribe psychiatric drugs for too short a time or at doses too low to work.

The power of groups

It was 60 years ago that a businessman and a physician, both

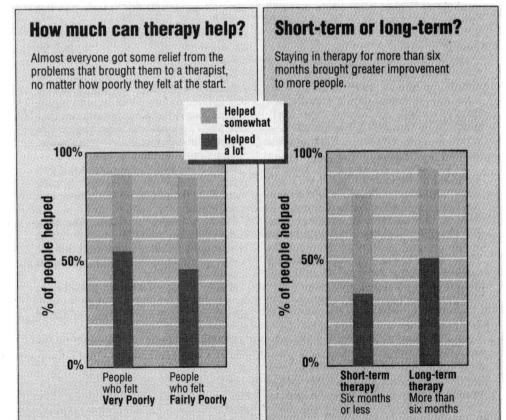

How much can therapy help?

Almost everyone got some relief from the problems that brought them to a therapist, no matter how poorly they felt at the start.

Helped somewhat
Helped a lot

% of people helped

100%

50%

0%

People who felt **Very Poorly**
People who felt **Fairly Poorly**

Short-term or long-term?

Staying in therapy for more than six months brought greater improvement to more people.

% of people helped

100%

50%

0%

Short-term therapy Six months or less
Long-term therapy More than six months

WHAT WORKS BEST?

THE RIGHT TREATMENTS FOR YOUR TROUBLES

Until a decade or so ago, any evidence that psychotherapy worked came from the testimonials of therapists and their patients. But today, controlled studies have shown that psychotherapy does make a difference: People with a broad range of problems can usually benefit from psychological treatment. More important, for certain conditions researchers have homed in on specific therapies and drugs that can bring swift improvement for the majority of sufferers.

Here is a summary of the top treatment options for four common problems. It was compiled from the scientific literature by psychologist Martin Seligman and reviewed by psychiatrists Stewart Agras of Stanford University and Jesse Schomer of Cornell University, and by social worker Eleanor Bromberg of The Hunter School of Social Work in New York. (For a comprehensive look at treatments that work, see Seligman's book, "What You Can Change & What You Can't," Ballantine Books, New York, 1995.)

Depression

More than the passing blues, depression can sap you of pleasure, hope, and vitality, upend your eating and sleeping habits, and draw a veil of despair that lasts for months or years. In bipolar depression, also called manic-depression, the lows alternate with excessive, frenetic highs. Most of the time, depression can be cut short and considerably relieved.

With **cognitive therapy,** you learn to recognize and change the negative assumptions and beliefs that color your emotions and shape your world view. If, for example, you react to small setbacks by thinking you can't do anything right, you'll learn to focus on evidence to the contrary—your recent promotion at work, for instance. Cognitive therapy brings considerable relief to about 70 percent of depressed people. It takes about a month to start working, and typically involves a few months of weekly sessions.

Interpersonal therapy is just as effective and runs about as long, but focuses instead on the difficulties of personal relationships. You'll examine current conflicts and disappointments, learn how they sow depression, and work on successful ways of relating to other people.

Drug therapy is about as effective as these psychotherapies. Each of the three major classes of antidepressant drugs works equally well. People who don't respond to one type of drug may respond to another; overall, 60 percent to 80 percent of depressed people get marked relief within three to six weeks. However, the classes differ significantly in their adverse effects: Fluoxetine (*Prozac*) and related drugs tend to be better tolerated, though they frequently produce insomnia, restlessness, and sexual problems. The older, "tricyclic" antidepressants such as amitriptyline (*Elavil*) can cause drowsiness, tremor, weight gain, and heart-rhythm changes. For people with manic-depression, treatment with the drug lithium carbonate (*Escalith, Lithane*) is clearly the best route.

Electroconvulsive therapy is used for severely depressed people who can't take, or don't respond to, antidepressant drugs. Electrodes placed on the head transmit bursts of electricity believed to affect many of the same brain chemicals as antidepressant drugs. The "dosage" has been greatly reduced from the jolts used in the past. Repeated several times over the course of a week, ECT quickly relieves severe depression about 75 percent of the time. The downside is the risk of anesthesia and the side effects—temporary but disturbing—of memory loss and confusion.

Anxiety

Unlike ordinary worrying, clinical anxiety is irrational, freezes you into inaction, or dominates your life.

Tranquilizers such as diazepam (*Valium*) and alprazolam (*Xanax*) can provide quick relief, but the benefit ends when the drug is stopped. Extended use may result in tolerance, which diminishes the benefit, and also produces dependency, making it hard to quit.

Everyday anxiety often yields to self-help techniques. Simple forms of **meditation** can be useful. So can various forms of **relaxation,** such as progressive relaxation. Some therapists teach these techniques, or you can check a local YMCA, community hospital, or yoga institute for courses.

If your anxiety is intense and unyielding, it may need professional attention. Cognitive-behavioral therapy is often helpful; you'll learn to counter the irrational thoughts that provoke anxiety and to overcome fears.

Panic

A panic attack isn't easily forgotten. It produces chest pain, sweating, nausea, dizziness, and a feeling of overwhelming dread. Millions of people suffer such episodes repeatedly and unexpectedly.

Antidepressant drugs and the anti-anxiety drug *Xanax* can dampen or even prevent panic attacks in the majority of people. But side effects include drowsiness and lethargy, and panic rebounds about half the time when therapy is stopped.

An alternative approach is cognitive therapy, which provides relief to almost all panic sufferers. Treatment is based on the idea that panic occurs when a person mistakes normal symptoms of anxiety for symptoms of a heart attack, going crazy, or dying. The fear that something is wrong can escalate into a full-fledged panic attack. In cognitive therapy you'll learn to short-circuit that reaction by interpreting anxiety symptoms for what they are.

> Research has shown that many conditions can be helped by more than one kind of therapy.

Phobias

Strong, irrational fears affect more than 10 percent of American adults. Some fear specific objects, such as animals, snakes, or insects; even more can't bear crowded places or open spaces, a condition called agoraphobia. Still others with social phobia recoil from situations involving other people.

Two behavior therapies are now used, with considerable success, to treat phobias. In both, you'll have to confront what you most fear. The more gradual technique is **systematic desensitization:** After learning progressive relaxation, you'll construct a fear hierarchy with the most terror-inducing situation at the top. In the first of a series of steps, you'll go into a relaxed state, then vividly imagine the least fearsome situation—or face it in real life. Gradually you'll move up the hierarchy and face more frightening situations.

During **flooding,** the other therapy, you're thrown in immediately with the thing that scares you; a cat phobic, for instance, will sit in a room full of cats. The goal is to stay for an agreed-upon length of time while the anxiety ebbs.

Behavior therapy is most successful with object and social phobias, producing lasting results in the majority of cases in a matter of weeks or months. In agoraphobia, behavior therapy is best combined with an antidepressant drug to control panic.

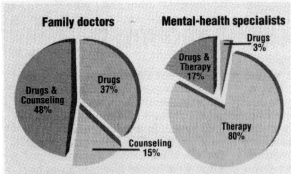

Family doctors

Drugs & Counseling 48%

Drugs 37%

Counseling 15%

Mental-health specialists

Drugs 3%

Drugs & Therapy 17%

Therapy 80%

Talk or drugs? Family doctors were much more likely to dispense mostly medication or a mix of drugs and talk. Very few mental-health therapists relied mainly on drugs; the vast majority provided psychotherapy.

struggling with alcoholism, realized they could stay sober by talking to one another. They talked to other alcoholics, too, and eventually worked out the system of long-term recovery known as Alcoholics Anonymous, or AA. Today there are over a million active AA members in the U.S., and attending an AA group is often recommended as part of professional treatment. The AA format has also been adopted by dozens of other self-help groups representing a wide spectrum of dysfunctional behavior, from Gamblers Anonymous to Sex and Love Addicts Anon. Support groups also bring together people who are dealing with medical illness or other trials.

One-third of our survey respondents went to a group, often in addition to individual psychotherapy. Overall, they told us, the groups seemed to help.

Readers who went to AA voiced overwhelming approval. Virtually all endorsed AA's approach to treatment, and most said their struggle with addiction had been largely successful. In keeping with AA's principle that recovery is a lifelong process, three-quarters of our readers had been in the group for more than two years, and most were still attending. Most of those who had dropped out said they'd moved on because their problems had improved.

Certainly, not everyone who goes to AA does as well; our sampling method probably over-represented long-term, and thus successful, AA members. AA's own surveys suggest that about half of those who come to the program are gone within three months. Studies that follow people who have undergone treatment for alcoholism find that AA is

no more or less effective than other programs: A year after entering treatment, about half the participants are still in trouble.

Nevertheless, AA has several components that may maximize the chance of success. In general, most alcoholics do well while they are being actively treated. In AA, members are supposed to attend 90 meetings in the first 90 days, followed by three meetings a week for life.

Drugs, pro and con

For decades, drug therapy to treat problems such as depression carried a raft of unpleasant, sometimes dangerous side effects. Then came *Prozac* (fluoxetine), launched in 1988. Safer and easier to take than previous antidepressants, *Prozac* and other drugs in its class—including sertraline (*Zoloft*) and paroxetine (*Paxil*)—have radically changed the treatment of depression. Along the way, people have claimed that *Prozac* seems to relieve a growing list of other complaints—from eating disorders to shyness, to most recently, premenstrual syndrome.

In our survey, 40 percent of readers who sought professional help received psychiatric drugs. And overall, about 60 percent of readers who took drugs said the medication helped a lot.

However, many of our readers did well with psychotherapy alone; in fact, people who received only psychotherapy improved as much as those who got therapy plus drugs.

For many people, having the option of talk therapy is important because every psychiatric drug has potential side effects that some individuals find hard to tolerate. Almost half of all our respondents on medication reported problems with the drug. Drowsiness and a feeling of disorientation were the most common complaints, especially among people taking the older antidepressants such as amitriptyline (*Elavil*).

Although the problems associated with psychiatric drugs are well-known, 20 percent of readers said their provider never discussed them —a disturbing lapse in communica-

tion. Equally disturbing was the finding that 40 percent of the people taking antianxiety drugs had done so for more than a year—25 percent for more than two years—even though long-term use results in habituation, requiring larger and larger doses.

Antianxiety medications such as *Xanax* and *Valium* can provide relief if used for a short time during a particularly stressful period, such as the death of a parent. But they haven't been well tested for generalized anxiety—a kind of chronic, excessive worrying combined with physical and emotional symptoms— and therapists have found them only erratically effective.

Xanax is approved by the U.S. Food and Drug Administration for panic disorder, which causes repeated bouts of unbearable anxiety; studies show that it acts quickly to reduce panic attacks. But after two months, *Xanax* apparently performs little better than a placebo. (See CONSUMER REPORTS, January 1993.) The reason many people take antianxiety drugs for so long is that they're extremely hard to kick; if the drug is stopped, symptoms return in full force.

How long will it take?

When a person needs psychotherapy, how much do they need? That has become a critical question— both for clinicians and for the insurers that pay for therapy. And it's a hard one to answer.

Nationally, most people who get therapy go for a relatively short time— an average of four to eight sessions. It's not clear, however, whether people stop going because they have been helped enough, because they don't think the therapy is working, or because they've run out of money. Controlled studies of specific kinds of therapy usually cover only 12 to 20 visits. While brief therapy often

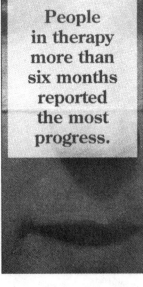

People in therapy more than six months reported the most progress.

helps, there's no way to tell from such studies whether 30 or 40 sessions, or even more, would be even more effective.

For the people in our survey, longer psychotherapy was associated with better outcomes. Among people who entered therapy with similar levels of emotional distress, those who stayed in treatment for more than six months reported greater gains than those who left earlier. Our data suggest that for many people, even a year's worth of therapy with a mental-health specialist may be very worthwhile. People who stayed in treatment for more than two years reported the best outcomes of all. However, these people tended to have started out with more serious problems.

We also found that people got better in three distinct ways, and that all three kinds of improvement increased with additional treatment. First, therapy eased the problems that brought people to treatment. Second, it helped them to function better, improving their ability to relate well to others, to be productive at work, and to cope with everyday stress. And it enhanced what can be called "personal growth." People in therapy had more confidence and self-esteem, understood themselves better, and enjoyed life more.

Despite the potential benefit of long-term therapy, many insurance plans limit mental-health coverage to "medically necessary" services—which typically means short-term treatment aimed at symptom relief. If you want to stay in therapy longer, you may have to pay for it yourself.

Our findings complement recent work by psychologist Kenneth Howard of Northwestern University. By following the progress of 854 psychotherapy patients, Howard and his associates found that recovery followed a "dose-response" curve, with the greatest response occurring early on. On average, 50 percent of people recovered after 11 weekly therapy sessions, and 75 percent got better after about a year.

Recommendations

Emotional distress may not always require professional help. But when problems threaten to become overwhelming or interfere with everyday life, there's no need to feel defeated.

Our survey shows there's real help available from every quarter—family doctors, psychotherapists, and self-help groups. Both talk therapy and medication, when warranted, can bring relief to people with a wide range of problems and deep despair.

With such clear benefits to be had, the strict limits on insurance coverage for mental-health care are cause for concern. As the debate over health care continues, we believe

that improving mental-health coverage is important.

If you want to see a therapist, you should approach therapy as an active consumer. In our survey, the more diligently a person "shopped" for a therapist—consulting with several candidates, checking their experience and qualifications, and speaking to previous clients—the more they ultimately improved. Once in treatment, those who formed a real partnership with their therapist —by being open, even with painful subjects, and by working on issues between sessions—were more likely to progress.

When you look for a therapist, competence and personal chemistry should be your priorities. You'll be sharing your most intimate thoughts and feelings, so it's important to choose someone who puts you at ease.

Many people first consult their family doctor, who has already won their confidence and trust. If you decide to stay with your physician for treatment, bear in mind that the approach will probably be medically based and relatively short.

If you would prefer to work with a therapist, ask your doctor for a referral. Other good referral sources are national professional associations or their local or state chapters. For information or referrals you can call the American Psychiatric Association, at 202 682-6220; the American Psychological Association, 202 336-5800; the National Association of Social Workers, 800 638-8799, ext. 291; the American Association for Marriage and Family Therapy, 800 374-2638; and the American Psychiatric Nurses Association, 202 857-1133. Also contact local universities, hospitals, and psychotherapy and psychoanalytic training institutes. For general information on mental illness, call the National Alliance for the Mentally Ill, 800 950-6264.

Family and friends may also know of reputable therapists; try to get several names to consider. Our readers who located therapists through personal or professional references felt better served than those who relied on ads, their managed care company's roster, or local clinics.

THE TYPES OF THERAPIES AND THERAPISTS

If you're considering mental-health treatment, you're facing a wide choice of therapies and practitioners. Many therapists favor a particular theoretical approach, though often they use a combination.

In **psychoanalysis**, Freud's classical technique employing a couch and free association, patients explore and confront troubling childhood experiences. In **psychodynamic therapy**, the emphasis is on discovering unconscious conflicts and defense mechanisms that hinder adult behavior. The goal of **interpersonal therapy** is to enhance relationships and communication skills. **Cognitive therapy** is aimed at helping people recognize and change distorted ways of thinking. **Behavioral therapy** seeks to replace harmful behaviors with useful ones.

As for choosing a therapist, be careful. Anyone can legally be called a psychotherapist, whether or not he or she has received the training and supervision needed to competently practice. Look for someone licensed or certified in one of the following fields:

■ **Psychiatrists** are physicians who have completed three years of residency training in psychiatry following four years of medical school and a one-year internship. All are trained in psychiatric diagnosis and pharmacotherapy, but only some residency

programs provide extensive experience in outpatient psychotherapy.

■ **Psychoanalysts** have a professional degree in psychiatry, psychology, or social work, plus at least two years of extensive supervised training at a psychoanalytic institute.

■ **Psychologists** with the credential Ph.D., Psy.D., or Ed.D. are licensed professionals with doctoral-level training, typically including a year of clinical internship in a mental-health facility and a year of supervised post-doctoral experience.

■ **Social workers** typically train in a two-year master's degree program that involves fieldwork in a wide range of human services, including mental health settings. Those who seek state certification or licensing as a clinical social worker need two years of supervised post-grad experience and must pass a statewide exam.

■ **Marriage and family therapists** may have a master's or doctoral degree from an accredited graduate training program in the field, or may have another professional degree with supervised experience in the specialty.

■ **Psychiatric nurses** are registered nurses who work in mental-health settings, often as part of a therapeutic team. Advanced practice nurses have a master's degree and can provide psychotherapy.

A Buyer's Guide to
Psychotherapy

How does a consumer, shopping for answers to life's dilemmas, know whose wisdom to buy? Hire a therapist who leads a life that seems desirable to you, insists psychiatrist Frank Pittman III, M.D.

For 33 years as a psychotherapist, I've sold myself by the hour. People pay to talk to me about themselves. They come singly, in pairs, and in small groups. Some of them ask me to help them figure out what they could do differently to make their life and relationships work better. Other just bitch and moan and demand pity.

I sell them my time and whatever wisdom I have developed. If they expect their insurance to pay for it, I may apply a psychiatric diagnosis to them as well. If their brain chemistry is too messed up for them to think through their situation and to do whatever needs to be done, I sometimes prescribe medicine to fix the problem in their brain so they can then go on to fix the problems in their life. I also give them my humor; I try to make an hour with me entertaining as well as enlightening. I feel honored that they have brought their pain to me. The least I can do is make the removal of their pain as painless as possible.

I used to be proud of what I did. That has changed. Perhaps it was the unsettling experience of trying to explain to friends from abroad—for whom American psychotherapy is a foreign culture—how perennial psychotherapy customer Woody Allen could have undergone therapy for most of his life and still not have seen anything incestuous in his sexual relationship with his de facto stepdaughter, the sister of his children. When asked about his analyst's reaction, Allen is rumored to have said, "It didn't come up. It wasn't a relevant issue for my therapy."

Most humiliating for a respectable psychotherapist is the recently popular application of the format and jargon of psychotherapy to people's search for a victim identity. The victim identity is like a doctor's excuse from a gym class or history exam, only it is an excuse from life itself. People who want to be victims may nurture their inner child, may style themselves as adult children of imperfect parenting, or may announce that they are survivors of real or imagined unpleasant experiences. Either way, they resign from the adult world, eschew responsibility for their conduct in relationships, and whimper that the world owes them a life.

Values and Psychotherapy

There *is* such a thing as mental illness. It is real and it is horrible, whether it occurs as schizophrenia or mania or depression. Treating real mental illness may be the major professional expertise of mental health professionals, but it is a minor activity of psychotherapists. Most psychotherapy is about values—about the value dilemmas of sane and ordinary people trying to lead a life amidst great personal, familial, and cultural confusion. The therapists who do psychotherapy effectively do so because they understand value conflicts and they convey, without having to preach about it, values that work.

Psychotherapy is a process in which people in pain and/or turmoil purchase the time and expertise of a therapist who helps them: 1) define the problem; 2) figure out what normal people might

do under these circumstances; 3) expose the misinformation, the misplaced loyalty, or the uncomfortable emotion that keeps the customer from doing the sensible thing; and 4) provide the customer with the courage (or fear of the therapist's disapproval) to change—that is, to do what needs to be done.

Psychotherapists vary widely in the rapidity with which they provide their customers with answers to the questions being raised, and the degree to which they take credit for providing the answers. Some will simply tell people what to do; others will make the customer guess for a few years before subtly signaling they've finally gotten it right.

Most therapists work hard at trying to get people to do what we think is right and to take credit for it themselves. The trick is to keep pushing and hinting without seeming so bossy, controlling, or disapproving that we run them out of therapy before they have changed their behavior or solved their problems. It's not an easy job and, while it doesn't require brilliance or magic or even a loving nature, it takes both talent and skill—the talent to keep the customer in therapy long enough for it to work and the skill to define the problems and solutions to the dilemmas of human existence.

Psychotherapy ordinarily offers a safe and accepting format for helping people come to grips with their emotions and then go ahead and do sensible things with their lives, whether they feel like it or not. It's a process by which people identify and talk about what they feel,

Reprinted with permission from *Psychology Today*, January/February 1994, pp. 50-53, 74, 76-78, 80-81. © 1994 by Sussex Publishers, Inc.

rather than act on their emotions and do what they feel like doing. In the process, there may be a transfer of sanity and reality testing from therapist to patient. The therapist's calm may soothe the frantic patient. Sometimes the therapist is the one who must get frantic in order to alarm an inappropriately calm patient who fails to see the dangers in his or her actions.

Either way, psychotherapy involves applying the value system of the therapist to the dilemmas of the clients. The most important work of psychotherapy takes place inside the therapist's head as he or she thinks through the patient's snag points in dealing with this latest bump along the road of life.

When you go to a psychiatrist for medication or shock treatment, or to a psychologist for psychological testing, it may not matter very much what sort of person the professional is. But if you're choosing to bring a psychotherapist into your life as a consultant, his or her value system is more important to you than training, credentials, or even a professional degree.

The Myth of Therapeutic Neutrality

Whatever psychotherapy is, it is not about therapeutic neutrality. Therapeutic neutrality is a stance inherited from classical psychoanalysis, in which the silent, passive analyst refuses to react or comment on what the patient is saying or doing, thus encouraging the patient to regress into a "transference neurosis" on the analyst. Needless to say, such unresponsiveness brings forth all manner of crazy emotional responses. Except in classical psychoanalysis, neutrality is not only rude and inappropriate, it also makes you crazy.

Even is a therapist *could* be neutral about the issues at hand—impossible!—that neutrality would at best bring the therapy to a limping halt and at worst seem to be an endorsement of the client's persistence to barrel the wrong way down a one-way street. (For a therapist to feign neutrality about someone racing for disaster is not neutral; it is sadistic.)

Yet therapists try to make themselves less threatening by pretending to be neutral about anything that borders on a moral issue. We therapists are trained to pretend to have no value systems at all and no sense of direction about the client's life, except for such benign virtues as unlimited patience, accurate empathy, steady optimism, nonpossessive warmth, and unconditional positive regard for whoever has rented the couch for that hour. Some therapists are opinionated people, with clearly established values, but they try to maintain their cramped neutral stances by detaching from patients and their dilemmas.

THE BLAMING BLIGHT

One of the horrors of psychotherapy is the affirmation clients may feel from their seemingly neutral therapists that they are "okay" even when they are doing terrible things to themselves and their loved ones. Some therapists listen without comment to tales of violence, substance abuse, infidelity, even incest. Their silence is tacit approval. Some therapists do worse than silently accept whatever the customer says or does; some actively affirm that the customer is always right. Therapists, as they ingratiate themselves to their customers, may actually provide "interpretations" to relieve clients of the guilt they need in order to keep them from hurting others and bringing disaster upon themselves.

Therapists may actually encourage customers to feel better about themselves by blaming their lives on other people, on the nature of human existence, or on the peculiar mores of the society around them. Repeatedly, men who are being unfaithful or violent are told by therapists that they are working out their anger at their mothers, while women who are being dishonest or mean are told they are battling patriarchy. Everyone gets distracted from the impact of the betrayal or the power play upon the marriage.

It used to be stylish for therapists to help people blame their lives on their mothers or on their wives—whoever loved them too possessively. Lately, the style has been to blame everything on fathers, husbands, or men in general—whoever failed to love them enough. There are therapists who are expert at finding errors made by parents and grant the now-grown children the right to consider themselves adult children of imperfect parenting. People who center their lives around blaming their parents aren't free to be adults and parents themselves. This blaming of others may relieve pain briefly, but it is not therapeutic; it does not lead to empowerment or control over one's life and behavior.

If people can't remember being victimized, some therapists specialize in uncovering forgotten abuse of various sorts. Forgotten incest is especially popular. I

don't know whether it does more harm to forget abuse or to remember it, but I'm sure that much of the incest gradually remembered in therapy or under hypnosis is a dutiful fabrication of dependent people trying to please a victimizing therapist.

THERAPY IS AN ADVERSARIAL PROCESS

Therapists should of course help people step out of their crippling state of victimhood. Good therapy is not a chaste love affair between buyer and seller of psychotherapeutic services. The therapist and the customer don't even have to like one another. The therapy may be working best when you don't like your therapist, when you get the firm impression that your therapist doesn't like you very much either, and when you are being told that you have to do something you don't want to do if you are ever to feel good about yourself.

In fact, the therapist is hired to scrutinize you sharply and find something about you that is unlikable and unworkable, and then to help you isolate and discard the offending behavior. If the therapist sees everything the way you do, the therapist would be in the same fix you're in. And if the therapist thinks you're wonderful the way you are and just wants you to realize it, the love affair that results is different from therapy. Therapy is an inherently adversarial process, not an alliance to buffer innocent victims against a world that isn't gentle enough.

THE WORLD TURNS

We are all given faulty instruction books by our parents. For the past 200 years, the old patriarchal system of gender role assignments has been eroding, too slowly of course, but still with disorienting speed. Each generation faces a new world in which girls have more options and more challenges in life and boys have less deference and less expectation that they will automatically sacrifice their lives for the masculine mystique.

While this is liberating for both men and women, it is also disorienting. Each generation of boys and girls must redefine for themselves and for one another what it expects of men and women. Boys and girls, to become men and women in a new world, must challenge, reject, and selectively rebel against their parents' values, which is frightening and can feel painfully disloyal.

Boys and girls don't have to fix their parents and don't have to cut off from them. They make the best use of their parents' values when they study their parents closely and question them about how they came to hold the values they hold, as well as how they find them to be working.

There are other aspects of us besides gender that are affected by the rapid changes in society. Social, cultural, and economic expectations change. We are now in a period of economic reversal. In many families the younger generation won't have it as cushy as their parents did, and may remain dependent on them.

Most younger people have moved part or all the way from their patriarchal roots and are enjoying greater range in their gender expression. Yet even the most progressive and open-minded of men and women may still carry within them, unchallenged, some of the models of marriage from their parents' or great-great-grandparents' generation, with the responsibilities, expectations, and privileges of a "head of the household" and his little "helpmate." Gender equality in marriage, championed by most (but not all) marriage therapists, may feel foreign operationally to many men and women. Those who recoil from equality may seek out a patriarchal therapist, perhaps a fundamentalist Christian counselor, who will try to protect them from having to challenge the model they learned growing up. Intellectually, they may want an equal relationship, but they feel deprived if they don't also have the loving domesticity of an idealized old-fashioned mother or the imperturbable strength of an idealized old-fashioned father. They just want the world to slow down until they can catch up.

THUS COME THE THERAPISTS

The world is changing so rapidly that people don't have to be mentally ill to be out of their minds some of the time, behaving inappropriately much of the time and a little bit disoriented all of the time. Therapists claim to have expertise in dealing with mental illness but also in dealing with the problems of living, in finding happiness and security in a rapidly changing world. Therapists, in effect, claim to have wisdom about human existence.

Actually, some probably do and some definitely don't. Therapists don't come into the business with any more wisdom than anyone else, though an inordinate number of them come from messed-up families that have made them wiser and more alert than those who slide into adulthood without enough trauma to trigger development of an armamentarium of coping skills.

But after meddling intimately in a few lives, the therapist changes. If the therapist is paying close attention to what is going on inside the client and inside the therapist, and having success in understanding people and in helping them change, the experience of doing therapy should make the therapist increasingly aware of various layers of emotional, interpersonal, and social reality. The therapist must either get callous, get depressed, or get wise. The most experienced therapist is not necessarily the best, but the happiest experienced therapists are undoubtedly the wisest, since the therapy they do works and the wisdom they get from doing therapy helps them shape values that work in their own lives.

THINKING LIKE A THERAPIST

I know as a therapist I don't have to have all the right answers to life's questions. But I do have to have some. I'm likely to have better answers than the people who are stuck. If I don't, at least I have different ones, which may be just as good in moving someone out of the fix they're stuck in. It takes only a little wisdom to provide hope that there are other ways to do things.

I try to explain to therapists who are overwhelmed by what they see in their offices that there are no techniques and no solutions that will solve these problems. But there are ways in which the therapist can think about the issues, ways in which the therapist can reframe the problem, that permits it to be either accepted or solved, not perhaps in the way that anyone would *want* to solve it, but at least in a way that permits life to go on. I try to teach therapists how to think about human dilemmas in a way that is therapeutic.

THE DANGERS OF EMOTION WORSHIP

Some therapists can't think therapeutically because they let feelings take priority, as if all actions must be emotionally coherent. These therapists assume that when people follow their feelings purely and clearly, they will get to the desired destination. In his book, *Another Roadside Attraction*, Tom Robbins says "Living from your feelings is like nailing a chiffon pie to the wall."

When therapists give their primary attention in therapy to how people feel, they convey the notion that feelings are the most important determinant of action. They distract customers from their exercises in reality testing, their efforts to ex-

plore and observe, and to understand the workings of the world around them. Instead, they turn their patients' attention inward, as if they were doping them up on hallucinogens. Such therapists seem to believe that the secrets of the universe, the true and accurate instruction book of life, are inside the increasingly muddled heads of their customers.

This might have made some sense back in Freud's day, when people were not accustomed to thinking, much less talking, about how they felt. But no one has an inner emotional life any more, since any feeling, before it is fully formed, is spilled out to the world on Sally, Oprah, or Phil. Introspectiveness does not lead to workable relationships because romantics spend their time thinking about how they want the people around them to be in order to make their dreams come true, rather than attempting to understand what their loved ones are like and why they are like that. Unceasing introspectiveness leads to narcissism and ultimately to loneliness and very few invitations to dinner with others.

If your therapist seems to give a great deal more weight to your feelings than to the feelings of the people who share your life, you may have to keep your attention focused on how you might be affecting them rather than just on how they are affecting you. You may even need to remind your therapist that acting on your impulses may not necessarily be good for your loved ones.

The most dangerous extreme of emotion worship is romanticism. Romantics are eager to sacrifice their lives, or the lives of their loved ones, in pursuit of emotional coherence. For romantics, life is inherently tragic. Romantic therapists may encourage the notion that following your emotions will give you the power to overcome reality, time, or gravity. Married people in affairs may think that, if they love each other enough, they can leave their mates and children and, after stepping over their bodies in their walk down the aisle, live happily ever after.

BEWARE OF CONSPIRATORIAL THERAPISTS

A few years ago, I wrote a book about the disruptive effect of infidelity and secrets, and found myself attacked by prominent marriage therapists. They explained that infidelity was normal behavior but too emotionally provocative to bring up in therapy, especially since it was no doubt the

Most psychotherapy is not about mental illness but about values—about the value dilemmas of sane and ordinary people trying to lead a life amidst great personal, familial, and cultural confusion.

fault of the marriage partner who was being betrayed, and who could thus not be told about it. My male colleagues explained that women who had been betrayed would just get "stirred up" and ruin the therapy with a lot of anger. My female colleagues explained that men shouldn't be told bad news since they would just get violent. Both explained that it was necessary to lie to people of other genders. Those therapists who were still speaking to me after the book came out offered to teach me their techniques for keeping the cuckold so disoriented about what was going on in the marriage and in therapy that the infidelity wouldn't have to be dealt with at all, and could continue untouched by the therapy.

To me it is arrogant of therapists to conspire with one member of a family or a couple to keep others in the family disoriented about matters that are crucial to their orientation and understanding of their life. Infidelity scares therapists. Couples therapists who conspire to keep sexual secrets are showing tremendous disrespect for the cuckold who is being betrayed, first by a spouse and then by the therapist.

Men have come in, referred by their divorce attorneys, asking for a course of ersatz marriage counseling that will look good in the divorce case and distract their wives from realizing that there is a secret affair going on. They hope that I can sufficiently confuse and disorient the wife, and make her think she is in some way responsible for the failure of the marriage. Then they can get by with a less expensive divorce settlement. Most therapists would refuse such a mission, but some enjoy the chance to champion a client against enemies.

What Makes A Good Therapist?

1. A good therapist has got to like doing therapy. A wise old therapist friend acknowledged that those of us who become psychotherapists are people who need more hours of therapy each day than we can afford to buy for ourselves. I don't mean that therapists have more mental illness than other people, but that they get more out of therapy. Good therapists are good patients, people who enjoy swimming in emotions without drowning in them. They feel refreshed after an emotional workout.

2. Good therapists have got to be optimistic, believing that life is a comedy, not a tragedy, even if you can't get out of it alive. They can't be afraid of failures and embarrassment and pain, or even of tragedies. Good therapists aren't protective of their clients. Therapists can't do good therapy when they are afraid of losing their customers, of having customers commit suicide or sue them.

3. Good therapists have got to be eager detectives and explorers, people who like to solve mysteries and figure out how life works. They have a homing device that leads them quickly and directly to the aspects of the situation that don't make sense. Sherlock Holmes and Sigmund Freud had more in common than cocaine. Good therapists don't take things at face value, they don't assume they understand everything from the beginning, and they certainly don't assume that everyone is alike and that one solution fits all. They have to be eager to understand the intricacies of a new situation. Good therapists are excited by each new client, and learn something new from each.

4. Good therapists certainly have to be warm—they may not be especially loving or nurturing, but they delight in intimacy. They must be able to understand and share experiences: their own, those of their customers, and those of the people whose lives are touched by their customers. Good therapists are not quite like good parents, who are massively invested in those they would raise—that position is inevitably too possessive. They are more like aunts and uncles, offering an alternate view of reality while invested in the outcome, but not so possessive that their own identity is at stake.

5. Good therapists have got to have a sense of humor. Without it, they may try to protect their customers from the cruelties of life—those unpleasant but necessary experiences that give people chances to expand consciousness and build character. Of course, good patients have to have a good sense of humor too. Good therapy is fun, and spoils both therapist and patient for the sort of cautious, polite interaction that takes place at social occasions.

6. Above all, good therapists have got to be fairly sane—not rigidly, anxiously, cautiously sane, but able to see fairly clearly how the world works. It also helps if therapists are happy people, not stuck in happiness like manics or TV weather forecasters, but able to experience a full range of human emotions.

A buyer of psychotherapy should not use a therapist as an instrument for inflicting harm on loved ones, for dispensing misinformation or concealing information that will drive his or her partner too crazy to understand what's going on. A therapist is not supposed to be your champion, but your critic. A therapist is not like a lawyer. The lawyer is out to prove you innocent of any wrongdoing; thereby the lawyer saves your skin. The therapist is out to show you how you screwed up and brought disaster

upon yourself; thereby the therapist saves your life. Your therapist, in pleading your case to the people in your life, will emphasize your guilt, not your innocence. Your lawyer wants to confuse the judge and the jury so you will never have to deal with those people again. The therapist wants to reveal the truth and enlighten the people in your life, so you can honestly and intimately deal with those people forever after.

As a therapy consumer, you may be tempted to see the therapist as a judge rather than as a defense attorney, and ask the therapist to take your side and declare you to be right. That would be a misunderstanding of the function of the therapist, which is to understand the ways in which you are wrong.

Foolish therapy customers have been known to hit their relatives with actual extracted or invented quotes from the therapist that are critical of the relatives and defensive of the patient. This can effectively sabotage couples or family therapy, where the therapist knows the relatives being criticized. When the relatives are criticized in absentia by a therapist, they understandably go on the defensive and will actively undercut the therapy. What a waste of a therapist!

WHAT'S YOUR THERAPIST'S VIEW OF MARRIAGE?

Some therapists believe in marriage so strongly they see singlehood as a state of emotional deprivation that is the cause of all the pain in the life of single people. Such therapists may rush people into ill-advised marriages, some of which will work and some of which won't.

Other therapists distrust marriage so totally they see it as a dangerously oppressive state of exploitation and impending doom. They assume that any pain a married person suffers is brought on by the marriage. These therapists likely experienced disappointment in their marriages or their parents' marriages.

In between are therapists who idealize marriage, and give full support to perfect marriages and short shrift to those with problems. Some therapists, especially those who didn't come in from the Sixties in time, still believe that mental health comes from running away from home, and if people are too old to run away from their parents, they can run away from their marriage.

They don't understand that the struggle of marriage is second only to the raising of children as the central maturing experience of life. As with the combat of war, you win the important victory, the one over yourself and your fears, simply by not running away.

Married people would do well to stick with therapists who believe in marriage. But such therapists must believe in divorce too, not as a path to happiness and a more perfect partner next time (second marriages have an even higher divorce rate than first ones, and third marriages are probably uninsurable), but as an escape from the unendurable, like recurrent violence, chronic alcoholism, or philandering. Therapists should make customers contemplating divorce aware of the devastating impact on the children and the shock waves that will continue for generations.

A therapist who endorses divorce too glibly or dismisses marriage too offhandedly is dangerous. But so is a therapist who does not empower you to leave a truly abusive marital situation. Knowing you can leave, and convincing your abusive partner that you can leave, perhaps by actually leaving for a time, may be more helpful than divorce. The point of therapy should not be to protect you from unpleasantness and disappointment, but to empower you to take charge of your life and your marriage. You must realize your marriage is not the property of your partner, but is yours. And you have a say in how it goes and whether it goes. You must not be bullied into it. Or out of it.

Patterns of Symptomatic Recovery in Psychotherapy

Stephen Mark Kopta, Kenneth I. Howard, Jenny L. Lowry, and Larry E. Beutler

Using the psychotherapy dosage model in which effect was probability of recovery, this study compared treatment response rates for psychological symptoms. Symptom checklists were administered to 854 psychotherapy outpatients at intake and during treatment. Sixty-two symptoms were grouped into 3 classes on the basis of probit analysis results. Chronic distress symptoms demonstrated the fastest average response rate, whereas characterological symptoms demonstrated the slowest. Acute distress symptoms showed the highest average percentage of patients recovered across doses. A typical outpatient needed about a year of psychotherapy to have a 75% chance of symptomatic recovery. The model holds promise for establishing guidelines for the financing of psychotherapy.

Howard, Kopta, Krause, and Orlinsky (1986) introduced a psychotherapy dosage model in which *dose* was measured by the number of sessions and the *effect* of treatment was measured by the percentage of patients improved or the normalized probability of improvement for one patient. For a sample of individual psychotherapy outpatients, using traditional measures of improvement, when effect was plotted against dose, Howard et al. found a positive relationship characterized by a negatively accelerated curve; that is, the more psychotherapy, the greater the probability of improvement, with diminishing returns at higher doses (see Figure 1). They also performed a meta-analysis on 15 samples of outpatient data. Submitting the data from

each sample to probit analysis, which provides a log-normal transformation of the curvilinear function, a linear dose–effect relationship was estimated so that after 8 weekly sessions, 53% of the patients improved; after 26 sessions, 74%; and after 52 sessions, 83%.

For the dosage model, the psychotherapy session is the unit of treatment and it is assumed that the number of sessions is stochastically related to exposure to the active ingredients (e.g., interpretations, reinforcements, empathic reflections) in any type of psychotherapy; that is, the more sessions the patient experiences, the higher the dose of active ingredients to which he or she is exposed. We make the analogy of number of sessions as dose in psychotherapy to the use of weight in milligrams as the dosage unit in pharmacological treatments.

Jacobson, Follette, and Revenstorf (1984) proposed that improvement reaches clinical significance when a patient recovers to the point where he or she is more similar to normal functional persons than to his or her dysfunctional peers. Applying the psychotherapy dosage model and using Jacobson et al.'s (1984) standard of clinical significance, one can estimate probabilities of when normal functioning is achieved for specific doses of psychotherapy. In other words, one can then estimate how much treatment is enough.

The purpose of this study was to discover the rates at which different psychological symptoms remit to normal levels during psychotherapy. We were also interested in exploring the related issue of defining, in general, how much psychotherapy might be enough for a typical patient.

Individual psychotherapy outpatients completed the Symptom Checklist-90—Revised (*SCL–90–R*; Derogatis, 1983) or a briefer version before their first therapy session and at least at one other point during treatment. Applying probit analysis to the data, dose–effect relations were calculated for the items (i.e., symptoms) of the *SCL–90–R*. Effect was operationalized as the probability that a given symptom score was derived from a normal, functional population. After inspection of the treatment response rates, the symptoms were empirically grouped (highest rates to lowest rates) into three classes: acute distress, chronic distress, and characterological symptoms, respectively. Then, comparisons between the classes were made, using percentage of patients recovered across doses as the dependent variable.

Editor's Note. Clara E. Hill served as the guest editor for this article. An outside action editor was used for processing this article to minimize any conflict of interest induced by Larry E. Beutler's role as Editor of the *Journal of Consulting and Clinical Psychology.*

Stephen Mark Kopta, Department of Psychology, University of Evansville; Kenneth I. Howard, Department of Psychology, Northwestern University; Jenny L. Lowry, Department of Psychology, St. Louis University; Larry E. Beutler, Graduate School of Education, University of California, Santa Barbara.

An earlier version of this article was presented at the 23rd Annual Meeting of the Society for Psychotherapy Research, Berkeley, California, in June 1992.

This research was supported by National Institute of Mental Health Grants R01 MH 42901 and 1 K05 MH00924-01A1, awarded to Kenneth I. Howard, and three University of Evansville Undergraduate Research Grants, awarded to Stephen Mark Kopta.

We thank Mary Smith of Ravenswood Hospital Community Mental Health Center, Richard Paul of Southwestern Indiana Mental Health Center, and Jay Lebow, formerly of DuPage County Health Department, Mental Health Division, as well as the staff of all five participating mental health centers for their cooperation. Our thanks also goes to Leonard Derogatis for providing *SCL–90–R* item endorsement frequencies from his normal, functional sample. We are grateful to Bruce Briscoe for his computer work, Zoran Martinovich for his statistical consultation, and to the undergraduate research assistants: Mary Jane Manford, Tina Hooper, Patrick Richardson, Anna Davis, and Jennifer Hill.

Correspondence concerning this article should be addressed to Stephen Mark Kopta, Department of Psychology, University of Evansville, 1800 Lincoln Avenue, Evansville, Indiana 47722.

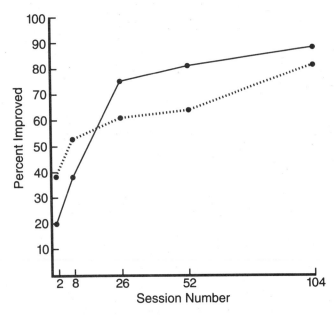

Figure 1. Note. From "The Dose–Effect Relationship in Psychotherapy," by Kenneth I. Howard, Stephen Mark Kopta, Merton S. Krause, and David E. Orlinsky, 1986, *American Psychologist, 41,* p. 160. Copyright 1986 by the American Psychological Association. Relation of number of sessions of psychotherapy and percentage of patients improved. (Objective ratings at termination are shown by the solid line; subjective ratings during therapy are shown by the broken line.)

Method

Patients

The sample consisted of adult outpatients (18 years or older) who were in individual psychotherapy at five mental health centers (see Table 1). The initial sample consisted of 854 patients. After the selection process (described later), as many as 685 patients were included in a data analysis for a given symptom. All patients experienced time-unlimited therapy; frequency of sessions was usually once a week. None of the patients experienced primarily behavioral therapy and few were given any significant psychopharmacological treatment. Table 1 presents demographic, diagnostic, and treatment details of the sample, broken down by site. The therapists or intake interviewers determined diagnoses through clinical interviews using the criteria of the *Diagnostic and Statistical Manual of Mental Disorders* (3rd edition, American Psychiatric Association [APA], 1980; 3rd edition, revised [*DSM–III–R*], APA, 1987).

Therapists

The psychotherapists were 141 psychologists, psychiatrists, and social workers, or trainees in these fields. They identified their theoretical orientations as follows: psychodynamic (71%), eclectic (15%), and other (14%; e.g., cognitive–behavioral, client-centered, etc.). Thirty-five percent indicated 5 or more years of experience practicing psychotherapy, whereas 65% noted less than 5 years experience. Fifty-six percent were female, with the mean age for all therapists of 33 years ($SD = 6.4$ years).

Materials

Symptom distress was measured with the *SCL–90–R* or one of three brief versions of this instrument, which have proven to be reliable and valid self-report measures (e.g., Derogatis, 1983). The *SCL–90–R* consists of 90 items or symptoms that were originally factor analyzed into nine symptom dimensions: Anxiety, Depression, Hostility, Interpersonal Sensitivity, Obsessive–Compulsive, Paranoid Ideation, Phobic Anxiety, Psychoticism, and Somatization (Derogatis, 1983). The three brief versions of the *SCL–90–R* included the 53-item Brief Symptom Inventory (at University of Arizona Health Science Center, $n = 63$; Derogatis & Spencer, 1983), a 47-item version (at Northwestern Memorial Hospital, $n = 263$), and a 61-item version (at Southwestern Indiana Mental Health Center, $n = 51$). Patients rated symptom distress on a 0 (*not at all*) to 4 (*extremely*) scale. Most of the items omitted from the brief versions were those that were endorsed (i.e., rated 1, 2, 3, or 4) by fewer than 55% of the patients in Derogatis's (1983) psychiatric outpatient sample ($N = 1,002$).

Procedure

After signing a consent form, patients completed one of four versions of the *SCL–90–R* before the first psychotherapy session (intake) and at

Table 1
Treatment, Demographic, and Diagnostic Information of the Entire Sample

| Site | Patients | | | Sessions | | Diagnosis (%) | | | | |
	n	Female (%)	Age (M)	Median	Range	Anxiety	Depression	Personality disorder	Psychosis	Other
DuPage County Health Department	40	70	28	6	1–40	18	44	7	1	30
Northwestern Memorial Hospital	336	68	32	4	1–52	17	60	4	4	14
Ravenswood Hospital	310	74	35	16	1–52	22	37	12	1	28
Southwestern Indiana Mental Health Center	51	72	31	3	1–25	21	36	10	1	32
University of Arizona Health Science Center	117	72	39	18	3–52	20	70	0	0	10

Table 2
Dose–Effect Relations for Acute Distress Symptoms: Percentage Recovered at Selected Sessions

Symptom (dimension, n)	No. of sessions							ED50
	0	2	4	8	13	26	52	
Temper outbursts (HS, 305)	50	56	59	62	65	68	72	1
Feeling the need to check and double check (OC, 102)	43	56	61	68	73	79	84	2
Numbness or tingling (SM, 100)	43	59	66	73	78	85	90	3
Doing things slowly (OC, 107)	42	56	62	70	74	81	86	2
Headaches (SM, 234)	39	51	57	63	68	75	81	3
Loss of interest in sex (DP, 292)	33	43	47	53	57	62	68	6
Heart racing (AN, 109)	33	55	65	75	81	89	95	2
Having ideas that others do not share (PI, 230)	32	45	51	58	63	71	77	5
Having trouble remembering (OC, 157)	30	44	51	58	64	72	79	5
Feeling restless (AN, 242)	30	43	50	57	63	71	77	5
Feeling fearful (AN, 444)	29	42	47	55	60	67	74	6
Don't get credit (PI, 312)	29	39	51	53	59	67	74	7
Worrying about sloppiness (OC, 201)	27	44	53	62	69	77	85	4
Nausea (SM, 215)	27	44	53	62	69	78	86	4
Feeling that everything is an effort (DP, 308)	26	39	46	54	60	68	76	7
Being critical of others (IS, 258)	25	41	48	57	63	71	79	6
Hopelessness about the future (DP, 481)	25	37	44	51	57	65	72	8
Crying easily (DP, 287)	24	41	50	61	68	83	86	5
Feeling trapped (DP, 336)	24	37	43	51	56	65	72	9
Feeling weak in body (SM, 119)	24	44	55	66	74	83	93	4
Mean ED50								5

Note. ED50 = median effective dose: Entries represent the session number at which 50% of patients are estimated to show clinically significant improvement. Symptom Checklist 90–Revised symptom dimensions are as follows: HS = Hostility, OC = Obsessive–Compulsive, SM = Somatization, DP = Depression, AN = Anxiety, PI = Paranoid Ideation, IS = Interpersonal Sensitivity. For all values, clinical significance cutoff point was 1.

least at one other point during the course of treatment. Administration points varied according to site. At Northwestern Memorial Hospital, Ravenswood Hospital, and Southwestern Indiana Mental Health Center, the symptom checklists were completed by patients at pretreatment (intake), during treatment (at selected points), and posttreatment (at termination). At DuPage County Health Department and the University of Arizona Health Science Center, the checklists were completed at pretreatment and posttreatment only.

For each symptom, a patient was included in the data analyses if he or she indicated that the symptom earned a score of 2 (*moderate*) or more on a rating of distress at intake; that is, symptoms were considered to be present for a patient if the distress rating was 2 or greater. In turn, the therapists were queried by questionnaire or verbally on their theoretical orientation, years of experience, age, and sex.

Results

The formula used to determine the presence of clinically significant improvement (i.e., recovery) followed the recommendations by Jacobson and Truax (1991) for the situation in which norms from a functional sample are available and it is assumed that the variances of the functional and dysfunctional populations are unequal. The functional sample, which was obtained from a diverse community in an Eastern state, was provided by Derogatis ($N = 974$; Derogatis, 1989).

A patient was judged to have reached reliable, clinically significant improvement, based on Jacobson and Truax's (1991) procedure, if both the clinical significance cutoff point and the reliable change index were surpassed. The clinical significance cutoff point represents a discrete point that separates the dysfunctional and functional populations. It was calculated by using Jacobson and Truax's c formula:

$$CS = \frac{s_0 M_1 + s_1 M_0}{s_0 + s_1},$$

where M_1 is the pretreatment mean of the patient sample, M_0 is the mean of the normal sample obtained from Derogatis (1989), and the standard deviations of the patient and normal samples are S_1 and S_0, respectively.

Patients rated each symptom on a discrete scale ranging from 0 to 4. The formula suggested by Jacobson and Truax (1991) revealed that a positive change of two points or more indicated that reliable change had occurred ($p < .05$). A score of either 0 (*not at all*) or 1 (*a little bit*) was considered to be asymptomatic for purposes of analysis. Cutoff points for the symptoms are presented in Tables 2, 3, and 4.

The pool of items was first reduced to prevent the instability of symptoms receiving few endorsements from inadvertently

Table 3
Dose–Effect Relations for Chronic Distress Symptoms: Percentage Recovered at Selected Sessions

Symptom (dimension, n)	No. of sessions							ED50
	0	2	4	8	13	26	52	
Lonely with people (PS, 312)[a]	24	26	36	43	48	57	65	16
Feelings easily hurt (IS, 395)[a]	22	35	42	50	56	65	73	9
Feeling something bad (AN, 131)[b]	21	32	38	45	50	58	66	14
Scared for no reason (AN, 133)[b]	20	30	35	41	46	53	61	20
Trouble concentrating (OC, 498)[a]	19	33	41	50	56	66	75	9
Feeling tense (AN, 641)[a]	19	30	35	42	48	56	64	17
Low in energy (DP, 456)[a]	18	31	38	47	53	63	72	11
Self-consciousness (IS, 286)[a]	18	32	40	50	57	67	76	9
Feelings of guilt (354)[a]	18	33	42	52	60	71	80	8
Repeated thoughts (OC, 537)[a]	17	32	42	52	60	71	80	8
Difficulty with decisions (OC, 466)[a]	17	31	38	48	55	66	76	10
Terror or panic (AN, 112)[b]	17	31	38	46	53	63	72	11
Feeling blue (DP, 634)[a]	16	29	40	47	54	64	74	11
Others not sympathetic (IS, 401)[a]	16	33	43	54	63	74	84	7
Feeling worthless (DP, 441)[b]	16	33	44	56	65	77	86	7
Poor appetite (104)[b]	14	26	32	45	48	58	68	16
Feeling lonely (DP, 573)[a]	14	26	32	41	48	53	68	16
Thoughts of death (141)[a]	14	31	42	53	62	75	84	8
Feeling blocked (OC, 389)[a]	13	25	33	42	50	60	71	14
Shy with opposite sex (IS, 112)[b]	13	22	28	35	41	50	60	27
Worry too much (DP, 685)[a]	11	21	27	35	41	51	61	25
Blaming yourself (DP, 571)[a]	11	26	35	46	54	66	77	11
Feeling no interest (DP, 253)[a]	11	23	21	30	47	57	67	17
Uneasy in crowds (PH, 100)[b]	11	22	29	37	44	55	65	20
Nervous when alone (PH, 174)[b]	10	20	26	35	42	52	63	23
People dislike you (IS, 124)[b]	10	21	28	36	43	54	65	20
Avoid things, places because frightened (PH, 211)[b]	9	21	28	39	47	60	72	16
Mean ED50								14

Note. ED50 = median effective dose. Entries represent the session number at which 50% of patients are estimated to show clinically significant improvement. Symptom Checklist 90–Revised symptom dimensions: PS = Psychoticism, IS = Interpersonal Sensitivity, AN = Anxiety, OC = Obsessive–Compulsive, DP = Depression, PH = Phobic Anxiety. Absence of acronym indicates that the symptom is not associated with any symptom dimension.
[a] Clinical significance cutoff point was 1.   [b] Clinical significance cutoff point was 0.

affecting the grouping. Only those symptoms that were indicated as being present (i.e., rated as 2 or greater) at intake for 100 or more patients were included in the subsequent analyses. The 64 items that met this criterion were analyzed by using probit analysis (Finney, 1971).

In the probit analysis procedure, dose was the session number at which a symptom checklist was administered. Each symptom of each patient was classified as a dichotomous variable, *recovered* or *not recovered,* depending on whether or not the symptom change achieved clinical significance. Probit analysis produces linear regression coefficients ($y = a + bx$), where y is effect (i.e., normalized probability of clinically significant improvement) and x is the log of dose. The log-normal transformation produces a linear function from the negatively accelerated curve (see Figure 1). As few patients ($n = 35$) received more than 52 sessions, data points greater than 52 sessions were omitted from the analyses to stabilize the regression estimates.

For each of the 64 included symptoms, the percentage of patients who recovered with selected doses of psychotherapy were calculated. The treatment response rates were consistent with Howard et al.'s (1986) previous findings that improvement is proportionally greater early in treatment, with diminishing returns of benefit at higher dose levels. Two symptoms (i.e., nervousness or shakiness inside, $n = 513$; feeling inferior to others, $n = 249$) did not demonstrate the positive, monotonic trends shown by the other symptoms. Instead, these symptoms were characterized by modest negative trends indicating that if they did not remit early in treatment, they were increasingly unlikely to do so as treatment proceeded.

We examined the treatment response rates of the remaining 62 symptoms and performed an empirical grouping that resulted in three symptom classes. On the basis of response rates (highest to lowest), the classes were named acute distress, chronic distress, and characterological, respectively.

The median effective dose (ED50) was calculated for each symptom. This criterion is the dosage at which 50% of patients are estimated to have responded to treatment; it is often used as the standard expression of treatment effectiveness in biological assay research (Finney, 1971).

A probability for the dose of zero sessions was also calculated. It represented the extrapolated estimate of the percentage of patients who would have improved after making an initial con-

Table 4
Dose–Effect Relations for Characterological Symptoms: Percentage Recovered at Selected Sessions

Symptom (dimension, n)	No. of sessions							ED50
	0	2	4	8	13	26	52	
People can't be trusted (PI, 289)[a]	25	33	38	43	47	53	59	19
Overeating (124)[a]	40	45	47	50	51	54	57	9
Urges to harm someone (HS, 113)[b]	25	33	37	41	45	51	56	24
Awakening early (278)[a]	40	42	46	48	50	52	55	14
Restless sleep (459)[a]	28	36	38	42	46	50	55	25
People take advantage (PI, 383)[a]	29	32	36	40	43	47	52	37
Urges to break things (HS, 161)[b]	26	33	36	40	45	48	52	36
Feeling watched (PI, 170)[b]	15	23	28	33	38	45	52	44
Others to blame (PI, 241)[b]	11	19	24	30	35	43	51	48
Something wrong with mind (PS, 304)[b]	12	16	24	30	34	41	49	56
Shouting/throwing (HS, 171)[b]	36	38	40	41	41	43	45	>104
Easily annoyed (HS, 586)[b]	28	33	35	37	39	41	44	>104
Never close to others (PS, 233)[b]	10	16	20	24	28	34	41	>104
Frequent arguments (HS, 262)[b]	22	25	26	28	30	31	33	>104
Trouble falling asleep (338)[a]	16	18	21	23	25	27	30	>104
Mean ED50								>104

Note. ED50 = median effective dose. Entries represent the session number at which 50% of patients are estimated to show clinically significant improvement. Symptom Checklist 90–Revised symptom dimensions: PI = Paranoid Ideation, HS = Hostility, PS = Psychoticism. Absence of acronym indicates that the symptom is not associated with any symptom dimension.
[a] Clinical significance cutoff point was 1.   [b] Clinical significance cutoff point was 0.

tact with the clinic but before attending the first session. Because an analysis could not be conducted when treatment length (dose) was actually equal to zero, a constant of one was added to each dose before the probit analysis and then subtracted from the dose after the analysis was completed.

Acute Distress Symptoms

As presented in Table 2, a visual inspection suggested two criteria that differentiated symptoms that remitted early from those that remitted later: (a) remission rates of 24% or greater after the initial contact for an appointment but before the first session, and (b) an ED50 of fewer than 10 sessions. These symptoms were characterized primarily by anxiety, depression, somatization, and obsessive–compulsive (compulsive component) symptoms as well as other symptoms of intense emotionality (e.g., temper outbursts). We identified this group of symptoms as reflecting *acute distress.*

These symptoms responded well to psychotherapy over the course of 52 sessions as estimates of clinically significant improvement ranged from 68% to 95% of the patients at 52 once-weekly sessions. Their mean ED50 dosage was 5 sessions.

Chronic Distress Symptoms

The symptoms presented in Table 3 exhibited response rates of 22% or less (except for *lonely with people,* 24%) to the initial contact for therapy but demonstrated impressive responsiveness over the course of treatment. We identified these symptoms as reflecting *chronic distress.* They included anxiety, phobic anxiety, depression, obsessive–compulsive (obsessive component),

and interpersonal sensitivity symptoms. These symptoms were usually characterized by anxiety (e.g., scared for no reason, or feeling tense), mood (e.g., feeling blue, or feeling worthless), and cognitive disturbance (e.g., having difficulty with decisions, or worrying too much) as well as interpersonal problems (e.g., feelings easily hurt, feeling self-conscious, or others not sympathetic).

Sixty percent to 86% of the patients achieved remission of these symptoms at 52 sessions. They represent symptoms that are unlikely to respond to simply soothing reassurance, empathy, or advice but do recover at a satisfactory rate over 52 sessions. Their ED50s were within 7 to 27 sessions, with a mean ED50 of 14 sessions.

Characterological Symptoms

Symptoms that responded slowly to psychotherapy included items from the Hostility, Paranoid Ideation, and Psychoticism subscales (see Table 4), along with symptoms of sleep disturbance and overeating. Because these symptoms failed to remit among many patients during the course of 52 sessions, we viewed them as characterological in nature.

A visual inspection suggested the following two criteria that distinguished characterological symptoms from acute distress and chronic distress symptoms: (a) Clinical significance was reached at 52 sessions by 59% or fewer of the patients; (b) The ED50 was greater than 18 sessions, or probability increases for achieving clinical significance from the initial contact for treatment (0 sessions) to 52 sessions was less than .18, or both. Six of these symptoms demonstrated less than a 50% chance of recovery after 52 sessions: shouting or throwing things, easily annoyed, frequent arguments, trouble falling asleep, something wrong with your mind, and never close to others.

Validating Symptom Classes

To validate the three symptom clusters, we subjected cluster scores to statistical analysis. First, length of therapy was transformed into natural logs of session number plus one. Percentage recovered data were analyzed with a polynomial trend analysis such that polynomial contrast codes reflected actual distances with respect to the transformed session numbers. Recovery rates were compared among the three symptom classes over time, using a trend analysis.

On average, symptoms in the acute distress class showed a higher overall percentage recovered across doses than symptoms in the chronic distress class, $F(1, 59) = 56.56, p < .001$, and symptoms in the characterological class, $F(1, 59) = 98.11$, $p < .001$. In addition, symptoms in the chronic distress class showed a higher overall percentage recovered across doses than symptoms in the characterological class, $F(1, 59) = 13.43, p < .01$. There was a general tendency for symptoms in the acute distress class to recover at a slower rate than symptoms in the chronic distress class, $F(1, 59) = 8.06, p < .01$, and at a faster rate than symptoms in the characterological class, $F(1, 59) =$

$55.21, p < .001$. Finally, symptoms in the chronic distress class recovered at a faster rate than those in the characterological class, $F(1, 59) = 107.30, p < .001$.

Figure 2 presents the plots of the percentage of patients recovered as a function of number of therapy sessions for the three symptom classes. Percentages, derived from the probit analyses (see Tables 2, 3, and 4), were averaged across symptoms within a class at selected dosage points (i.e., sessions 0, 2, 4, etc.). Although acute distress and characterological symptoms demonstrated higher recovery levels at the beginning of treatment (at 0 sessions), chronic distress symptoms tended to remit at a faster rate once formal therapy began (sessions 2, 4, 8, etc.). After two sessions, with regard to percentage of patients recovered, chronic distress symptoms, on average, surpassed characterological symptoms across the remaining 50 sessions.

How Much Is Enough?

An issue of concern in this project was, in general, how much treatment is sufficient to produce meaningful benefit. To answer this question, we selected the symptoms that were (a) most frequently present in the sample (i.e., where at least 50% of the patients reported the symptom as present), and (b) present in the acute and chronic distress symptom groups because these symptoms had proven to be reasonably responsive to psycho-

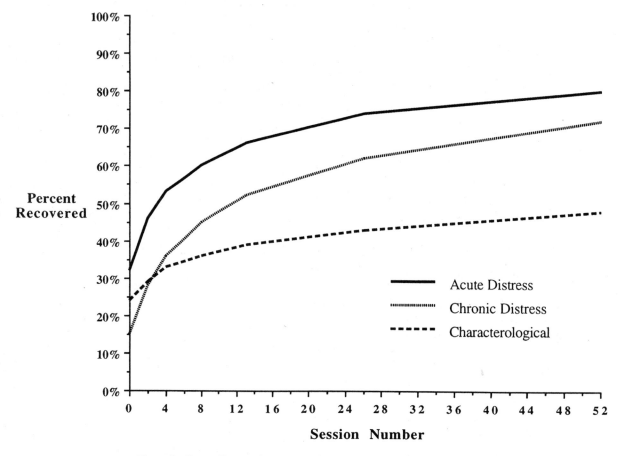

Figure 2. Dose–effect relations, averaged across symptoms, for acute, chronic, and characterological symptom classes ($N = 854$).

therapy within 52 sessions. As shown in Table 5, there were 18 symptoms that met these criteria.

Following the logic of Howard et al. (1986), we selected the point at which 75% (ED75) of patients had obtained clinical significance as a rational criterion of *sufficient*. Averaging the ED75 dosages across these symptoms, it was estimated that 58 sessions—a little more than a year of once-weekly therapy—produced recovery among 75% of patients (see Table 5). The estimated mean ED50 dosage was much lower for these symptoms, however. Fifty percent of patients recovered by the end of 11 sessions or about 2.5 months of once-weekly treatment.

Differential Dropout Process

An important methodological issue on which the aforementioned conclusions depend is the assumption that symptom severity was not associated with length of treatment. To rule out the possibility that a differential dropout rate across sessions might have accounted for the results, we correlated the pretherapy Global Severity Index score (GSI; total distress score divided by the number of symptoms) of the symptom checklist with the final dose at termination. The correlation was nonsignificant ($r = .06$, $p > .05$).

Representativeness of the Sample

Symptom distress levels of our sample were similar to Derogatis's psychiatric outpatient sample; the pretherapy GSI mean and standard deviation for our sample was 1.52 and .74, respectively, versus 1.26 and .68 for Derogatis's sample. Thus, in light of these findings and the fact that our data were collected from

mental health centers at several locations in the United States, our sample is very representative of the general outpatient psychiatric population.

Discussion

Results of this study provide support for the differential responsiveness of psychological symptoms to the psychotherapy process. By using a clinical significance criterion with the dosage model, we have introduced an approach that holds promise for estimating how much psychotherapy is enough.

For this study, we were not seeking to delineate the *true* effectiveness of treatment by controlling for placebo or spontaneous remission processes; our interest here was to describe the sequence of symptomatic recovery of patients who were actually engaged in psychotherapy. The benefits of psychotherapy above placebo or spontaneous remission processes have been consistently documented in several research reviews (e.g., Lambert & Bergin, 1994; Shapiro & Shapiro, 1982).

As shown in Tables 2, 3, and 4, symptoms associated with the same symptom dimension responded to treatment at noticeably different rates. For example, some anxiety, depression, and obsessive–compulsive symptoms responded rapidly (the acute category) and others responded slowly (the chronic distress category) to treatment. Symptoms associated with psychoticism were grouped into the chronic distress and characterological classes; paranoid ideation and hostility symptoms fell into the acute distress and characterological classes. These findings, based on treatment response rates rather than factor analysis, contradict the conclusion (e.g., Cyr, McKenna-Foley, & Peacock, 1985) that the *SCL–90–R* measures only a single global distress factor. Although a single factor score may describe responses at any point in time, the current findings indicate that discrete symptoms have remarkably different prognostic values. Furthermore, had we used the nine symptom dimensions provided by Derogatis (1983), it would have obscured very different treatment response rates for symptoms within the same dimension.

Admittedly, the grouping of symptoms was not always uniform and some symptoms were difficult to classify into one of our three clusters. Still, a common pattern of symptomatic recovery is apparent and appears to be characterized by different rates of response to psychotherapy. This process is summarized in Figure 2.

For the characterological symptoms, the DSM–III–R (APA, 1987) associates the hostility, paranoid ideation, and psychoticism symptoms in this group with the more severe personality disorders of paranoid, schizoid, schizotypal, and borderline. As the characterological symptoms responded poorly to the first 52 sessions of psychotherapy, a longer time frame of individual therapy appears to be necessary. It is unfortunate that our results provide no information on symptomatic recovery beyond 52 sessions of treatment.

With regard to estimating how much is enough, two qualifications to these findings should be noted. First, the ED75 and ED50 levels were arbitrarily selected as examples for discussion of this issue. Second, the dosage estimates of 58 sessions (for ED75) and 11 sessions (for ED50) relate to a prototypal outpatient who suffers from the most frequently treated symptoms

Table 5

ED75 Dosage for Acute and Chronic Distress Symptoms That Were Most Frequently Endorsed as Present (Rated 2 or Higher)

Symptom (dimension)	ED75
Crying easily (DP)	22
Feeling worthless (DP)	24
Repeated thoughts (OC)	34
Feeling critical of others (IS)	35
Feeling guilty	36
Blaming self (DP)	45
Having trouble concentrating (OC)	50
Having difficulty making decisions (OC)	50
Feeling blue (DP)	55
Feeling fearful (AN)	56
Feelings easily hurt (IS)	62
Feeling trapped (DP)	66
Feeling low in energy (DP)	66
Hopeless about the future (DP)	67
Feeling blocked (OC)	70
Feeling lonely (DP)	86
Feeling tense (AN)	106
Worry too much (DP)	120
Mean ED75	58

Note. ED75 = Session number at which 75% of patients are estimated to show clinically significant improvement. Symptom Checklist 90–Revised symptom dimensions: DP = Depression, OC = Obsessive-Compulsive, IS = Interpersonal Sensitivity, AN = Anxiety.

responsive to psychotherapy; some patients, depending on their specific symptom patterns, would require more sessions to reach normal functioning and others may need less treatment.

The findings of this study present an interesting contrast to those of Howard et al. (1986). Their dosage estimates for various improvement rates for a typical patient were considerably lower than the estimates presented here (e.g., for the 75% improvement level, approximately 26 sessions versus 58 sessions). An explanation for these differences lies in the fact that Howard et al., using a variety of traditional measures, investigated general improvement that did not require a return to normal functioning. Thus, it makes sense that fewer sessions are needed to simply improve rather than to recover.

In spite of the large sampling base of the data, the generalizability of our results is limited in several respects. This study did not control for the differential response rates between the same symptoms within different syndromes or diagnostic classes. There remains little understanding of improvement patterns for symptoms within the context of other symptoms. Evidence suggests that for certain types of patients, the same symptoms respond differently to psychotherapy. As noted earlier, Pilkonis and Frank (1988) found that unipolar depressed patients with personality disorder improved more slowly than similarly depressed patients with no personality disorder. Understanding symptomatic improvement patterns within the context of diagnostic categories or syndromes ought to be a priority for future investigators.

With regard to outcome criteria, there are findings that suggest that reduction in symptom distress follows certain change processes and precedes others. Howard, Lueger, Maling, and Martinovich (1993) reported that the psychotherapy recovery process demonstrates a stepwise pattern in which subjective well-being, then symptoms, and finally general life functioning improve sequentially. According to this three-phase model, symptomatic recovery is the intermediate phase of a complete recovery process. Thus, the model indicates that perhaps a more definitive assessment of outcome (and of how much is enough) should involve instruments measuring life functioning areas such as interpersonal and work functioning.

We believe the dosage model holds promise for helping to establish needed empirical guidelines for financing psychotherapy. With the dosage model, financing or dosage guidelines could be based on empirically determined probabilities of effectiveness. To be sure, when resources are limited, any selected probability criterion should take into account the humane consideration to provide the patient with a reasonable chance for recovery as well as the cost-containment demands and cost-effectiveness factors.

We do not believe that the specific dose–effect estimates presented here should be used as firm clinical standards. Further research with careful attention to the issues noted earlier is needed. However, our findings represent a significant step toward understanding the complex process of symptomatic recovery in psychotherapy. This research also provides a rational, empirical approach to designing reimbursement policies for managed mental health care systems and insurance programs.

References

American Psychiatric Association. (1980). *Diagnostic and statistical manual of mental disorders* (3rd ed.). Washington, DC: Author.

American Psychiatric Association. (1987). *Diagnostic and statistical manual of mental disorders* (3rd ed., rev.). Washington, DC: Author.

Cyr, J. J., McKenna-Foley, J. M., & Peacock, E. (1985). Factor structure of the SCL–90–R: Is there one? *Journal of Personality Assessment, 49,* 571–578.

Derogatis, L. R. (1983). *SCL–90–R: Administration, scoring, and procedural manual—II.* Baltimore, MD: Clinical Psychometric Research.

Derogatis, L. R. (1989). [Item endorsement frequencies for the SCL–90–R from a community population.] Unpublished raw data from Clinical Psychometric Research, Baltimore, MD.

Derogatis, L. R., & Spencer, P. M. (1983). The *Brief Symptom Inventory: Administration, scoring, and procedures manual—I.* Baltimore, MD: Clinical Psychometric Research.

Finney, D. J. (1971). *Probit analysis* (3rd ed.). Cambridge, England: Cambridge University Press.

Howard, K. I., Kopta, S. M., Krause, M. S., & Orlinsky, D. E. (1986). The dose–effect relationship in psychotherapy. *American Psychologist, 41,* 159–164.

Howard, K. I., Lueger, R. J., Maling, M. S., & Martinovich, Z. (1993). A phase model of psychotherapy outcome: Causal mediation of change. *Journal of Consulting and Clinical Psychology, 61,* 678–685.

Jacobson, N. S., Follette, W. C., & Revenstorf, D. (1984). Psychotherapy outcome research: Methods for reporting variability and evaluating clinical significance. *Behavior Therapy, 15,* 336–352.

Jacobson, N. S., & Truax, P. (1991). Clinical significance: A statistical approach to defining meaningful change in psychotherapy research. *Journal of Consulting and Clinical Psychology, 59,* 12–19.

Lambert, M. J., & Bergin, A. E. (1994). The effectiveness of psychotherapy. In A. E. Bergin & S. L. Garfield (Eds.), *Handbook of psychotherapy and behavior change* (4th ed.). New York: Wiley.

Pilkonis, P. A., & Frank, E. (1988). Personality pathology in recurrent depression: Nature, prevalence, and relationship to treatment response. *American Journal of Psychiatry, 145,* 435–441.

Shapiro, D. A., & Shapiro, D. (1982). Meta-analysis of comparative therapy outcome studies: A replication and refinement. *Psychological Bulletin, 92,* 581–604.

Received April 12, 1993
Revision received December 8, 1993
Accepted February 2, 1994

What You Can Change & What You Cannot Change

There are things we can change about ourselves and things we cannot. Concentrate your energy on what is possible—too much time has been wasted.

Martin E. P. Seligman, Ph.D.

This is the age of psychotherapy and the age of self-improvement. Millions are struggling to change: We diet, we jog, we meditate. We adopt new modes of thought to counteract our depressions. We practice relaxation to curtail stress. We exercise to expand our memory and to quadruple our reading speed. We adopt draconian regimens to give up smoking. We raise our little boys and girls to androgyny. We come out of the closet or we try to become heterosexual. We seek to lose our taste for alcohol. We seek more meaning in life. We try to extend our life span.

Sometimes it works. But distressingly often, self-improvement and psychotherapy fail. The cost is enormous. We think we are worthless. We feel guilty and ashamed. We believe we have no will-power and that we are failures. We give up trying to change.

On the other hand, this is not only the age of self-improvement and therapy, but also the age of biological psychiatry. The human genome will be nearly mapped before the millennium is over. The brain systems underlying sex, hearing, memory, left-handedness, and sadness are now known. Psychoactive drugs quiet our fears, relieve our blues, bring us bliss, dampen our mania, and dissolve our delusions more effectively than we can on our own.

Our very personality—our intelligence and musical talent, even our religiousness, our conscience (or its absence), our politics, and our exuberance—turns out to be more the product of our genes than almost anyone would have believed a decade ago. The underlying message of the age of biological psychiatry is that our biology frequently makes changing, in spite of all our efforts, impossible.

But the view that all is genetic and biochemical and therefore unchangeable is also very often wrong. Many people surpass their IQs, fail to "respond" to drugs, make sweeping changes in their lives, live on when their cancer is "terminal," or defy the hormones and brain circuitry that "dictate" lust, femininity, or memory loss.

The ideologies of biological psychiatry and self-improvement are obviously colliding. Nevertheless, a resolution is apparent. There are some things about ourselves that can be changed, others that cannot, and some that can be changed only with extreme difficulty.

What can we succeed in changing about ourselves? What can we not? When can we overcome our biology? And when is our biology our destiny?

I want to provide an understanding of what you can and what you can't change about yourself so that you can concentrate your limited time and energy on what is possible. So much time has been wasted. So much needless frustration has been endured. So much of therapy, so much of child rearing, so much of self-improving, and even some of the great social movements in our century have come to nothing because they tried to change the unchangeable. Too often we have wrongly thought we were weak-willed failures, when the changes we wanted to make in ourselves were just not possible. But all this effort was necessary: Because there have been so many failures, we are now able to see the boundaries of the unchangeable; this in turn allows us to see clearly for the first time the boundaries of what *is* changeable.

With this knowledge, we can use our precious time to make the many rewarding changes that are possible. We can live with less self-reproach and less remorse. We can live with greater confidence. This knowledge is a new understanding of who we are and where we are going.

CATASTROPHIC THINKING: PANIC

S. J. Rachman, one of the world's leading clinical researchers and one of the founders of behavior therapy, was on the phone. He was proposing that I be the "discussant" at a conference about panic disorder sponsored by the National Institute of Mental Health (NIMH).

"Why even bother, Jack?" I responded. "Everyone knows that panic is biological and that the only thing that works is drugs."

"Don't refuse so quickly, Marty. There is a breakthrough you haven't yet heard about."

Breakthrough was a word I had never heard Jack use before.

"What's the breakthrough?" I asked.

"If you come, you can find out."

So I went.

I had known about and seen panic patients for many years, and had read the literature with mounting excitement during

From *Psychology Today,* May/June 1994, pp. 34-41, 70, 72-74, 84. Excerpted from *What You Can Change and What You Can't* by Martin E. P. Seligman. © 1993 by Martin E. P. Seligman. Reprinted by permission of Alfred A. Knopf, Inc.

So much child rearing, therapy, and self-improvement have come to nothing.

the 1980s. I knew that panic disorder is a frightening condition that consists of recurrent attacks, each much worse than anything experienced before. Without prior warning, you feel as if you are going to die. Here is a typical case history:

The first time Celia had a panic attack, she was working at McDonald's. It was two days before her 20th birthday. As she was handing a customer a Big Mac, she had the worst experience of her life. The earth seemed to open up beneath her. Her heart began to pound, she felt she was smothering, and she was sure she was going to have a heart attack and die. After about 20 minutes of terror, the panic subsided. Trembling, she got in her car, raced home, and barely left the house for the next three months.

Since then, Celia has had about three attacks a month. She does not know when they are coming. She always thinks she is going to die.

Panic attacks are not subtle, and you need no quiz to find out if you or someone you love has them. As many as five percent of American adults probably do. The defining feature of the disorder is simple: recurrent awful attacks of panic that come out of the blue, last for a few minutes, and then subside. The attacks consist of chest pains, sweating, nausea, dizziness, choking, smothering, or trembling. They are accompanied by feelings of overwhelming dread and thoughts that you are having a heart attack, that you are losing control, or that you are going crazy.

THE BIOLOGY OF PANIC

There are four questions that bear on whether a mental problem is primarily "biological" as opposed to "psychological":

- Can it be induced biologically?
- Is it genetically heritable?
- Are specific brain functions involved?
- Does a drug relieve it?

Inducing panic. Panic attacks can be created by a biological agent. For example, patients who have a history of panic attacks are hooked up to an intravenous line. Sodium lactate, a chemical that nor-

mally produces rapid, shallow breathing and heart palpitations, is slowly infused into their bloodstream. Within a few minutes, about 60 to 90 percent of these patients have a panic attack. Normal controls—subjects with no history of panic—rarely have attacks when infused with lactate.

Genetics of panic. There may be some heritability of panic. If one of two identical twins has panic attacks, 31 percent of the cotwins also have them. But if one of two fraternal twins has panic attacks, none of the cotwins are so afflicted.

Panic and the brain. The brains of people with panic disorders look somewhat unusual upon close scrutiny. Their neurochemistry shows abnormalities in the system that turns on, then dampens, fear. In addition, the PET scan (positron-emission tomography), a technique that looks at how much blood and oxygen different parts of the brain use, shows that patients who panic from the infusion of lactate have higher blood flow and oxygen use in relevant parts of their brain than patients who don't panic.

Drugs. Two kinds of drugs relieve panic: tricyclic antidepressants and the antianxiety drug Xanax, and both work better than placebos. Panic attacks are dampened, and sometimes even eliminated. General anxiety and depression also decrease.

Since these four questions had already been answered "yes" when Jack Rachman called, I thought the issue had already been settled. Panic disorder was simply a biological illness, a disease of the body that could be relieved only by drugs.

A few months later I was in Bethesda, Maryland, listening once again to the same four lines of biological evidence. An inconspicuous figure in a brown suit sat hunched over the table. At the first break, Jack introduced me to him—David Clark, a young psychologist from Oxford. Soon after, Clark began his address.

"Consider, if you will, an alternative theory, a cognitive theory." He reminded all of us that almost all panickers believe that they are going to die during an attack. Most commonly, they believe that they are having heart attacks. Perhaps, Clark suggested, this is more than just a mere symptom. Perhaps it is the root cause. Panic may simply be the *catastrophic misinterpretation of bodily sensations.*

For example, when you panic, your heart starts to race. You notice this, and you see it as a possible heart attack. This makes you very anxious, which means

What Can We Change?

When we survey all the problems, personality types, patterns of behavior, and the weak influence of childhood on adult life, we see a puzzling array of how much change occurs. From the things that are easiest to those that are the most difficult, this rough array emerges:

Panic	Curable
Specific Phobias	Almost Curable
Sexual Dysfunctions	Marked Relief
Social Phobia	Moderate Relief
Agoraphobia	Moderate Relief
Depression	Moderate Relief
Sex Role Change	Moderate
Obsessive–Compulsive Disorder	Moderate Mild Relief
Sexual Preferences	Moderate Mild Change
Anger	Mild, Moderate Relief
Everyday Anxiety	Mild Moderate Relief
Alcoholism	Mild Relief
Overweight	Temporary Change
Posttraumatic Stress Disorder (PTSD)	Marginal Relief
Sexual Orientation	Probably Unchangeable
Sexual Identity	Unchangeable

your heart pounds more. You now notice that your heart is *really* pounding. You are now *sure* it's a heart attack. This terrifies you, and you break into a sweat, feel nauseated, short of breath—all symptoms of terror, but for you, they're confirmation of a heart attack. A full-blown panic attack is under way, and at the root of it is your misinterpretation of the symptoms of anxiety as symptoms of impending death.

We are now able to see the boundaries of the unchangeable.

I was listening closely now as Clark argued that an obvious sign of a disorder, easily dismissed as a symptom, is the disorder itself. If he was right, this was a historic occasion. All Clark had done so far, however, was to show that the four lines of evidence for a biological view of panic could fit equally well with a misinterpretation view. But Clark soon told us about a series of experiments he and his colleague Paul Salkovskis had done at Oxford.

First, they compared panic patients with patients who had other anxiety disorders and with normals. All the subjects read the following sentences aloud, but the last word was presented blurred. For example:

dying
If I had palpitations, I could be *excited*

choking
If I were breathless, I could be *unfit*

When the sentences were about bodily sensations, the panic patients, but no one else, saw the catastrophic endings fastest. This showed that panic patients possess the habit of thinking Clark had postulated.

Next, Clark and his colleagues asked if activating this habit with words would induce panic. All the subjects read a series of word pairs aloud. When panic patients got to "breathlessness-suffocation: and "palpitations-dying," 75 percent suffered a full-blown panic attack right there in the laboratory. No normal people had panic attacks, no recovered panic patients (I'll tell you more in a moment about how they got better) had attacks, and only 17 percent of other anxious patients had attacks.

The final thing Clark told us was the "breakthrough" that Rachman had promised.

"We have developed and tested a rather novel therapy for panic," Clark continued in his understated, disarming way. He explained that if catastrophic misinterpretations of bodily sensation are the cause of a panic attack, then changing the tendency to misinterpret should cure the disorder. His new therapy was straightforward and brief:

Patients are told that panic results when they mistake normal symptoms of mounting anxiety for symptoms of heart attack, going crazy, or dying. Anxiety itself, they are informed, produces shortness of breath, chest pain, and sweating. Once

Issues of the soul can barely be changed by psychotherapy or drugs.

they misinterpret these normal bodily sensations as an imminent heart attack, their symptoms become even more pronounced because the misinterpretation changes their anxiety into terror. A vicious circle culminates in a full-blown panic attack.

Patients are taught to reinterpret the symptoms realistically as mere anxiety symptoms. Then they are given practice right in the office, breathing rapidly into a paper bag. This causes a buildup of carbon dioxide and shortness of breath, mimicking the sensations that provoke a panic attack. The therapist points out that the symptoms the patient is experiencing— shortness of breath and heart racing—are harmless, simply the result of overbreathing, not a sign of a heart attack. The patient learns to interpret the symptoms correctly.

"This simple therapy appears to be a cure," Clark told us. "Ninety to 100 percent of the patients are panic free at the end of therapy. One year later, only one person had had another panic attack."

This, indeed, was a breakthrough: a simple, brief psychotherapy with no side effects showing a 90-percent cure rate of a disorder that a decade ago was thought to be incurable. In a controlled study of 64 patients comparing cognitive therapy to drugs to relaxation to no treatment, Clark and his colleagues found that cognitive therapy is markedly better than drugs or relaxation, both of which are better than

Self-Analysis Questionnaire
Is your life dominated by anxiety? Read each statement and then mark the appropriate number to indicate *how you generally feel*. There are no right or wrong answers.

1. I am a steady person.

Almost never	Sometimes	Often	Almost always
4	3	2	1

2. I am satisfied with myself.

Almost never	Sometimes	Often	Almost always
4	3	2	1

3. I feel nervous and restless.

Almost never	Sometimes	Often	Almost always
1	2	3	4

4. I wish I could be as happy as others seem to be.

Almost never	Sometimes	Often	Almost always
1	2	3	4

5. I feel like a failure.

Almost never	Sometimes	Often	Almost always
1	2	3	4

6. I get in a state of tension and turmoil as I think over my recent concerns and interests.

Almost never	Sometimes	Often	Almost always
1	2	3	4

7. I feel secure.

Almost never	Sometimes	Often	Almost always
4	3	2	1

(continued)

nothing. Such a high cure rate is unprecedented.

How does cognitive therapy for panic compare with drugs? It is more effective and less dangerous. Both the antidepressants and Xanax produce marked reduction in panic in most patients, but drugs must be taken forever; once the drug is stopped, panic rebounds to where it was before therapy began for perhaps half the patients. The drugs also sometimes have severe side effects, including drowsiness, lethargy, pregnancy complications, and addictions.

After this bombshell, my own "discussion" was an anticlimax. I did make one point that Clark took to heart. "Creating a cognitive therapy that works, even one that works as well as this apparently does, is not enough to show that the *cause* of panic is cognitive." I was niggling. "The biological theory doesn't deny that some other therapy might work well on panic. It merely claims that panic is caused at the bottom by some biochemical problem."

Two years later, Clark carried out a crucial experiment that tested the biological theory against the cognitive theory. He gave the usual lactate infusion to 10 panic patients, and nine of them panicked. He did the same thing with another 10 patients, but added special instructions to allay the misinterpretation of the sensations. He simply told them: "Lactate is a natural bodily substance that produces sensations similar to exercise or alcohol. It is normal to experience intense sensations during infusion, but these do not indicate an adverse reaction." Only three out of the 10 panicked. This confirmed the theory crucially.

The therapy works very well, as it did for Celia, whose story has a happy ending. She first tried Xanax, which reduced the intensity and the frequency of her panic attacks. But she was too drowsy to work, and she was still having about one attack every six weeks. She was then referred to Audrey, a cognitive therapist who explained that Celia was misinterpreting her heart racing and shortness of breath as symptoms of a heart attack, that they were actually just symptoms of mounting anxiety, nothing more harmful. Audrey taught Celia progressive relaxation, and then she demonstrated the harmlessness of Celia's symptoms of overbreathing. Celia then relaxed in the presence of the symptoms and found that they gradually subsided. After several more practice sessions, therapy terminated. Celia has gone two years without another panic attack.

8. I have self-confidence.

Almost never	Sometimes	Often	Almost always
4	3	2	1

9. I feel inadequate.

Almost never	Sometimes	Often	Almost always
1	2	3	4

10. I worry too much over something that does not matter.

Almost never	Sometimes	Often	Almost always
1	2	3	4

To score, simply add up the numbers under your answers. Notice that some of the rows of numbers go up and others go down. The higher your total, the more the trait of anxiety dominates your life. If your score was:

10–11, you are in the lowest 10 percent of anxiety.

13–14, you are in the lowest quarter.

16–17, your anxiety level is about average.

19–20, your anxiety level is around the 75th percentile.

22–24 (and you are male) your anxiety level is around the 90th percentile.

24–26 (and you are female) your anxiety level is around the 90th percentile.

25 (and you are male) your anxiety level is at the 95th percentile.

27 (and you are female) your anxiety level is at the 95th percentile.

Should you try to change your anxiety level? Here are my rules of thumb:

• If your score is at the 90th percentile or above, you can probably improve the quality of your life by lowering your general anxiety level—regardless of paralysis and irrationality.

• If your score is at the 75th percentile or above, and you feel that anxiety is either paralyzing you or that it is unfounded, you should probably try to lower your general anxiety level.

• If your score is 18 or above, and you feel that anxiety is unfounded and paralyzing, you should probably try to lower your general anxiety level.

EVERYDAY ANXIETY

Attend to your tongue—right now. What is it doing? Mine is swishing around near my lower right molars. It has just found a minute fragment of last night's popcorn (debris from *Terminator 2*). Like a dog at a bone, it is worrying the firmly wedged flake.

Attend to your hand—right now. What's it up to? My left hand is boring in on an itch it discovered under my earlobe.

Your tongue and your hands have, for the most part, a life of their own. You can bring them under voluntary control by consciously calling them out of their "default" mode to carry out your commands:

Anxiety scans your life for imperfections. When it finds one, it won't let go.

"Pick up the phone" or "Stop picking that pimple." But most of the time they are on their own. They are seeking out small imperfections. They scan your entire mouth and skin surface, probing for anything going wrong. They are marvelous, nonstop grooming devices. They, not the more fashionable immune system, are your first line of defense against invaders.

Anxiety is your mental tongue. Its default mode is to search for what may be about to go wrong. It continually, and without your conscious consent, scans your life—yes, even when you are asleep, in dreams and nightmares. It reviews your work, your love, your play—until it finds an imperfection. When it finds one, it worries it. It tries to pull it out from its hiding place, where it is wedged inconspicuously under some rock. It will not let go. If the imperfection is threatening enough, anxiety calls your attention to it by making you uncomfortable. If you do not act, it yells more insistently—disturbing your sleep and your appetite.

You can reduce daily, mild anxiety. You can numb it with alcohol, Valium, or marijuana. You can take the edge off with meditation or progressive relaxation. You can beat it down by becoming more conscious of the automatic thoughts of danger that trigger anxiety and then disputing them effectively.

But do not overlook what your anxiety is trying to do for you. In return for the pain it brings, it prevents larger ordeals by making you aware of their possibility and goading you into planning for and forestalling them. It may even help you avoid them altogether. Think of your anxiety as the "low oil" light flashing on the dashboard of your car. Disconnect it and you will be less distracted and more comfortable for a while. But this may cost you a burned-up engine. Our *dysphoria,* or bad feeling, should, some of the time, be tolerated, attended to, even cherished.

GUIDELINES FOR WHEN TO TRY TO CHANGE ANXIETY

Some of our everyday anxiety, depression, and anger go beyond their useful function. Most adaptive traits fall along a normal spectrum of distribution, and the capacity for internal bad weather for everyone some of the time means that some of us may have terrible weather all of the time. In general, when the hurt is pointless and recurrent—when, for example, anxiety insists we formulate a plan but no plan will work—it is time to take action to relieve the hurt. There are three hallmarks indicating that anxiety has become a burden that wants relieving:

First, is it *irrational?*

We must calibrate our bad weather inside against the real weather outside. Is what you are anxious about out of proportion to the reality of the danger? Here are some examples that may help you answer this question. All of the following are not irrational:

• A fire fighter trying to smother a raging oil well burning in Kuwait repeatedly wakes up at four in the morning because of flaming terror dreams.

• A mother of three smells perfume on her husband's shirts and, consumed by jealousy, broods about his infidelity, reviewing the list of possible women over and over.

• A student who had failed two of his midterm exams finds, as finals approach, that he can't get to sleep for worrying. He has diarrhea most of the time.

The only good thing that can be said about such fears is that they are well-founded.

In contrast, all of the following are irrational, out of proportion to the danger:

• An elderly man, having been in a fender bender, broods about travel and will no longer take cars, trains, or airplanes.

• An eight-year-old child, his parents having been through an ugly divorce, wets his bed at night. He is haunted with visions of his bedroom ceiling collapsing on him.

• A housewife who has an MBA and who accumulated a decade of experience as a financial vice president before her twins were born is sure her job search will be fruitless. She delays preparing her résumés for a month.

The second hallmark of anxiety out of control is *paralysis.* Anxiety intends action: Plan, rehearse, look into shadows for lurking dangers, change your life. When anxiety becomes strong, it is unproductive; no problem-solving occurs. And when anxiety is extreme, it paralyzes you. Has your anxiety crossed this line? Some examples:

• A woman finds herself housebound because she fears that if she goes out, she will be bitten by a cat.

• A salesman broods about the next customer hanging up on him and makes no more cold calls.

• A writer, afraid of the next rejection slip, stops writing.

The final hallmark is *intensity.* Is your life dominated by anxiety? Dr. Charles Spielberger, one of the world's foremost

'Dieting below your natural weight is a necessary condition for bulimia. Returning to your natural weight will cure it.'

testers of emotion, has developed well-validated scales for calibrating how severe anxiety is. To find out how anxious *you* are, use the self-analysis questionnaire.

LOWERING YOUR EVERYDAY ANXIETY

Everyday anxiety level is not a category to which psychologists have devoted a great deal of attention. Enough research has been done, however, for me to recommend two techniques that quite reliably lower everyday anxiety levels. Both techniques are cumulative, rather than one-shot fixes. They require 20 to 40 minutes a day of your valuable time.

The first is *progressive relaxation,* done once or, better, twice a day for at least 10 minutes. In this technique, you tighten and then turn off each of the major muscle groups of your body until you are wholly flaccid. It is not easy to be highly anxious when your body feels like Jell-O. More formally, relaxation engages a response system that competes with anxious arousal.

The second technique is regular *meditation.* Transcendental meditation ™ is one useful, widely available version of this. You can ignore the cosmology in which it is packaged if you wish, and treat it simply as the beneficial technique it is. Twice a day for 20 minutes, in a quiet setting, you close your eyes and repeat a *mantra* (a syllable whose "sonic properties are known") to yourself. Meditation works by blocking thoughts that produce anxiety. It complements relaxation, which blocks the motor components of anxiety but leaves the anxious thoughts untouched.

Done regularly, meditation usually induces a peaceful state of mind. Anxiety at other times of the day wanes, and hyperarousal from bad events is dampened. Done religiously, TM probably works better than relaxation alone.

There's also a quick fix. The minor tranquilizers—Valium, Dalmane, Librium, and their cousins—relieve everyday anxiety. So does alcohol. The advantage of all these is that they work within minutes and

193

require no discipline to use. Their disadvantages outweigh their advantages, however. The minor tranquilizers make you fuzzy and somewhat uncoordinated as they work (a not uncommon side effect is an automobile accident). Tranquilizers soon lose their effect when taken regularly, and they are habit-forming—probably addictive. Alcohol, in addition, produces gross cognitive and motor disability in lockstep with its anxiety relief. Taken regularly over long periods, deadly damage to liver and brain ensue.

If you crave quick and temporary relief from acute anxiety, either alcohol or minor tranquilizers, taken in small amounts and only occasionally, will do the job. They are, however, a distant second-best to progressive relaxation and meditation, which are each worth trying before you seek out psychotherapy or in conjunction with therapy. Unlike tranquilizers and alcohol, neither of these techniques is likely to do you any harm.

Weigh your everyday anxiety. If it is not intense, or if it is moderate and not irrational or paralyzing, act now to reduce it. In spite of its deep evolutionary roots, intense everyday anxiety is often changeable. Meditation and progressive relaxation practiced regularly can change it forever.

DIETING: A WAIST IS A TERRIBLE THING TO MIND

I have been watching my weight and restricting my intake—except for an occasional binge like this—since I was 20. I weighed about 175 pounds then, maybe 15 pounds over my official "ideal" weight. I weigh 199 pounds now, 30 years later, about 25 pounds over the ideal. I have tried about a dozen regimes—fasting, the Beverly Hills Diet, no carbohydrates, Metrecal for lunch, 1,200 calories a day, low fat, no lunch, no starches, skipping every other dinner. I lost 10 or 15 pounds on each in about a month. The pounds always came back, though, and I have gained a net of about a pound a year—inexorably.

This is the most consistent failure in my life. It's also a failure I can't just put out of mind. I have spent the last few years reading the scientific literature, not the parade of best-selling diet books or the flood of women's magazine articles on the latest way to slim down. The scientific findings look clear to me, but there is not yet a consensus. I am going to go out on a limb, because I see so many signs all pointing in one direction. What I have concluded will, I believe, soon be the consensus of the scientists. The conclusions surprise me. They

will probably surprise you, too, and they may change your life.

Her[e] is what the picture looks like to me:

- Dieting doesn't work.
- Dieting may make overweight worse, not better.
- Dieting may be bad for health.
- Dieting may cause eating disorders—including bulimia and anorexia.

ARE YOU OVERWEIGHT?

Are you above the ideal weight for your sex, height, and age? If so, you are "overweight." What does this really mean? Ideal weight is arrived at simply. Four million people, now dead, who were insured by the major American life-insurance companies, were once weighed and had their height measured. At what weight on average do people of a given height turn out to live longest? That weight is called ideal. Anything wrong with that?

You bet. The real use of a weight table, and the reason your doctor takes it seriously, is that an ideal weight implies that, on average, if you slim down to yours, you will live longer. This is the crucial claim. Lighter people indeed live longer, on average, than heavier people, but how much longer is hotly debated.

But the crucial claim is unsound because weight (at any given height) has a normal distribution, *normal* both in a statistical sense and in the biological sense. In the biological sense, couch potatoes who overeat and never exercise can legitimately be called overweight, but the buxom, "heavy-boned" slow people deemed overweight by the ideal table are at their natural and healthiest weight. If you are a 155-pound woman and 64 inches in height, for example, you are "overweight" by around 15 pounds. This means nothing more than that the average 140-pound, 64-inch-tall woman lives somewhat longer than the average 155-pound woman of your height. It does not follow that if you slim down to 125 pounds, *you* will stand any better chance of living longer.

In spite of the insouciance with which dieting advice is dispensed, no one has properly investigated the question of whether slimming down to "ideal" weight produces longer life. The proper study would compare the longevity of people who are at their ideal weight without dieting to people who achieve their ideal weight by dieting. Without this study the common medical advice to diet down to your ideal weight is simply unfounded.

This is not a quibble; there is evidence

that dieting damages your health and that this damage may shorten your life.

MYTHS OF OVERWEIGHT

The advice to diet down to your ideal weight to live longer is one myth of overweight. Here are some others:

- *Overweight people overeat.* Wrong. Nineteen out of 20 studies show that obese people consume no more calories each day than nonobese people. Telling a fat person that if she would change her eating habits and eat "normally" she would lose weight is a lie. To lose weight and stay there, she will need to eat excruciatingly less than a normal person, probably for the rest of her life.
- *Overweight people have an overweight personality.* Wrong. Extensive research on personality and fatness has proved little. Obese people do not differ in any major personality style from nonobese people.
- *Physical inactivity is a major cause of obesity.* Probably not. Fat people are indeed less active than thin people, but the inactivity is probably caused more by the fatness than the other way around.
- *Overweight shows a lack of willpower.* This is the granddaddy of all the myths. Fatness is seen as shameful because we hold people responsible for their weight. Being overweight equates with being a weak-willed slob. We believe this primarily because we have seen people decide to lose weight and do so in a matter of weeks.

But almost everyone returns to the old weight after shedding pounds. Your body has a natural weight that it defends vigorously against dieting. The more diets tried, the harder the body works to defeat the next diet. Weight is in large part genetic. All this gives the lie to the "weak-willed" interpretations of overweight. More accurately, dieting is the conscious will of the individual against a more vigilant opponent: the species' biological defense against starvation. The body can't tell the difference between self-imposed starvation and actual famine, so it defends its weight by refusing to release fat, by lowering its metabolism, and by demanding food. The harder the creature tries not to eat, the more vigorous the defenses become.

BULIMIA AND NATURAL WEIGHT

A concept that makes sense of your body's vigorous defense against weight loss is *natural weight.* When your body screams "I'm hungry," makes you lethargic, stores fat, craves sweets and renders them more delicious than ever, and makes you obsessed with food, what it is defending is your natural weight. It is signaling that you have dropped into a range it will not accept. Natural weight prevents you from gaining too much weight or losing too much. When you eat too much for too long, the opposite defenses are activated and make long-term weight gain difficult.

There is also a strong genetic contribution to your natural weight. Identical twins reared apart weigh almost the same throughout their lives. When identical twins are overfed, they gain weight and add fat in lockstep and in the same places. The fatness or thinness of adopted children resembles their biological parents—particularly their mother—very closely but does not at all resemble their adoptive parents. This suggests that you have a genetically given natural weight that your body wants to maintain.

The idea of natural weight may help cure the new disorder that is sweeping young America. Hundreds of thousands of young women have contracted it. It consists of bouts of binge eating and purging alternating with days of undereating. These young women are usually normal in weight or a bit on the thin side, but they are terrified of becoming fat. So they diet. They exercise. They take laxatives by the cup. They gorge. Then they vomit and take more laxatives. This malady is called *bulimia nervosa* (bulimia, for short).

Therapists are puzzled by bulimia, its causes, and treatment. Debate rages about whether it is an equivalent of depression, or an expression of a thwarted desire for control, or a symbolic rejection of the feminine role. Almost every psychotherapy has been tried. Antidepressants and other drugs have been administered with some effect but little success has been reported.

I don't think that bulimia is mysterious, and I think that it will be curable. I believe that bulimia is caused by dieting. The bulimic goes on a diet, and her body attempts to defend its natural weight. With repeated dieting, this defense becomes more vigorous. Her body is in massive revolt—insistently demanding food, storing fat, craving sweets, and lowering metabolism. Periodically, these biological defenses will overcome her extraordinary willpower (and extraordinary it must be to even approach an ideal weight, say, 20 pounds lighter than her natural weight). She will then binge. Horrified by what this will do to her figure, she vomits and takes laxatives to purge calories. Thus, bulimia is a natural consequence of self-starvation to lose weight in the midst of abundant food.

The therapist's task is to get the patient to stop dieting and become comfortable with her natural weight. He should first convince the patient that her binge eating is caused by her body's reaction to her diet. Then he must confront her with a question: Which is more important, staying thin or getting rid of bulimia? By stopping the diet, he will tell her, she can get rid of the uncontrollable binge–purge cycle. Her body will now settle at her natural weight, and she need not worry that she will balloon beyond that point. For some patients, therapy will end there because they would rather be bulimic than "loathsomely fat." For these patients, the central issue—ideal weight versus natural weight—can now at least become the focus of therapy. For others, defying the social and sexual pressure to be thin will be possible, dieting will be abandoned, weight will be gained, and bulimia should end quickly.

These are the central moves of the cognitive-behavioral treatment of bulimia. There are more than a dozen outcome studies of this approach, and the results are good. There is about 60 percent reduction in binging and purging (about the same as with antidepressant drugs). But unlike drugs, there is little relapse after treatment. Attitudes toward weight and shape relax, and dieting withers.

Of course, the dieting theory cannot fully explain bulimia. Many people who diet don't become bulimic; some can avoid it because their natural weight is close to their ideal weight, and therefore the diet they adopt does not starve them. In addition, bulimics are often depressed, since binging-purging leads to self-loathing. Depression may worsen bulimia by making it easier to give in to temptation. Further, dieting may just be another symptom of bulimia, not a cause. Other factors aside, I can speculate that dieting below your natural weight is a necessary condition for bulimia, and that returning to your natural weight and accepting that weight will cure bulimia.

OVERWEIGHT VS. DIETING: THE HEALTH DAMAGE

Being heavy carries some health risk. There is no definite answer to how much, because there is a swamp of inconsistent findings. But even if you could just wish pounds away, never to return, it is not certain you should. Being somewhat above your "ideal" weight may actually be your healthiest natural condition, best for your particular constitution and your particular metabolism. Of course you can diet, but

the odds are overwhelming that most of the weight will return, and that you will have to diet again and again. From a health and mortality perspective, should you? *There is, probably, a serious health risk from losing weight and regaining it.*

In one study, more than five thousand men and women from Framingham, Massachusetts, were observed for 32 years. People whose weight fluctuated over the years had 30 to 100 percent greater risk of death from heart disease than people whose weight was stable. When corrected for smoking, exercise, cholesterol level, and blood pressure, the findings became more convincing, suggesting that weight fluctuation (the primary cause of which is presumably dieting) may itself increase the risk of heart disease.

If this result is replicated, and if dieting is shown to be the primary cause of weight cycling, it will convince me that you should not diet to reduce your risk of heart disease.

DEPRESSION AND DIETING

Depression is yet another cost of dieting, because two root causes of depression are failure and helplessness. Dieting sets you up for failure. Because the goal of slimming down to your ideal weight pits your fallible willpower against untiring biological defenses, you will often fail. At first you will lose weight and feel pretty good about it. Any depression you had about your figure will disappear. Ultimately, however, you will probably not reach your goal; and then you will be dismayed as the pounds return. Every time you look in the mirror or vacillate over a white chocolate mousse, you will be reminded of your failure, which in turn brings depression.

On the other hand, if you are one of the fortunate few who can keep the weight from coming back, you will probably have to stay on an unsatisfying low-calorie diet for the rest of your life. A side effect of prolonged malnutrition is depression. Either way, you are more vulnerable to it.

If you scan the list of cultures that have a thin ideal for women, you will be struck by something fascinating. All thin-ideal cultures also have eating disorders. They also have roughly twice as much depression in women as in men. (Women diet twice as much as men. The best estimate is that 13 percent of adult men and 25 percent of adult women are now on a diet.) The cultures without the thin ideal have no eating disorders, and the amount of depression in women and men in these cultures is the same. This suggests that around the world, the thin ideal and dieting not only cause eating disorders, but they may also cause women to be more depressed than men.

THE BOTTOM LINE

I have been dieting off and on for 30 years because I want to be more attractive, healthier, and more in control. How do these goals stack up against the facts?

Attractiveness. If your attractiveness is a high-enough priority to convince you to diet, keep three drawbacks in mind. First, the attractiveness you gain will be temporary. All the weight you lose and maybe more will likely come back in a few years. This will depress you. Then you will have to lose it again and it will be harder the second time. Or you will have to resign yourself to being less attractive. Second, when women choose the silhouette figure they want to achieve, it turns out to be thinner than the silhouette that men label most attractive. Third, you may well become bulimic particularly if your natural weight is substantially more than your ideal weight. On balance, if short-term attractiveness is your overriding goal, diet. But be prepared for the costs.

Health. No one has ever shown that losing weight will increase my longevity. On balance, the health goal does not warrant dieting.

Control. For many people, getting to an ideal weight and staying there is just as biologically impossible as going with much less sleep. This fact tells me not to diet, and defuses my feeling of shame. My bottom line is clear: I am not going to diet anymore.

DEPTH AND CHANGE: THE THEORY

Clearly, we have not yet developed drugs or psychotherapies that can change all the problems, personality types, and patterns of behavior in adult life. But I believe that success and failure stems from something other than inadequate treatment. Rather, it stems from the depth of the problem.

We all have experience of psychological states of different depths. For example, if you ask someone, out of the blue, to answer quickly, "Who are you?" they will usually tell you—roughly in this order—their name, their sex, their profession. whether they have children, and their religion or race. Underlying this is a continuum of depth from surface to soul—with all manner of psychic material in between.

I believe that issues of the soul can barely be changed by psychotherapy or by drugs. Problems and behavior patterns somewhere between soul and surface can be changed somewhat. Surface problems can be changed easily, even cured. What is changeable, by therapy or drugs, I speculate, varies with the depth of the problem.

My theory says that it does not matter *when* problems, habits, and personality are acquired; their depth derives only from their biology, their evidence, and their power. Some childhood traits, for example, are deep and unchangeable but not because they were learned early and therefore have a privileged place.

Rather, those traits that resist change do so either because they are evolutionarily prepared or because they acquire great power by virtue of becoming the framework around which later learning crystallizes. In this way, the theory of depth carries the optimistic message that we are not prisoners of our past.

When you have understood this message, you will never look at your life in the same way again. Right now there are a number of things that you do not like about yourself and that you want to change: your short fuse, your waistline, your shyness, your drinking, your glumness. You have decided to change, but you do not know what you should work on first. Formerly you would have probably selected the one that hurts the most. Now you will also ask yourself which attempt is most likely to repay your efforts and which is most likely to lead to further frustration. Now you know your shyness and your anger are much more likely to change than your drinking, which you now know is more likely to change than your waistline.

Some of what does change is under your control, and some is not. You can best prepare yourself to change by learning as much as you can about what you can change and how to make those changes. Like all true education, learning about change is not easy; harder yet is surrendering some of our hopes. It is certainly not my purpose to destroy your optimism about change. But it is also not my purpose to assure everybody they can change in every way. My purpose is to instill a new, warranted optimism about the parts of your life you can change and so help you focus your limited time, money, and effort on making actual what is truly within your reach.

Life is a long period of change. What you have been able to change and what has resisted your highest resolve might seem chaotic to you: for some of what you are never changes no matter how hard you try, and other aspects change readily. My hope is that this essay has been the beginning of wisdom about the difference.

Cognitive-Behavioral Therapy Today

Robert M. Goisman

Cognitive-behavioral therapy (CBT) is an increasingly popular set of treatment methods based on cognitive theory and behavioral principles. One of these principles is classical conditioning — the pairing of existing patterns of stimulus and response with new stimuli to create new responses. A second is operant conditioning, or patterning reward and punishment to alter behavior. A third is social learning, which includes learning by observation, role-playing, rehearsal, and training in problem-solving strategies and social skills.

There are several reasons for the growing reputation of CBT. First, its brevity and relatively low cost are valued in an era of managed care and reduced availability of insurance. Second, psychiatrists have been abandoning a diagnostic system that once implicitly favored psychodynamic theory and therapy. Third, tests of psychotherapy outcome are increasingly demanded, and they are best conducted with treatments for which precise descriptive manuals are available. Last — and to the point — CBT has repeatedly been proven to be effective in the treatment of many psychiatric disorders.

Cognitive-behavioral therapists use a variety of techniques, but they all have certain things in common. They devote most of their attention to well-defined, measurable aspects of behavior. They are more interested in the reasons that a problem is persisting than in its original causes. They often plan therapy sessions in detail and assign homework to reinforce skills learned in therapy and promote their use in real life.

Four disorders for which CBT is commonly used are anxiety, depression, borderline personality, and schizophrenia.

Anxiety: The groundbreaking work of Wolpe, Lazarus, and their colleagues in the 1950s led to a simple, direct, and rapid treatment for phobias. Exposure and cognitive correction are the major features of this treatment. Exposure, a form of classically based deconditioning, means approaching the feared object and staying in contact with it until habituation develops and the anxiety fades. Desensitization is a slow, stepwise form of exposure in which fear is eliminated by gradual adaptation, just as allergic reactions are eliminated by gradually increasing doses of an allergenic substance. Desensitization may be performed either in the imagination or, more commonly today, in real life (in vivo).

In flooding, another kind of exposure therapy, the patient approaches the object of a phobia quickly and maintains prolonged contact. This technique is demanding but effective for carefully selected, high-

From *Harvard Mental Health Letter,* May 1997, pp. 4-7. © 1997 by the President and Fellows of Harvard College. Reprinted by permission.

ly motivated patients. Implosion, a rapid approach to internal rather than external stimuli, is sometimes used to treat posttraumatic stress disorder; for example, a veteran might be asked to record an account of his wartime experience and listen to the tape repeatedly until it no longer arouses anxiety.

Two further variations on this theme are interoceptive exposure and exposure with response prevention. Interoceptive exposure is used to treat panic disorder. The patient deliberately induces the physical symptoms of panic in the presence of the therapist, perhaps by hyperventilating to produce shortness of breath or exercising to raise the heart rate. When these sensations are evoked voluntarily in a comfortable atmosphere without intense emotion, they lose their association with panic anxiety. This technique can be combined with cognitive methods that attack the catastrophic thoughts accompanying panic: "My heart is beating too fast — I must be having a heart attack," or "I am so anxious that I will surely go crazy." The patient is taught to recognize these thoughts and prepare rebuttals to them.

Exposure with response prevention is used mainly in the treatment of obsessive-compulsive disorder. Patients are asked to "contaminate" themselves — for example, by touching something that may be dirty — and then avoid repetitive handwashing and other rituals of decontamination. The "dirty" object is analogous to the object of a phobia, and preventing the ritual is analogous to maintaining contact with something that inspires fear. Learning to tolerate the resulting anxiety reduces the patient's need to perform the ritual.

Depression: Aaron Beck and others have shown how to relieve depression by changing a patient's thinking. The therapist assumes that certain kinds of thought can cause depression: "If I am not perfect, then I am a failure", or "Everyone must like me or I will die lonely and unmourned." These broad thought patterns, known as schemas, show their influence through misinterpretations of everyday events that take the form of automatic thoughts. The underlying source of schemas and automatic thoughts is a bias in favor of self-deprecating and pessimistic explanations — what Beck calls the "cognitive triad": negative views of oneself, the world, and the future. The overall aim of therapy is to recognize and correct this bias and its consequences.

The therapist usually begins with behavioral exercises, since overt behavior is often easier to change than thinking habits. Goals are set early, and exercises are designed to meet them. A typical behavioral exercise is monitoring one's moods to increase positive reinforcement (reward, pleasurable occasions). Another exercise, graded task assignment, breaks down seemingly overwhelming projects into small increments so that they can be accomplished one step at a time. Role-playing is used for improving assertiveness, among many other purposes.

Most of the exercises are cognitive. The depressed patient records episodes of acute unhappiness, noting when and where they occur, what thoughts accompany them, and how persuasive those thoughts are. The patient then learns to exchange the thoughts for less depressing and more rational ones. At first the process may seem purely intellectual, but eventually it takes on emotional significance as well.

For example, the patient might be a depressed woman who is convinced that her boss has deliberately ignored her in the hall. Her schema may be: "If my work isn't perfect, then I'm worthless"; the automatic thought may be: "She didn't look at me because she thinks my work is poor." These misinterpretations prevent the patient from considering that her boss may just have had something else on her mind. The therapist helps the patient to test the evidence by asking such questions as "How do you know your boss thought your work was bad?" and "What other explanation might there be?" Eventually they go on to examine the underlying bias that leads to such distortions.

CBT is now a standard treatment for major depression and dysthymia (milder chronic depression). Recently it has been used to treat bipolar (manic-depressive) disorder, with an emphasis on asking the patient to evaluate manic thoughts and behavior while in a normal mood. Good results have been reported, but more studies are needed.

Borderline personality: Borderline patients pose special challenges for psychotherapy because their moods, thinking, behavior, self-image, and personal relations are extremely unstable. Suicide attempts, self-mutilation, and early morning phone calls sometimes deter clinicians from working with them despite their great need. A psychodynamic understanding of these patients can be illuminating, and biological treatment of their mood disorders is sometimes indispensable. But psychodynamic psychotherapy alone is unreliable and may take too long; medication is not consistently effective and may be risky because of the patient's tendency to take overdoses.

The prospects for treating borderline personality have improved with the advent of dialectical behavior therapy (DBT), a method devised by Marsha

Linehan. She uses operant conditioning, cognitive therapy, feminist political theory, and Zen Buddhism in a form of individual and group treatment that is aimed most directly at reducing parasuicidal behavior (self-mutilation) but also improves the lives of these patients in many other ways.

DBT is usually conducted for a year in one weekly two-and-a-half-hour session of group therapy and one of individual therapy. The curriculum is mapped out in detail and repeated in its entirety after six months. (Repetition is necessary because many borderline patients have been sexually abused as children, and the abuse makes them vulnerable to dissociative symptoms that limit their capacity to retain therapeutic gains.) The group is analogous to a classroom and individual therapy sessions to a tutorial. The individual therapists meet with group leaders for an hour a week to consult, exchange impressions, coordinate their work, and check one another for fidelity to the philosophy and technique of DBT. Patients must quit if they miss more than four consecutive sessions; they are not accepted for DBT unless their individual therapists agree to attend the consultation group meetings.

The group therapy curriculum is divided into several units that are specified in a workbook: mindfulness skills, interpersonal effectiveness, regulation of emotions, and acceptance of reality and tolerance of distress. In each unit the basic concepts are introduced, and patients perform exercises that include writing, reading, mood-monitoring, and role-playing. Therapists constantly emphasize the acquisition and improvement of social skills. The curriculum begins with the least emotionally fraught material, but toward the end patients are learning how to handle crises in their lives without self-destructive behavior.

Patients who call the therapist in a crisis are asked, not how or why it happened, but what they have done in such situations in the past and what they might do now. That way, callers are taught how to solve their problems instead of being rewarded simply for venting feelings or seeking comfort from the therapist. For similar reasons, when a patient has to be hospitalized, the therapist does not visit the hospital but expresses interest in resuming their meetings after the patient is discharged.

This treatment can be expensive and requires considerable preparation, but research funded by the National Institute of Mental Health has shown that it pays for itself by reducing the number of visits to psychiatric and medical emergency rooms. Studies now under way are testing the effectiveness of DBT in the treatment of drug abusers and mentally ill patients in day hospitals.

Schizophrenia: The behavioral treatment of psychotic patients has a long history. Early attempts were made to reduce their symptoms by ignoring psychotic talk and paying attention to rational communication instead. In a tradition derived from B. F. Skinner's work on operant conditioning, schizophrenic patients have benefited from token economy programs in which vouchers are given for approved behavior. Another derivative of Skinner's work is contingency management — the use of privileges to influence the behavior of hospitalized patients.

In recent years Robert Liberman and his colleagues at UCLA have developed a more sophisticated behavioral approach to hospitalized psychotic patients. Liberman regards schizophrenia as a catastrophic illness which, like a stroke, can cause the patient to lose acquired social skills and interfere with the acquisition of new ones. After the hallucinations and delusions of acute psychosis are treated with drugs, Liberman begins psychological and social rehabilitation in groups resembling classes that meet for an hour several times a week. The curriculum includes the nature of psychiatric illness, the uses and side effects of psychiatric drugs, the avoidance of alcohol and street drugs, conversational skills, the constructive use of free time, strategies for living outside a psychiatric hospital, and ways to cope with persistent symptoms and detect an impending relapse. Patients watch videotapes and undertake role-playing and written exercises; they may also be assigned homework. The results are fewer relapses, less drug and alcohol abuse, and sometimes less need for medication. The National Alliance for the Mentally Ill, a major support group for patients with serious mental illness, has endorsed this approach because it educates patients about the symptoms of schizophrenia and reduces the social stigma attached to it by treating it as a medical illness. Thus CBT, from its beginnings as a technique focused on simple phobias, has grown into a sophisticated body of theory and practice used to treat a wide range of conditions. Some that I have not discussed in detail are sexual dysfunctions, alcohol abuse, autism, and mental retardation. Today, cognitive and behavioral methods are also being combined with psychodynamic therapy and medication. Although formal studies of this combination treatment have just begun, it appears to be sometimes more effective than any single treatment and may represent an important new direction for psychiatry.

Robert M. Goisman, M.D., is Director of Outpatient Training and Research and of Medical Student Education at the Massachusetts Mental Health Center, Boston, and Assistant Professor of Psychiatry at Harvard Medical School.

Biological Therapies

Just as mental health practitioners face a wide range of disorders and are constantly searching for new and effective treatments, so recent developments in understanding the biological influences in various disorders have spurred a growing interest in biological therapies. However, the use of such treatments actually has a long past; for example, the first psychosurgical procedures were done in the 1930s.

Which biological therapy is most effective, and for whom should it be used? Do biological therapies have advantages over psychological therapies? What are the side effects of various drug treatments? Can psychological and biological therapies be combined effectively? These important questions must be addressed by both patients and physicians when considering the use of any biological treatment for mental disorders.

Researchers have been making remarkable discoveries that increase our understanding of the biological factors involved in many mental disorders. For example, we now have a clearer understanding of the brain circuits responsible for fear. Discoveries like this have led to several new drugs such as Prozac; however, we should be cautious about accepting claims for such treatments. The report by Sharon Begley focuses our attention on the need to be careful in our evaluation of new drugs.

One reason to be concerned about the use of new drugs is that most drugs have side effects. Many side effects may not be recognized in short-term trials. Serious questions need to be asked about using drugs for everything, including changing one's personality. The rapid increase in the use of drugs such as Ritalin to treat attention deficit hyperactivity disorder raises several issues related to drug treatment. The possible side effects are one concern, especially in a population of children.

Psychosurgery is an irreversible and highly controversial treatment for mental disorders. It has been used in the past for a number of disorders, including schizophrenia. The rare psychosurgical treatments available today bear almost no resemblance to the procedures of the 1930s and 1940s. However, occasional psychosurgical procedures using stereotactic instruments are still done today. Among the reasons for this surgical procedure are attempts to reduce violent seizures associated with epilepsy, as described by Joann Ellison Rodgers.

Looking Ahead: Challenge Questions

What limitations, if any, should be put on the use of drugs for purposes other than their approved uses?

Should there be safeguards to ensure that nondrug treatments are used before drugs are prescribed for mental disorders, especially among children? Why or why not?

Why do drugs often have side effects that are not recognized at first?

How can patients who suffer from serious mental disorders give true informed consent for procedures such as psychosurgery?

UNIT 8

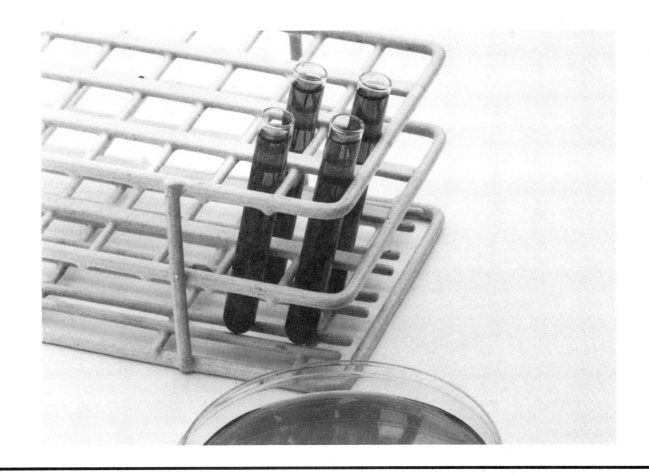

One pill makes you larger, And one pill makes you small . . .

BEYOND PROZAC: Scientific insights into the brain are raising the prospect of made-to-order, off-the-shelf personalities

Sharon Begley

. . . That was 1960s pharmacology. In that turned-on, tuned-out decade, the pharmacopeia of mind-altering drugs was about as subtle as a sledgehammer—uppers replaced sleep, downers offered calm, hallucinogens projected visions of marmalade skies into the brain. Many of them were illegal, and all of them threatened to stop the heart, blow out neurons or cause permanent addiction. This is 1990s pharmacology: suffering stage fright before delivering a speech? Pop a little orange pill. Moping around in the winter doldrums? Try a white one. Want to boost your self-esteem, focus better on your work, tame the impulse to shop till you drop, shrug off your spouse's habit of littering the floor with underwear, overcome your shyness or keep yourself from blurting out your deepest secrets to the first stranger who comes along? Science has, or soon will have, just the legal, doctor-prescribed pill for you.

It's gone beyond Prozac. That antidepressant has spawned a culture of pill poppers: people who do not suffer from severe depression (for which the Food and Drug Administration approved Prozac in 1987) but who find that the little green and white capsule makes them more cheerful, more mellow, more self-assured. Now the same scientific insights into the brain that led to the development of Prozac are raising the prospect of nothing less than made-to-order, off-the-shelf personalities. For good or ill, research that once mapped the frontiers of disease—indentifying the brain chemistry involved in depression, paranoia and schizophrenia—is today closing in on the chemistry of normal personality. As a result, researchers are on the verge of "chemical attempts to modify character," writes neuropsychiatrist Richard Restak in the soon-to-be-published "Receptors." Most of the new drugs will be aimed not so much at 'patients' as at people who are already functioning on a high level . . . enriching [their] memory, enhancing intelligence, heightening concentration, and altering for the good people's internal moods."

That prospect has brought psychopharmacology—the science of drugs that affect the mind—to "the brink of revolution," as

psychiatrist Stuart Yudofsky of Baylor University puts it. It is a revolution propelled by three advances. First came the theory that every memory, every emotion, every aspect of temperament originates in molecules called neurotransmitters. These chemical signals course through specialized circuits in the brain. Research on brain chemistry starting in the 1940s produced lithium, Valium and other psychoactive drugs, which correct chemical imbalances responsible for grave mental illness. Second, "brain mapping" pinpoints which areas of gray matter become active during particular thoughts or mental states. PET (positron emission tomography), for instance, is a sort of sonogram of the brain that can, among other things, trace sad thoughts to parts of the frontal cortex. Finally, researchers are identifying which neurotransmitters travel those circuits. For example, too much of the neurotransmitter dopamine in the brain's emotion centers, and too little in the seat of reason (diagram, "Mapping the Mind"), seems to cause suspiciousness—raving paranoia and maybe even a habit of wondering if the plumber overcharged you.

Major mental illness wasn't always linked to personality disorders. But according to the model of the mind emerging in the 1990s, mental disease differs from endearing quirks only in degree. Personality disorders arise from *subtle* disturbances in the same systems that produce serious mental illnesses, argues Dr. Larry Siever of Mount Sinai School of Medicine in New York. "Someone just barely able to restrain his impulsive actions wouldn't [seem] psychotic," says Siever. "But he could act rashly"—habitually ducking into a movie instead of going to work, or buying unseen property in Florida on a whim.

As neuroscientists learn what chemicals cause which personality traits, the temptation to fool around with nature will be irresistible. The drugs that perform the mental makeovers are supposed to have no serious side effects and not cause addiction. But more than 40 years of psychoactive drugs has proved that nothing is without hazard (at first, Valium, cocaine, and nicotine were not thought to be addictive, either). "If someone takes a drug every day for four years because it makes him feel or work better, something may happen that we don't know about,"

 From *Newsweek*, February 7, 1994, pp. 36-40. © 1994 by Newsweek, Inc. All rights reserved. Reprinted by permission.

warns psychiatrist Solomon Snyder of Johns Hopkins University. That caution, however, has a difficult time standing up against the Faustian power of the new drugs. "For the first time in human history," says Restak, "we will be in a position to design our own brain." Some of the targets:

SHYNESS AND HYPERSENSITIVITY

Of all the traits that bedevil humans, shyness may be the most hard-wired into the brain. About 20 percent of people start life with neurochemistry that predisposes them to be shy, concludes Harvard University psychologist Jerome Kagan; the other 80 percent become shy or outgoing because of life's experiences. Now scientists may have figured out how biology becomes destiny. An inhibited child seems to be born with what amounts to a hairtrigger brain circuit: compared with other children, it takes much less to stimulate his amygdala, a small cashew-shaped structure deep in the brain that helps control heart rate and perspiration. No wonder shy infants squirm and cry: even mild stress makes their hearts pound and their palms sweat. In addition, inhibited children may have excessive levels of the neurotransmitter norepinephrine, a cousin of the fight-or-flight chemical adrenaline: just walking into kindergarten for the first time produces as much stress as a gladiator's facing the lions. "I think the time will come when we will know exactly the chemical profile of the temperamentally fearful child," says Kagan. "Then pharmacologists could work on very specific cures."

In some people, shyness is not a primary trait but instead a means of coping. "So much of social interaction is based on unspoken rhythms and pacing," says Mount Sinai's Siever, "that people who don't get those beats often feel left out and alienated"—like the woman who can't tell from body language that the man she's chatting with wants to flee. Society perceives her as slightly strange; she responds by withdrawing. Siever suspects that suspiciousness and an inability to process the information contained in the rhythms and cues of social interactions arise from an oversupply of dopamine in the brain's emotion-control room and a shortage in the more rational cortex.

One jobless, fiftyish man seemed to fit this description perfectly. He lived alone, filled his days with crossword puzzles and TV, and "worried that others were making fun of him,"

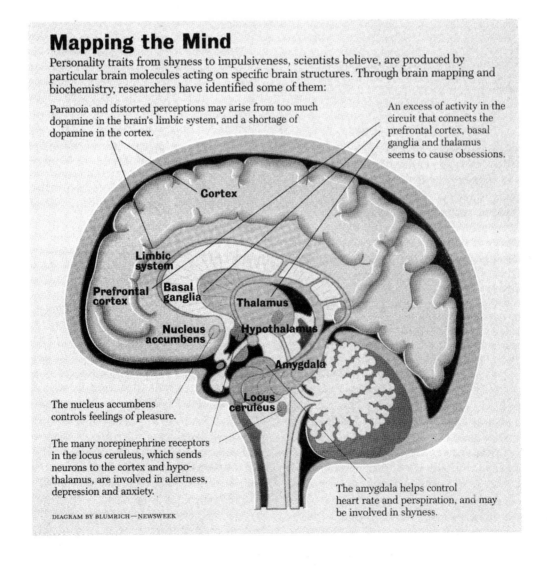

Mapping the Mind

Personality traits from shyness to impulsiveness, scientists believe, are produced by particular brain molecules acting on specific brain structures. Through brain mapping and biochemistry, researchers have identified some of them:

Paranoia and distorted perceptions may arise from too much dopamine in the brain's limbic system, and a shortage of dopamine in the cortex.

An excess of activity in the circuit that connects the prefrontal cortex, basal ganglia and thalamus seems to cause obsessions.

Cortex

Limbic system

Prefrontal cortex

Basal ganglia

Thalamus

Nucleus accumbens

Hypothalamus

Amygdala

Locus ceruleus

The nucleus accumbens controls feelings of pleasure.

The many norepinephrine receptors in the locus ceruleus, which sends neurons to the cortex and hypo-thalamus, are involved in alertness, depression and anxiety.

DIAGRAM BY BLUMRICH—NEWSWEEK

The amygdala helps control heart rate and perspiration, and may be involved in shyness.

says Siever. Like all of Siever's patients, he was seriously ill. Siever suspected, based on biochemical tests, that the man's inability to understand social cues stemmed from a dopamine imbalance. The antidepressant Wellbutrin, which stokes the cortex with dopamine, seemed to help: the man felt sharper and "more activated" (though a back disability kept him from working). Still, scientists caution that what works on the seriously ill might have no effect on someone who decides to cure her lack of social grace with a pill when all she needs is a crash course in etiquette.

Shyness can also grow in the shadow of hypersensitivity, the tendency to fall into a deep funk over even an innocuous rejection. For years, psychiatrist Donald Klein of Columbia-Presbyterian Medical Center in New York had noticed something strange about this funk: it closely resembled the reaction of an amphetamine user suffering withdrawal symptoms. That sparked a bold theory. "The brain is normally making its own stimulant," which keeps people on an even keel, and even makes them outgoing, says Klein. Some people who embarrass easily and cower at the very thought of rejection may do so because their brain does not pump out enough stimulants. They become physically pained by rejection just as a speed freak is physically pained by going cold turkey. "Recently we have shown that we can treat this by preserving the balance of stimulants in the brain and so blocking the withdrawal symptoms," says Klein. He and Columbia's Michael Liebowitz give hypersensitive patients Nardil, the trade name for a substance that blocks the destruction of the brain's natural uppers. As a result, it restores a healthy chemical balance in the hypersensitive mind. "With pills twice a day you usually see results in six weeks," says Klein.

IMPULSIVENESS AND OBSESSION

Just about everyone has, at one time or another, succumbed to the impulse to buy those goodies at the supermarket checkout. In more severe forms, such impulsive behavior expresses itself as kleptomania and other mental illnesses whose sufferers act first and think second. But mild or severe, impulsivity may arise from the inability to learn that behaviors have consequences, like punishment, and so must be controlled or modified.

Depending on where the impulsivity comes from, psychopharmacologists may soon know how to stifle it. As a teenager, did you repeatedly stay out until dawn despite getting grounded for it every time? Are you prone to doing what gets you fired? The problem may stem from too little serotonin, the chemical whose job it is to censor behavior that previously led to punishment, says Siever. Shortages of serotonin in the frontal lobes and in the brain's limbic system, where emotions come from, also seem to lift the lid off impulses. In this case, the dearth of serotonin seems to have the same effect as a shortage of ink in which to write life's lessons: the person is unable to connect disagreeable consequences with what provoked them. Or the problem may simply be an inept working memory. (*But Mom, I forgot you wanted me home!*) Working memory stores information while the mind considers whether it is worth keeping and how to file it. Working memory falters without enough dopamine.

There's a final suspect in impulsivity. Noticing everything can be as debilitating as noticing nothing. Norepinephrine tells the mind what's important by, in effect, putting a chemical red flag on it to say, "Look at this!" In normal people that system kicks in when, for instance, a lion is charging. But in people with too much norepinephrine *everything* gets pumped up. Every perceived slight from a co-worker demands a response, every twinge of desire becomes an irresistible urge to buy.

If impulsives think about their actions too little, obsessives think about them too much. When Mother double-checks that the sleeping children are indeed breathing, and when she's a stickler about dirt on the carpets or grime in the kitchen, she is being mildly compulsive; when she checks 100 times, vacuums 20 times a day and goes through Fantastik like an alcoholic through rotgut, she is manifesting obsessive-compulsive disorder. Sufferers seem unable to get a sense of completeness from any action, like scrubbing the bathtub a mere once. Brain imaging is now showing such obsession in living color. PET scans of a patient touched with a dirty rag—cleanliness is a typical obsession—show a response like a broken record. Signals travel between three structures in the brain stem—the prefrontal cortex, the basal ganglia and the thalamus—endlessly. In normal people, the signal stops after one orbit thanks to a new message, screaming, "*The floor is clean already!*" "Lots of people have milder variants of this," says neuroscientist Lewis Baxter of the University of California, Los Angeles. "They check the stove two times, though not 102. They say that intellectually they know the stove is OK, but they can't get the *emotional* boost that says, 'Hey, it's working'." Baxter believes that even mild compulsiveness might succumb to drugs that change the brain's regulation of serotonin. In fact, Prozac is about to be approved for use against obsessive-compulsive behavior. The great unknown is whether Prozac and other powerful drugs will work on milder forms of severe disorders.

ANXIETY AND CONCENTRATION

The neural pathways to anxiety exist because early humans who got a little nervous at the sight of, say, a crouching saber tooth had a survival edge over more laid-back tribesmen. Now, in the age of anxiety, many people would just as soon give back this legacy of natural selection. At the National Institute of Mental Health, Philip Gold is figuring out how. He traces stress to the circuit responsible for the fight-or-flight response. In the chronically anxious, he says, "it turns on, but it doesn't turn off." Antidepressants called tricyclics, which throttle back levels of the fight-or-flight norepinephrine, seem to still the perpetual arousal in the circuit.

A *shortage* of norepinephrine seems to rob people of the ability to pay attention to what's important, and only to what's important. Sally Jackson, the fortysomething owner of a Boston public-relations firm, knows the problem well. She had often felt unfocused, so last winter she began taking Ritalin, a stimulant that increases the availability of norepinephrine. Although Ritalin is best known as the controversial medication for children diagnosed with attention-deficit disorder (ADD, alias hyperactivity), adults are now taking the yellow pills to improve their concentration. "Without it, I would sit at my desk for hours and get nothing done," says Jackson, who believes she has ADD. "But once I started Ritalin, every proposal I wrote, we won the account. I'm better on deadline and it keeps me focused on one task at a time." She swallows one pill in the morning and another if she hits a 3 p.m. lull.

I MEDICATE, THEREFORE WHO AM I?

Prozac to cheer you up and Ritalin to focus are merely the most prominent new mind drugs. Anticonvulsants such as Dilantin, prescribed for epileptics, turn out to reduce stress in some people. Beta blockers are heart drugs: they lower blood pressure and heart rate. But doctors figured out an entirely new use for them: combating stage fright. The drugs block receptors for norepinephrine; with less adrenaline igniting their brain circuits, people like oboist Stuart Dunkel, who plays for the Boston Opera, have no trouble calming performance anxiety. Before, complicated solos would make Dunkel's heart beat like a jackhammer and his breathing so shallow he couldn't sustain notes. With beta blockers, "there's a psychological release," he says. The drugs are not addictive, and Dunkel reports no side effects.

Other mind drugs are in the pipeline. One, with the tongue-tying name dexfenfluramine, seems to smooth out mood swings, especially those caused by winter doldrums and premenstrual syndrome. Naturally, it targets neurotransmitters: it keeps brain neurons bathed in serotonin longer than otherwise, explains Judith Wurtman of the Massachusetts Institute of Technology. Already used in Europe and South America as an anti-obesity drug (mood swings often trigger eating binges), dex-fenfluramine has been submitted to the FDA for approval. A few weeks ago researchers at UC Irvine announced the discovery of the first drug that seems to improve working memory. The discovery sprang from work on neurotransmitters and their receptors, the shapely molecules that neurotransmitters fit like keys in locks. Researchers led by Gary Lynch found that in rats, the drug BDP binds to receptors for the neurotransmitter glutamate, which triggers neuronal changes that constitute memory. As a result, it acts like the father who lowers the basketball net for his vertically challenged child, reducing the amount of stimulation neurons require to form memories. If BDP works in people, the history lesson that once took hours to learn would take mere minutes. An Irvine-based start-up, Cortex Pharmaceuticals, Inc., plans to test BDP's safety.

Who could criticize a drug that stamps the rules for long division into your child's head after a single lesson? As psychiatrist Daniel Luchins of the University of Chicago points out, society accepts plastic surgery (albeit with some jokes): "If we have something that made people unshy, are they obliged to stay shy because of some ethical concern? What's the difference between 'I'm unhappy because I don't like my looks' and 'I'm unhappy because I'm shy?' "

For openers, one's core being is defined more by character traits than by the shape of one's nose. Just ask Cyrano. And not everything we feel, let alone everything we are, is shaped by too much or too little of some polysyllabic brain chemical. Yet as society moves ever closer to minds-made-to-order, the pressure on those who cannot, or choose not to, give their brain a makeover becomes intense. Some colleagues, and competitors, of Ritalin-popping executives feel themselves at a disadvantage, like rules-respecting sprinters facing a steroid user. Will guidance counselors urge parents to give their kids memory pills before the SATs? Will supervisors "suggest" workers take a little something to sharpen their concentration? The prospect of pills to make the dour cheery, and the tense mellow, calls into question the very notion of the self—is it truly the "self" in any meaningful sense if it is as easy to change as a bust measurement? "The brain is where our soul and spirit lie," says Harvard's Kagan. "People are very threatened by this."

Perhaps most worrisome is the idea of sandpapering away personality traits that not only make us individuals, but which evolved for a good reason. Anxiety, for instance, "probably evolved in tandem with the evolution of the human brain," writes Restak. Blunting that edge has a price. And just as physical pain keeps us from burning our flesh, perhaps mental pain, like that brought on by the death of a child, serves a purpose—one that is defeated by a pill that soothes when one should instead be raging. Shyness has also served civilization well. Some of history's great thinkers and creators—T. S. Eliot, Emily Dickinson, Anton Bruckner—were shy. "Inhibited children tend to wander off into vocations like music, literature and philosophy," says Kagan. A society that uses drugs to induce conformity does so at its peril.

With DEBRA ROSENBERG in Boston, JOSHUA COOPER RAMO in New York and MARY HAGER in Washington

PROZAC. ZOLOFT. PAXIL. WELLBUTRIN.

Prescriptions for Happiness?

The biological approach to treating unhappiness is booming. But is it all it's cracked up to be? Two noted researchers demonstrate that the "scientific" studies that underpin claims of drug effectiveness are seriously flawed—undone by signals from our bodies. Perhaps the studies really prove the power of placebo—and the absurdity of drawing any line between what is biological and what is psychological.

Seymour Fisher, Ph.D., and Roger P. Greenberg, Ph.D.

The air is filled with declarations and advertisements of the power of biological psychiatry to relieve people of their psychological distress. *Some biological psychiatrists are so convinced of the superiority of their position that they are recommending young psychiatrists no longer be taught the essentials of doing psychotherapy. Feature stories in such magazines as* Newsweek *and* Time *have portrayed drugs like Prozac as possessing almost a mystical potency. The best-selling book* Listening to Prozac *by psychiatrist Peter Kramer, M.D., projects the idyllic possibility that psychotropic drugs may eventually be capable of correcting a spectrum of personality quirks and lacks.*

As longtime faculty members of a number of psychiatry departments, we have personally witnessed the gradual but steadily accelerated dedication to the idea that "mental illness" can be mastered with biologically based substances. Yet a careful sifting of the pertinent literature indicates that modesty and skepticism would be more appropriate responses to the research accumulated thus far.

In 1989, we first raised radical questions about such biological claims in a book, The Limits of Biological Treatments for Psychological Distress: Comparisons with Psychotherapy and Placebo *(Lawrence Erlbaum). Our approach has been to filter the studies that presumably anchor them through a series of logical and quantitative (meta-analytic) appraisals.*

How Effective Are Antidepressant Drugs?

Antidepressants, one of the major weapons in the biological therapeutic arsenal, illustrate well the largely unacknowledged uncertainty that exists in the biological approach to psychopathology. We suggest that, at present, no one actually knows how effective antidepressants are. Confident declarations about their potency go well beyond the existing evidence.

To get an understanding of the scientific status of antidepressants, we analyzed how much more effective the antidepressants are than inert pills called "placebos." That is, if antidepressants are given to one depressed group and a placebo to another group, how much greater is the recovery of those taking the active drug as compared to those taking the inactive placebo? Generous claims that antidepressants usually produce improvement in about 60 to 70 percent of patients are not infrequent, whereas placebos are said to benefit 25 to 30 percent. If antidepressants were, indeed, so superior to placebos, this would be a persuasive advertisement for the biological approach.

We found 15 major reviews of the antidepressant literature. Surprisingly, even the most positive reviews indicate that 30 to 40 percent of studies show no significant difference in response to drug versus placebo! The reviews indicate overall that one-third of patients do not improve with antidepressant treatment, one-third improve with placebos, and an additional third show a response to medication they

From *Psychology Today*, September/October 1995, pp. 32-37. © 1995 by Seymour Fisher and Roger P. Greenberg. Reprinted by permission.

would not have attained with placebos. In the most optimistic view of such findings, two-thirds of the cases (placebo responders and those who do not respond to anything) do as well with placebo as with active medication.

We also found two large-scale quantitative evaluations (meta-analyses) integrating the outcomes of multiple studies of antidepressants. They clearly indicated, on the average, quite modest therapeutic power.

We were particularly impressed by the large variation in outcomes of studies conducted at multiple clinical sites or centers. Consider a study that compared the effectiveness of an antidepressant among patients at five different research centers. Although the pooled results demonstrate that the drug was generally more effective than placebo, the results from individual centers reveal much variation. After six weeks of treatment, every one of the six measures of effectiveness showed the antidepressant (imipramine) to be merely equivalent to placebo in two or more of the centers. In two of the settings, a difference favoring the medication was detected on only one of 12 outcome comparisons.

In other words, the pooled, apparently favorable, outcome data conceal that dramatically different results could be obtained as a function of who conducted the study and the specific conditions at each locale. We can only conclude that a good deal of fragility characterized the apparent superiority of drug over placebo. The scientific literature is replete with analogous examples.

Incidentally, we also looked at whether modern studies, which are presumably better protected against bias, use higher doses, and often involve longer treatment periods, show a greater superiority of the antidepressant than did earlier studies. The literature frequently asserts that failures to demonstrate antidepressant superiority are due to such methodological failures as not using high enough doses, and so forth.

We examined this issue in a pool of 16 studies assembled by psychiatrists John Kane and Jeffrey Lieberman in 1984. These studies all compare a standard drug, such as imipramine or amitriptyline, to a newer drug and a placebo. They use clearer diagnostic definitions of depression than did the older studies and also adopt currently accepted standards for dosage levels and treatment duration. When we examined the data, we discovered that the advantage of drug over placebo was modest. Twenty-one percent more of the patients receiving

a drug improved as compared to those on placebo. Actually, most of the studies showed no difference in the percentage of patients significantly improved by drugs. There was no indication that these studies, using more careful methodology, achieved better outcomes than older studies.

Finally, it is crucial to recognize that several studies have established that there is a high rate of relapse among those who have responded positively to an antidepressant but then are taken off treatment. The relapse rate may be 60 percent or more during the first year after treatment cessation. Many studies also show that any benefits of antidepressants wane in a few months, even while the drugs are still being taken. This highlights the complexity of evaluating antidepressants. They may be effective initially, but lose all value over a longer period.

ARE DRUG TRIALS BIASED?

As we burrowed deeper into the antidepressant literature, we learned that there are also crucial problems in the methodology used to evaluate psychotropic drugs. Most central is the question of whether this methodology properly shields drug trials from bias. Studies have shown that the more open to bias a drug trial is, the greater the apparent superiority of the drug over placebo. So questions about the trustworthiness of a given drug-testing procedure invite skepticism about the results.

The question of potential bias first came to our attention in studies comparing inactive placebos to active drugs. In the classic double-blind design, neither patient nor researcher knows who is receiving drug or placebo. We were struck by the fact that the presumed protection provided by the double-blind design was undermined by the use of placebos that simply do not arouse as many body sensations as do active drugs. Research shows that patients learn to discriminate between drug and placebo largely from body sensations and symptoms.

A substance like imipramine, one of the most frequently studied antidepressants, usually causes clearly defined sensations, such as dry mouth, tremor, sweating, constipation. Inactive placebos used in studies of antidepressants also apparently initiate some body sensations, but they are fewer,

more inconsistent, and less intense as indicated by the fact that they are less often cited by patients as a source of discomfort causing them to drop out of treatment.

Vivid differences between the body sensations of drug and placebo groups could signal to patients as to whether they are receiving an active or inactive agent. Further, they could supply discriminating cues to those responsible for the patients' day-to-day treatment. Nurses, for example, might adopt different attitudes toward patients they identify as being "on" versus "off" active treatment and consequently communicate contrasting expectations.

THE BODY OF EVIDENCE

This is more than theoretical. Researchers have reported that in a double-blind study of imipramine, it was possible by means of side effects to identify a significant number of the patients taking the active drug. Those patients receiving a placebo have fewer signals (from self and others) indicating they are being actively treated and should be improving. By the same token, patients taking an active drug receive multiple signals that may well amplify potential placebo effects linked to the therapeutic context. Indeed, a doctor's strong belief in the power of the active drug enhances the apparent therapeutic power of the drug or placebo.

Is it possible that a large proportion of the difference in effectiveness often reported between antidepressants and placebos can be explained as a function of body sensation discrepancies? It is conceivable, and fortunately there are research findings that shed light on the matter.

Consider an analysis by New Zealand psychologist Richard Thomson. He reviewed double-blind, placebo-controlled studies of antidepressants completed between 1958 and 1972. Sixty-eight had employed an inert placebo and seven an active one (atropine) that produced a variety of body sensations. The antidepressant had a superior therapeutic effect in 59 percent of the studies using inert placebo—but in only one study (14 percent) using the active placebo. The active placebo eliminated any therapeutic advantage for the antidepressants, apparently because it convinced patients they were getting real medication.

Vivid differences between the body sensations of drug and placebo could signal to patients whether they are receiving an active or inactive agent.

A patient's attitude toward the therapist is just as biological in nature as a patient's response to an antidepressant drug.

How Blind Is Double-Blind?

Our concerns about the effects of inactive placebos on the double-blind design led us to ask just how blind the double-blind really is. By the 1950s reports were already surfacing that for psychoactive drugs, the double-blind design is not as scientifically objective as originally assumed. In 1993 we searched the world literature and found 31 reports in which patients and researchers involved in studies were asked to guess who was receiving the active psychotropic drug and who the placebo. In 28 instances the guesses were significantly better than chance—and at times they were surprisingly accurate. In one double-blind study that called for administering either imipramine, phenelzine, or placebo to depressed patients, 78 percent of patients and 87 percent of psychiatrists correctly distinguished drug from placebo.

One particularly systematic report in the literature involved the administration of alprazolam, imipramine, and placebo over an eight-week period to groups of patients who experienced panic attacks. Halfway through the treatment and also at the end, the physicians and the patients were asked to judge independently whether each patient was receiving an active drug or a placebo. If they thought an active drug was being administered, they had to decide whether it was alprazolam or imipramine. Both physicians (with an 88 percent success rate) and patients (83 percent) substantially exceeded chance in the correctness of their judgments. Furthermore, the physicians could distinguish alprazolam from imipramine significantly better than chance. The researchers concluded that "double-blind studies of these pharmacological treatments for panic disorder are not really 'blind.' "

Yet the vast majority of psychiatric drug efficacy studies have simply *assumed* that the double-blind design is effective; they did not test the blindness by determining whether patients and researchers were able to differentiate drug from placebo.

We take the somewhat radical view that this means most past studies of the efficacy of psychotropic drugs are, to unknown degrees, scientifically untrustworthy. At the least, we can no longer speak with confidence about the true differences in therapeutic power between active psychotropic drugs and placebos. We must suspend judgment until future studies are completed with more adequate controls for the defects of the double-blind paradigm.

Other bothersome questions arose as we scanned the cascade of studies focused on antidepressants. Of particular concern is how unrepresentative the patients are who end up in the clinical trials. There are the usual sampling problems having to do with which persons seek treatment for their discomfort, and, in addition, volunteer as subjects for a study. But there are others. Most prominent is the relatively high proportion of patients who "drop out" before the completion of their treatment programs.

Numerous dropouts occur in response to unpleasant side effects. In many published studies, 35 percent or more of patients fail to complete the research protocol. Various procedures have been developed to deal fairly with the question of how to classify the therapeutic outcomes of dropouts, but none can vitiate the simple fact that the final sample of fully treated patients has often been drastically reduced.

There are still other filters that increase sample selectivity. For example, studies often lose sizable segments of their samples by not including patients who are too depressed to speak, much less participate in a research protocol, or who are too disorganized to participate in formal psychological testing. We also found decisions not to permit particular racial or age groups to be represented in samples or to avoid using persons below a certain educational level. Additionally, researchers typically recruit patients whose depression is not accompanied by any other type of physical or mental disorder, a situation that does not hold for the depressed in the general population.

So we end up wondering about the final survivors in the average drug trial. To what degree do they typify the average individual in real life who seeks treatment? How much can be generalized from a sample made up of the "leftovers" from multiple depleting processes? Are we left with a relatively narrow band of those most willing to conform to the rather rigid demands of the research establishment? Are the survivors those most accepting of a dependent role?

The truth is that there are probably multiple kinds of survivors, depending upon the specific local conditions prevailing where the study was carried out. We would guess that some of the striking differences in results that appear in multicenter drug studies could be traced to specific forms of sampling bias. We do not know how psychologically unique the persons are who get recruited into, and stick with, drug research enterprises. We are not the first to raise this question, but we are relatively more alarmed about the potential implications.

Researcher Motivation And Outcome

We recently conducted an analysis that further demonstrates how drug effectiveness diminishes as the opportunity for bias in research design wanes. This analysis in which a newer antidepressant is compared (under double-blind conditions) with an older, standard antidepressant and a placebo. In such a context the efficacy of the newer drug (which the drug company hopes to introduce) is of central interest to the researcher, and the effectiveness of the older drug of peripheral import. Therefore, if the double-blind is breached (as is likely), there would presumably be less bias to enhance the efficacy of the older drug than occurred in the original trials of that drug.

We predicted that the old drug would appear significantly less powerful in the newer studies than it had in earlier designs, where it was of central interest of the researcher. To test this hypothesis, we located 22 double-blind studies in which newer antidepressants were compared with an older antidepressant drug (usually imipramine) and a placebo. Our meta-analysis revealed, as predicted, that the efficacy rates, based on clinicians' judgments of outcome, were quite modest for the older antidepressants. In fact, they were approximately one-half to one-quarter the average size of the effects reported in earlier studies when the older drug was the only agent appraised.

Let us be very clear as to what this signifies: When researchers were evaluating the antidepressant in a context where they were no longer interested in proving its therapeutic power, there was a dramatic decrease in that apparent power, as compared to an earlier context when they were enthusiastically interested in demonstrating the drug's potency. A change in researcher motivation was enough to change outcome. Obviously this means too that the present double-blind design for testing drug efficacy is exquisitely vulnerable to bias.

Another matter of pertinence to the presumed biological rationale for the efficacy of antidepressants is that no consistent links have been demonstrated between the concentration of drug in blood and its efficacy. Studies have found significant correlations for some drugs, but of low magnitude. Efforts to link plasma levels to therapeutic outcome have been disappointing.

Similarly, few data show a relationship between antidepressant dosage levels and their therapeutic efficacy. That is, large doses of the drug do not necessarily have greater effects than low doses. These inconsistencies are a bit jarring against the context of a biological explanatory framework.

We have led you through a detailed critique of the difficulties and problems that prevail in the body of research testing the power of the antidepressants. We conclude that it would be wise to be relatively modest in claims about their efficacy. Uncertainty and doubt are inescapable.

While we have chosen the research on the antidepressants to illustrate the uncertainties attached to biological treatments of psychological distress, reviews of other classes of psychotropic drugs yield similar findings. After a survey of anti-anxiety drugs, psychologist Ronald Lipman concluded there is little consistent evidence that they help patients with anxiety disorders: "Although it seems natural to assume that the anxiolytic medications would be the most effective psychotropic medications for the treatment of anxiety disorders, the evidence does not support this assumption."

Biological Versus Psychological?

The faith in the biological approach has been fueled by a great burst of research. Thousands of papers have appeared probing the efficacy of psychotropic drugs. A good deal of basic research has attacked fundamental issues related to the nature of brain functioning in those who display psychopathology. Researchers in these areas are dedicated and often do excellent work. However, in their zeal, in their commitment to the so-called biological, they are at times overcome by their expectations. Their hopes become rigidifying boundaries. Their vocabulary too easily becomes a jargon that camouflages over-simplified assumptions.

A good example of such oversimplification is the way in which the term "biological" is conceptualized. It is too often viewed as a realm distinctly different from the psychological. Those invested in the biological approach all too often practice the ancient Cartesian distinction between somatic-stuff and soul-stuff. In so doing they depreciate the scientific significance of the phenomena they exile to the soul-stuff category.

But paradoxically, they put a lot of interesting phenomena out of bounds to their prime methodology and restrict themselves to a narrowed domain. For example, if talk therapy is labeled as a "psychological" thing—not biological—this implies that biological research can only hover at the periphery of what psychotherapists do. A sizable block of behavior becomes off limits to the biologically dedicated.

In fact, if we adopt the view that the biological and psychological are equivalent (biological monism), there is no convincing real-versus-unreal differentiation between the so-called psychological and biological. It *all* occurs in tissue and one is not more "real" than the other. A patient's attitude toward the therapist is just as biological in nature as a patient's response to an antidepressant. A response to a placebo is just as biological as a response to an anti-psychotic drug. This may be an obvious point, but it has not yet been incorporated into the world views of either the biologically or psychologically oriented.

Take a look at a few examples in the research literature that highlight the overlap or identity of what is so often split apart. In 1992, psychiatrist Lewis Baxter and colleagues showed that successful psychotherapy of obsessive-compulsive patients results in brain imagery changes equivalent to those produced by successful drug treatment. The brain apparently responds in equivalent ways to both the talk and drug approaches. Even more dramatic is a finding that instilling in the elderly the illusion of being in control of one's surroundings (by putting them in charge of some plants) significantly increased their life span compared to a control group. What could be a clearer demonstration of the biological nature of what is labeled as a psychological expectation than the postponement of death?

Why are we focusing on this historic Cartesian confusion? Because so many who pursue the so-called biological approach are by virtue of their tunnel vision motivated to overlook the psychosocial variables that mediate the administration of such agents as psychotropic drugs and electroconvulsive therapy. They do not permit themselves to seriously grasp that psychosocial variables are just as biological as a capsule containing an antidepressant. It is the failure to understand this that results in treating placebo effects as if they were extraneous or less of a biological reality than a chemical agent.

Placebo Effects

Indeed, placebos have been shown to initiate certain effects usually thought to be reserved for active drugs. For example, placebos clearly show dose-level effects. A larger dose of a placebo will have a greater impact than a lower dose. Placebos can also create addictions. Patients will poignantly declare that they cannot stop taking a particular placebo substance (which they assume is an active drug) because to do so causes them too much distress and discomfort.

Placebos can produce toxic effects such as rashes, apparent memory loss, fever, headaches, and more. These "toxic" effects may be painful and even overwhelming in their intensity. The placebo literature is clear: Placebos are powerful body-altering substances, especially considering the wide range of body systems they can influence.

Actually, the power of the placebo complicates all efforts to test the therapeutic efficacy of psychotropic drugs. When placebos alone can produce positive curative effects in the 40 to 50 percent range (occasionally even up to 70–80 percent), the active drug being tested is hard-pressed to demonstrate its superiority. Even if the active drug exceeds the placebo in potency, the question remains whether the advantage is at least partially due to the superior potential of the active drug itself to mobilize placebo effects because it is an active substance that stirs vivid body sensations. Because it is almost always an inactive substance (sugar pill) that arouses fewer genuine body sensations, the placebo is less convincingly perceived as having therapeutic prowess.

Drug researchers have tried, in vain, to rid themselves of placebo effects, but these effects are forever present and frustrate efforts to demonstrate that psychoactive drugs have an independent "pure" biological impact. This state of affairs dramatically testifies that the labels "psychological" and "biological" refer largely to different per-

---

Administering a therapeutic drug is not simply a medical, biological act. It is also a complex social act, its effectiveness mediated by the patient's expectations.

If a stimulant drug is administered with the deceptive instruction that it is a sedative, it can initiate a physiological response characteristic of a sedative, such as decreased heart rate.

spectives on events that all occur in tissue. At present, it is somewhat illusory to separate the so-called biological and psychological effects of drugs used to treat emotional distress.

The literature is surprisingly full of instances of how social and attitudinal factors modify the effects of active drugs. Anti-psychotic medications are more effective if the patient likes rather than dislikes the physician administering them. An antipsychotic drug is less effective if patients are led to believe they are only taking an inactive placebo. Perhaps even more impressive, if a stimulant drug is administered with the deceptive instruction that it is a sedative, it can initiate a pattern of physiological response, such as decreased heart rate, that is sedative rather than arousing in nature. Such findings reaffirm how fine the line is between social and somatic domains.

What are the practical implications for distressed individuals and their physicians? Administering a drug is not simply a medical (biological) act. It is, in addition, a complex social act whose effectiveness will be mediated by such factors as the patient's expectations of the drug and reactions to the body sensations created by that drug, and the physician's friendliness and degree of personal confidence in the drug's power. Practitioners who dispense psychotropic medications should become thoroughly acquainted with the psychological variables modifying the therapeutic impact of such drugs and tailor their own behavior accordingly. By the same token, distressed people seeking drug treatment should keep in mind that their probability of benefiting may depend in part on whether they choose a practitioner they truly like and respect. And remember this: You are the ultimate arbiter of a drug's efficacy.

How to go about mastering unhappiness, which ranges from "feeling blue" to despairing depression, puzzles everyone. Such popular quick fixes as alcohol, conversion to a new faith, and other splendid distractions have proven only partially helpful. When antidepressant drugs hit the shelves with their seeming scientific aura, they were easily seized upon. Apparently serious unhappiness (depression) could now be chemically neutralized in the way one banishes a toothache.

But the more we learn about the various states of unhappiness, the more we recognize that they are not simply "symptoms" awaiting removal. Depressed feelings have complex origins and functions. In numerous contexts—for example, chronic conflict with a spouse—depression may indicate a realistic appraisal of a troubling problem and motivate a serious effort to devise a solution.

While it is true that deep despair may interfere with sensible problem-solving, the fact is that, more and more, individuals are being instructed to take antidepressants at the earliest signs of depressive distress and this could interfere with the potentially constructive signaling value of such distress. Emotions are feelings full of information. Unhappiness is an emotion, and despite its negativity, should not be classified single-mindedly as a thing to tune out. This in no way implies that one should submit passively to the discomfort of feeling unhappy. Actually, we all learn to experiment with a variety of strategies for making ourselves feel better, but the ultimate aim is long-term effective action rather than a depersonalized "I feel fine."

Seymour Fisher, Ph.D., [was] professor of psychology and coordinator of research training in the Department of Psychiatry and Behavioral Sciences at the University of New York Health Science Center, Syracuse.

Roger P. Greenberg, Ph.D., is professor and head of the Division of Clinical Psychology, as well as director of psychology internship training, at the University of New York Health Science Center, Syracuse.

More than 1 million American children take Ritalin regularly to help them with Attention Deficit Disorder, an increase of two and a half times since 1990. Do we have a miracle cure—or overmedicated kids?

Mother's Little Helper

I T IS ANOTHER MEDICATION morning at Winnebago Elementary School in the middle-class Chicago suburb of Bloomingdale. Three pings sound precisely over the intercom at 11:45 a.m. Principal Mark Wagener opens a locked file cabinet and withdraws a giant Tupperware container filled with plastic prescription vials. Nearly a dozen students scramble to the office for their Ritalin, a drug that calms the agitated by stimulating the brain. These children—all ages, mostly boys—have been diagnosed with Attention-Deficit/Hyperactivity Disorder, a complex neurological impairment that takes the brakes off brains and derails concentration.

THIS STORY WAS WRITTEN by LynNell Hancock and reported by Pat Wingert and Mary Hager in Washington, Claudia Kalb in Boston, Karen Springen in Chicago and Dante Chinni in New York.

The school nurse places the pills, one by one, in the children's mouths, a rite of safe passage before lunch. "Let me see . . . ," says nurse Pat Nazos, as she checks under each child's tongue for a stray, unswallowed capsule.

A decade ago, Wagener remembers, only two Winnebago students lined up for Ritalin. He is uncertain how many more "take their meds," as some students say. Some take time-released pills before school. Others take their doses at off-hours. One boy's jogging watch is timed to beep for Ritalin at 10 a.m. and 2 p.m. Like many administrators, Wagener is not sure what to make of it. Are doctors just catching this disabling affliction more often? Or has our culture gone so high-baud haywire that we have lost patience with the demanding quirks of our children? For some students, Wagener observes, Ritalin can make the crucial difference between failing a test or sitting still long enough to pass it. But for others, he laments, "they've just got an excuse to be bad."

The Ritalin riddle, a brain teaser for the '90s, confounds doctors, parents and, sometimes, children. The stimulant can be a godsend for those who truly need it. Pharmaceutically speaking, "Ritalin is one of the raving successes in psychiatry," says Dr. Laurence Greenhill of Columbia University medical school. Now it's a routinely prescribed drug at distinguished institutions from Johns Hopkins to the Mayo Clinic, a pill that allows children and a growing number of adults to focus their minds and rein in their rampaging attention spans.

But for those who don't need it, Ritalin and its generic twins can be useless, or can even backfire. There is no X-ray, no blood test, no CT scan to determine who needs it; diagnosing attention deficit remains as much art as science. There are no definitive long-term studies to reassure parents that this stimulant isn't causing some hidden havoc to their child. Critics dismiss the drug as just a behavioral "quick fix" for children forced to live in an impatient culture that feeds on deadlines, due dates, sound bites

From *Newsweek*, March 18, 1996, pp. 50-56. © 1996 by Newsweek, Inc. All rights reserved. Reprinted by permission.

and megabytes. "It takes time for parents and teachers to sit down and talk to kids," says Dr. Sharon Collins, a pediatrician in Cedar Rapids, Iowa, where reportedly 8 percent of the children are on Ritalin. "It takes less time to get a child a pill."

WHAT'S CLEAR AMID the debate is that a remarkable revolution has taken place in the care and treatment of America's children. ADHD has become America's No. 1 childhood psychiatric disorder. Experts believe that more than 2 million children (or 3 to 5 percent) have the disorder. According to an estimate by the National Institute of Mental Health, about one student in every classroom is believed to experience it. Since 1990, Dr. Daniel Safer of Johns Hopkins University School of Medicine calculates, the number of kids taking Ritalin has grown 2½ times. Among today's 38 million children at the ages of 5 to 14, he reports, 1.3 million take it regularly. Sales of the drug last year alone topped $350 million.

This is, beyond question, an American phenomenon. The rate of Ritalin use in the United States is at least five times higher than in the rest of the world, according to federal studies. It's so common in some upscale precincts that a mini black market has emerged in a handful of playgrounds and campuses. "Vitamin R"—one of its recreational names—sells for $3 to $15 per pill, to be crushed and snorted for a cheap and relatively modest buzz.

Ritalin is the brand name of the drug known as methylphenidate. Doctors have discovered that this and other stimulants work like an antenna adjuster for children

Ritalin's Rise

Created in 1955, Ritalin was classified as a controlled substance in 1971.

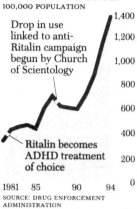

CONSUMPTION IN GRAMS PER 100,000 POPULATION

Drop in use linked to anti-Ritalin campaign begun by Church of Scientology

Ritalin becomes ADHD treatment of choice

1981 85 90 94

1,400
1,200
1,000
800
600
400
200
0

SOURCE: DRUG ENFORCEMENT ADMINISTRATION

whose brains crackle with static interference, as if a dozen stations are coming in on one channel. Technically, the stimulant appears to increase the level of dopamine in the frontal lobe of the brain, where it regulates attention and impulsivity. It is a powerful drug, and one that the U.S. Drug Enforcement Administration has classified as a Schedule II controlled substance, in the same category as cocaine, methadone and methamphetamine. Parent groups are now lobbying to ease the restrictions on Ritalin to avoid monthly doctor's visits. The DEA is opposing them, going so far last month as to enlist the help of the International Narcotics Control Board.

For all the success they've had in treating ADHD, many doctors are convinced that Ritalin is overprescribed. "I fear that

ADHD is suffering from the 'disease of the month' syndrome," says Dr. Peter S. Jensen, chief of the Child and Adolescent Disorders Research Branch of NIMH. Teachers—even in preschool—are known to pull parents of active kids aside and suggest Ritalin. Overwhelmed with referrals, school psychologists (averaging one for every 2,100 students) say they feel pressed to recommend pills first before they have time to begin an evaluation. Psychiatrists nationwide say that about half the children who show up in their offices as ADHD referrals are actually suffering from a variety of other ailments, such as learning disabilities, depression or anxiety—disorders that look like ADHD, but do not need Ritalin. Some seem to be just regular kids. A St. Petersburg, Fla., pediatrician says parents of normal children have actually asked him for Ritalin just to improve their grades. "When I won't give it to them, they switch doctors," says Dr. Bruce Epstein. "They can find someone who will."

Finding someone who will is distressingly easy. Doctors themselves admit their methods are too often hasty. Almost half the pediatricians surveyed for a recent report in the Archives of Pediatric and Adolescent Medicine said they send ADHD children home in an hour. With such a rapid turnaround, many doctors never talk to teachers, review the child's educational levels, nor do any kind of psychological work-up—all essential diagnostic elements (chart, "ADHD Checklist"). Most children only get a prescription.

Making matters worse is that, ADHD experts now say, most children need behavior-modification therapy and special help in school. But most of the surveyed pediatricians said they rarely recommend anything more than pills. "A lot of doctors," says

ADHD Checklist

Professionals will base their diagnosis of ADHD on the following guidelines. From each list, six or more of the following symptoms need to exist in a way that significantly impairs the child:

Inattention

✔ pays little attention to details; makes careless mistakes
✔ has short attention span
✔ does not listen when spoken to directly
✔ does not follow instructions; fails to finish tasks
✔ has difficulty organizing tasks
✔ avoids tasks that require sustained mental effort
✔ loses things
✔ is easily distracted
✔ is forgetful in daily activities

Hyperactivity, impulsivity

HYPERACTIVITY
✔ fidgets; squirms in seat
✔ leaves seat in classroom when remaining seated is expected
✔ runs about or climbs excessively at inappropriate times
✔ has difficulty playing quietly
✔ acts as if "driven by a motor"
✔ talks excessively
IMPULSIVITY
✔ blurts out answers before questions are completed

SOURCE: AMERICAN PSYCHIATRIC ASSOCIATION

The Road to Ritalin

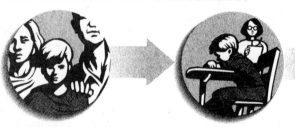

Step 1: Adult observations

PARENTS: Parents are often the first to notice extreme (with an emphasis on extreme) behavior: trouble following simple instructions and controlling temper; hyperactivity. Parents may compare observations with the child's teacher.

TEACHER: If the teacher thinks the student has unusual trouble sitting still or concentrating, a school psychologist may be called in (if one is available) to examine, test the child and gather behavioral history from the parents.

What the Doctor Ordered

In a recent survey, almost half of the pediatricians said they spent less than an hour evaluating children before prescribing Ritalin.

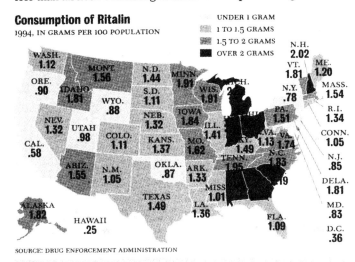

Consumption of Ritalin
1994, IN GRAMS PER 100 POPULATION

UNDER 1 GRAM
1 TO 1.5 GRAMS
1.5 TO 2 GRAMS
OVER 2 GRAMS

WASH. 1.12
ORE. .90
IDAHO 1.81
MONT. 1.56
N.D. 1.44
MINN. 1.91
WIS. 1.91
S.D. 1.11
WYO. .88
NEB. 1.32
IOWA 1.84
ILL. 1.41
NEV. 1.32
UTAH .98
COLO. 1.11
KANS. 1.37
MO. 1.82
KY. 1.49
W.VA. 1.13
VA. 1.74
CAL. .58
ARIZ. 1.55
N.M. 1.05
OKLA. .87
ARK. 1.33
TENN. 1.95
N.C. .83
MISS. 1.01
TEXAS 1.49
LA. 1.36
ALASKA 1.82
HAWAII .25
PA. 1.51
N.Y. .78
N.H. 2.02
VT. 1.81
ME. 1.20
MASS. 1.54
R.I. 1.34
CONN. 1.05
N.J. .85
DELA. 1.81
MD. .83
D.C. .36
FLA. 1.09

SOURCE: DRUG ENFORCEMENT ADMINISTRATION

Dr. F. Xavier Castellanos, an ADHD researcher at NIMH, "are lulled into complacency. They think that by giving a child Ritalin, the likelihood of helping him is high and the downside is low."

What is ADHD? The disorder is almost as elusive as its name. More than a century ago, these children were known as "fidgety Phils." In the '50s, they were "hyperkinetic." The term Attention Deficit Disorder was coined in 1980. "Hyperactivity" was added in 1987 to describe the vast majority. (Roughly 20 percent suffer ADD without the hyperactivity.) But the label still isn't quite right. "It's not that they are not paying attention," says Sally L. Smith, founder of The Lab School of Washington,

a private K–12 institution for children with learning disabilities. "They are paying *too* much attention, to *too* many things."

CHILDREN WITH ATTENtion problems are "lost in space and time," says Smith. Boys are afflicted up to three times as often as girls. They tend to be bright, but are poor students. These are the children who can't wait their turn. They blurt out answers before questions are asked. They can't stop wiggling their legs, tapping their pencils. They lose their bookbags, their homework,

their tempers . . . not sometimes, but *constantly*. Decades ago "these children were the outcasts, the losers, the zoned-out kids," says Castellanos. Many just left school. "I had an uncle who dropped out in the fourth grade," says Dr. Martha Denckla, director of cognitive neurology at Johns Hopkins. "The explanation was, 'Milton was not a student'." She is convinced he was ADHD. The difference is, today's schools can't afford to give up on them.

It's not that these kids are purposely defiant. They simply can't control themselves. Debbie Mans realized that her twin boys were more than just rambunctious when they reached preschool. Alex, the wilder of the two, couldn't handle being with 18 children in his nursery-school class. He would hit the kids, the teacher, and then hurl himself around the room. "The teachers told me he was everything from colorblind to dumb to just plain bad," says Mans.

She knew intelligence wasn't the issue: this was a boy who at the age of 3 could put a broken telephone back together. After taking a host of tests, Alex and his twin, Sam, were diagnosed with learning disabilities and ADHD. They had trouble following directions because they could neither perceive them properly nor pay attention long enough to try. The twins, now 7, were given Ritalin to help untangle the gibberish. It has, but no single pill will fix everything. Attention deficit is often only a fraction of a child's problems. Like the Mans twins, many have additional learning disabilities.

If doctors believe they have found a treatment, they do not pretend to fully comprehend the disorder. For now, scientists know ADHD is not the result of brain damage, wrong diet or bad parenting, as previously surmised. Instead, they have a

There are many different kinds of doctors and types of tests parents may choose if they suspect their child has ADHD.

Parents should explore as many options as possible before medication is tried. One ideal scenario:

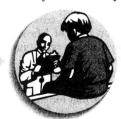  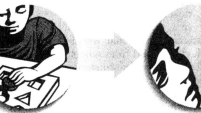

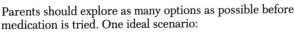

Step 2: Medical exam

PEDIATRICIAN: The doctor looks for physical conditions that can explain the child's problem: vision or hearing difficulties, allergies, etc. Should consult with other specialists, but too often writes a prescription instead.

Step 3: Specialists' observations

PSYCHIATRIST, NEUROLOGIST: This specialist looks for emotional disorders and evaluates the family situation. Takes testimony from other adults: teachers, scout leaders, etc. Does the child have ADHD or severe anxiety or depression?

DEVELOPMENTAL SPECIALIST: A speech pathologist or occupational therapist tests for even more subtle problems. Searches for learning disabilities and perception problems that can be marked by inattention.

Step 4: Treatment

For ADHD, treatment can include a program of behavior modification, imposing more structure and removing distractions; medication, usually Ritalin, to help the child focus. Doctors will monitor the child's progress.

new set of suspects. Dr. James Swanson, a psychologist at the University of California, Irvine, believes it may be the result of something gone awry in pregnancy, anything from fetal distress to alcohol or exposure to lead in utero. Dr. Lawrence Greenberg, a Minnesota ADHD specialist, estimates that as many as a quarter of surviving premature infants may have ADHD. Other researchers blame heredity. ADHD researcher Dr. Russell Barkley, of the University of Massachusetts, reports that nearly half the ADHD children have a parent, and more than one third have a sibling, with the disorder.

That's no surprise to the Schmidt family of Rochester, Minn. Over the past three years, all five have been diagnosed with attention deficit. The first case was Stephen, 8, who appeared to be hypersensitive and hard of hearing. "You would look straight at him, and say something, and he'd always say 'What?'" says Joan, 40, his mom. The psychiatrist determined that Stephen, Dennis, 37, and Daniel, 10, all had ADHD. Joan and her daughter, Maggie, 5, were found to have ADD, without the hyperactivity. One child takes Ritalin, another the antidepressant Wellbutrin. The rest take daily combinations of Ritalin for ADHD, plus antidepressants (Prozac, Wellbutrin or Paxil) for accompanying depression.

There are three distinctive signals of ADHD: inattention, impulsivity and hyperactivity. But all can be part of an ordinary child's modus operandi, too. Most kids get distracted during the day, do impulsive things and bounce off walls. So, how can doctors tell when the behavior means "normal kid" and when it means trouble?

Doctors should take family histories, observe behavior, give cognitive tests and a battery of behavioral exams. They rule out other diseases. And they ask questions. Dr. Edward Hallowell, a child psychiatrist and coauthor of "Driven to Distraction," asks: "How does he get dressed in the morning? How does he behave at dinner, in restaurants, with other kids?" Eventually physicians make a judgment. "Parents need to make sure their child has a full evaluation before the first pill is put in their child's mouth," says Dr. Stanley Greenspan, psychiatrist and author of "The Challenging Child."

Noticing ADD is even trickier. These children are the lethargic daydreamers, "little absent-minded professors," says Barkley in his book, "Taking Charge of ADHD." They neither finish their work nor cause a fuss. Many are girls. "People think children with ADD look like baby gorillas, ripping wallpaper off the wall," says Dr. Betsy Busch, a pediatrician in Chestnut Hill, Mass.

This would all be a lot easier if science could isolate a flaw in the brain to aid diagnosis. Several studies indicate that ADHD brains may look and function slightly differently from "normal" brains. PET (positron emission tomograph) scans indicate that ADHD brains use less glucose—meaning less energy—in the prefrontal-lobe control center for attention and impulsivity. Other tests show less electrical activity in the

---

To make an ADHD diagnosis, doctors take family histories, observe behavior, give abstract cognitive tests and ask questions. It would be a lot easier if science could isolate a flaw in the brain.

---

same zone directly behind the forehead. In the most recent study, NIMH researchers measured the brains of ADHD boys using an MRI (magnetic resonance imaging). Preliminary findings show slightly smaller areas in the frontal lobe in boys who have attention deficit than those who don't. These are important pieces to the puzzle, but pieces, nonetheless.

After the tests, the anxiety and the judgment comes the pill. It's ubiquitously called Ritalin, even though the patent expired 23 years ago and generic methylphenidate is widely sold. For Ciba-Geigy, the Swiss pharmaceutical giant which last week announced a proposed merger with Sandoz, another drug goliath, Ritalin remains a glittering profit center. And for patients, a benefit if not a panacea. NIMH experts report that this stimulant is a positive treatment for nine out of 10 ADHD children who require medication. (Two other stimulants, Dexedrine and Cylert, are prescribed less often.) Older children testify to its effects. "Ritalin is like my training wheels," says Dylan MaGowan, a junior at The Lab School of Washington. "It helps keep me on track."

Researchers believe methylphenidate juices up the central nervous system. The drug appears to have its own attention deficit, taking effect in 30 minutes and then petering out after three or four hours. Kids usually take five to 10 mg three times a day for prime-time schoolwork. They often take "drug holidays" on the weekends and every few months.

Most experts believe that Ritalin is risk-free, having witnessed no permanent dis- abilities. "Stimulants have been used since the late '30s," says the NIMH's Jensen, "with no evidence of long-term damage." But studies are still inconclusive. Adding a flurry of doubts to the debate, the Food and Drug Administration last month released a study of mice that found Ritalin may have the potential to cause a rare form of liver cancer. Since there has been no comparative rise in hepatoblastoma among those on the drug over the decades, the FDA still regards Ritalin as "safe and effective."

Another story emerges, however, when the drug is abused on the playground. High doses, snorted or injected, can become addictive. The DEA warns that the "smart drug" may become a problem "street drug" in the near future. But aside from one death due to Ritalin overdose last April, the numbers of abusers seem to be next to negligible. Scientists believe it will have a tough time making an appearance on the favorite-party-drug list. Ritalin is too complex to manufacture illegally. It doesn't create anything near the euphoria of cocaine. Kids on prescribed doses, more often than not, want to stop when they get older. They get tired of the hassle and are often embarrassed by being different. "It's the opposite reaction to addiction," says Denckla.

Some side effects have been spotted, even when correct doses are followed. Children often complain of loss of sleep, stomach pains and irritability, particularly when the dose is wearing off. The most distressing, though still fairly rare, problem is facial tics.

NINE-YEAR-OLD JOHN White, as he asks to be called, experienced the worst aspects of Ritalin, from conflicting diagnoses to near disaster. At first, nothing but a taste for Jarlsberg and an exceptional intelligence distinguished the child from others. Then he transferred to a more structured school in the middle of first grade. Within weeks the new teacher was complaining that John was talking out of turn; he wouldn't concentrate on his assignments. After a battery of tests, a neurologist declared him to be borderline ADHD. "I knew that if we didn't accept some kind of diagnosis, we wouldn't get help from the school," says his mother, Sarah.

Soon after his first Ritalin dose, John began losing his appetite. He stopped sleeping. He would explode with laughter one minute, shed tears the next. "It was scary," says Sarah. Then, the facial tics developed: eye tics, mouth tics, vocal tics. A hair-pulling habit—one that continued months after she pulled him off Ritalin— left a bald spot on the back of his head. Sarah enrolled him in biofeedback therapy and schooled her son at home for some months. Three years later John is thriving, Ritalin-free. "We choose to look at him as just a very bright child," says Sarah, "with some quirks."

When she talks about Ritalin, Sally Smith likes to hold up a ruler. "This is how much Ritalin does for you," says Smith, pointing to the one-inch mark. "Ritalin makes you available to learn. You and your parents and teachers have to work on all the rest." Smith's Lab School in Washington works with the most severe cases of ADHD and learning disabilities. And her staff has developed all sorts of clever strategies to help children get through their days. Teachers put down masking tape in the hallways so the kids will be reminded of where they should stand. Others will divide desk tops into different colored segments: one side for work, the other for storage. Children earn points for self-control and can cash them in for pizza slices or free time.

But The Lab School, and others like it, are extraordinary—and expensive. Most families can't afford $15,000-a-year tuitions. Experts believe that many kids are languishing in classes that are way too big, on medication that is not quite right. Peter Briger, 7, has spun through several different drugs and as many different classroom settings in the past six months. Ritalin didn't work. Cylert was no better. Now imipramine, an antidepressant, may be causing breathing problems. It does seem to calm him. Without special attention

The Medicine Cabinet

Doctors have more than one choice when prescribing for patients with ADHD.

Stimulants

These drugs enhance the flow of dopamine in the brain, which can increase impulse control and attention span.

Ritalin *(Methylphenidate)*
Dexedrine *(Dextroamphetamine)*
Cylert *(Pemoline)*

POSSIBLE SIDE EFFECTS: Insomnia, weight loss, irritability, nausea, dizziness, headaches.

Antidepressants

Besides treating depression, they can decrease hyperactivity and aggression in some patients.

Tofranil *(Imipramine)*
Norpramin *(Desipramine)*
Elavil *(Amitriptyline)*

POSSIBLE SIDE EFFECTS: Dizziness, drowsiness, dry mouth, excessive sweating, weight gain, fatigue. May also affect blood pressure and heart rate. Avoid if there is a family history of seizures or heart attack.

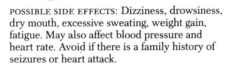

SOURCE: "THE HANDBOOK OF PSYCHIATRIC DRUGS," HENRY HOLT AND CO.; "BEYOND RITALIN," VILLARD BOOKS

from teachers, he has yet to demonstrate much focus. Peter spends half his day in Manhattan's PS 191 in a class of more than 20 second graders. On a typical day recently, he sat on top of his desk, headed for the drinking fountain and banged his head with a three-ring binder. His notebooks were filled with scribbles, decorated intermittently with half-written assignments. "He's lost so much time," says Millie Morales, the aunt who has cared for Peter since his mom died and his dad went to prison.

To researchers, it's a classic "pay now or pay more later" situation. "Studies indicate that those with untreated ADHD are more likely to become alcoholics, smokers or drug abusers than the general population," says Castellanos of NIMH. More than one third drop out of school, says Barkley of the University of Massachusetts. And, he says, about one tenth of ADHD adults attempt suicide.

In the end, what makes all this debate so urgent is its subject: the nation's children. The fear, simply put, is that too many who need help may be going unnoticed, untreated, while too many who don't are getting pills instead of proper care. But there is glory here, too. Children who otherwise would be cast aside are receiving world-class treatment. Obviously, we need more of the latter, less of the former. And to do that, parents, doctors, therapists and teachers need to exercise care. It may be a truism, but one that can too easily be forgotten in a rush to diagnosis.

PHARMACOTHERAPY FOR THE TREATMENT OF DEPRESSION

Michael E. Thase, M.D.
David J. Kupfer, M.D.*

Pharmacotherapy with antidepressants is the cornerstone of medical management of the depressive disorders. Many psychiatrists consider antidepressants, either alone or in combination with psychotherapy, to be the treatment of first choice for severe episodes of depression and the best way to prevent new episodes for people who have suffered recurrent bouts of depression.

Clinical depression does not present a single illness, like diphtheria, but a group of related disorders, like pneumonia or high blood pressure. These related depressive disorders are linked by changes in how the brain functions that often parallel the clinical symptoms. Antidepressants probably work by stabilizing or correcting changes in chemistry that accompany both the symptoms and disturbances of brain function. Traditionally, researchers have focused on two brain chemicals, or neurotransmitters, that play important roles in regulation of sleep, mood, appetite, energy, and the ability to enjoy. These neurotransmitters are norepinephrine and serotonin. However, the regulation of the brain's systems is wonderfully complex, and it is pretty clear that depression is **not** just a disorder caused by a simple imbalance of neurotransmitters.

Antidepressants do not "cure" depression but, when effective, they control the symptoms within two to six weeks. Antidepressants are not addictive or habit forming, and they are no more a "crutch" than high blood pressure medication. However, because we often artificially separate the function of the mind from that of the body and have a stigma against "mental illness," there are

About the authors: Michael E. Thase, M.D., is professor of psychiatry at the University of Pittsburgh School of Medicine and the Western Psychiatric Institute and Clinic. His research interests pertain to the assessment and treatment of mood disorders, including the short-term and prophylactic efficacy of pharmacotherapy and cognitive therapy in relationship to the psychobiologocial correlates of depression.

David J. Kupfer, M.D., is the Thomas Detre Professor and chairman of the Department of Psychiatry at the University of Pittsburgh School of Medicine and director of research at Western Psychiatric Institute and Clinic. Dr. Kupfer's research has focused primarily on the conceptualization, diagnosis, and treatment of mood disorders. He directs both the NIMH-funded Clinical Research Center for Affective Disorders and the Stanley Center for the Innovative Treatment of Bipolar Disorders.

many people who believe that taking antidepressants is a "cop-out." For most people who do not want to take medication, it is reasonable to try a modern form of psychotherapy, such as interpersonal or cognitive behavior therapy, before trying an antidepressant. However, for people with the **most** severe forms of depression, there is not much evidence that psychotherapy can substitute for antidepressant medication. Also, medication should be considered when two to three months of therapy have not led to much relief of symptoms.

Table 1 provides a summary of the types of antidepressant medications that are currently available. Until 1988, antidepressant pharmacotherapy was largely limited to two families of medications: the tricyclic antidepressants (TCAs) and the monoamine oxidase inhibitors (MAOIs). The TCAs are used more than the MAOIs. Although the MAOIs are effective, the need for a special diet (i.e., low in tyramine) to prevent hypertensive crises and concerns about side effects now limit their use.

We are in the middle of an exciting decade in which a number of new antidepressants have been introduced. Several have already passed Food and Drug Administration "muster," meaning that they have been shown to be superior to placebo and at least as effective as TCAs. Heralded by the introduction of fluoxetine (Prozac) in early 1988, these newer antidepressants offer significant advantages in terms of safety in overdose. For the average person, treatment with any of the newer agents also may have a lower "burden" of annoying side effects (e.g., dry mouth, blurry vision, constipation, weight gain, or over-sedation). In addition to their safety and tolerability, the class of antidepressants known as the serotonin selective reuptake inhibitors (SSRIs) are convenient to use because they can be taken once a day.

Fluoxetine, as said, belongs to this class of medication. More recently introduced members of this class include sertraline (Zoloft), paroxetine (Paxil), and fluvoxamine (Luvox). The SSRIs now are the leading class of newly prescribed antidepressants in the United States. Their impact in the treatment of depression is comparable with that following the introduction of Tagamet and Zantac for treatment of peptic ulcer.

From *The Decade of the Brain*, Summer 1996, pp. 5-6. © 1996 by the National Alliance for the Mentally Ill. Reprinted by permission.

TABLE 1. COMMONLY PRESCRIBED ANTIDEPRESSANTS

Class	Generic Name (Brand Name)	Typical (Maximal) Therapeutic Dosage (mg/day)	Comments
Tricyclics (TCAs)	Amitriptyline (Elavil) Imipramine (Tofranil) Doxepin (Sinequan) Nortriptyline (Pamelor/Aventyl) Desipramine (Norpramin)	100–200 (300) 100–200 (300) 100–200 (300) 50–100 (200)* 100–200 (300)	All TCAs may be fatal in overdoses of more than 1 week's supply. Most TCAs are available in generic form.
Phenylpiperazines	Trazodone (Desyrel) Nefazodone (Serzone)	150–300 (600) 200–400 (600)	Trazodone is available in generic form. Divided dosages of nefazodone are recommended.
Serotonin selective reuptake inhibitors (SSRIs)	Fluoxetine (Prozac) Sertraline (Zoloft) Paroxetine (Paxil)	10–20 (80) 50–100 (200) 20–30 (50)	None of the SSRIs are available in generic form.
Aminoketone	Bupropion (Wellbutrin)	150–300 (450)	Doses > 450 mg/d associated with risks of seizures. Divided dosages recommended
Bicyclic	Venlafaxine (Effexor)	75–225 (375)	May be particularly helpful for severe depressions. Divided daily dosages recommended.

Maximum dosage is typically defined by a serum drug level of > 150 ng/ml.

Despite their popularity and numerous advantages, SSRIs are not trouble-free. Common side effects include nausea, diarrhea, nervousness, tremor, insomnia, and headache. Some people will have trouble reaching orgasm. These side effects are often managed by reducing the dosage or switching to a different SSRI. Initial concerns that drugs like fluoxetine might trigger suicidal behavior have not been supported by scientific studies of large samples. On occasion, however, a state of severe restlessness may lead to worsening in SSRI-treated patients.

Any of the three SSRIs currently available would make a reasonable choice for first-line therapy. However, there are differences between these drugs that may affect your doctor's decision about which one to prescribe—and they are not interchangeable. When the SSRIs are not helpful, some doctors favor using the "old fashioned" tricyclics and others prefer different classes of newer medications. Importantly, people who failed to respond to one class of antidepressants still have a fifty-fifty chance of responding to a different type of medication. Nefazodone (Serzone) is a newer antidepressant that probably affects both serotonin and norepinephrine. Nefazodone, like most of the TCAs and trazodone, tends to be more sedating than the SSRIs, which may be an advantage for patients suffering from insomnia. Despite an otherwise generally comparable side effect profile, nefazodone is less likely to cause sexual problems than the SSRIs. Nefazodone's popularity may be inhibited a bit by the need for twice-daily dosing.

Venlafaxine (Effexor) also directly affects both norepinephrine and serotonin. Venlafaxine is a strong antidepressant, and it is often used ahead of the tricyclics for SSRI nonresponders. Venlafaxine should be taken in divided daily dosages and, at high dosages, it causes elevated blood pressure in about ten percent of patients. Otherwise, its side effects are similar to the SSRIs.

Bupropion (Wellbutrin) is distinctly different from the other new antidepressants with respect to both its chemical structure and presumed mode of action. Bupropion structurally resembles the catecholamines and amphetamines. It is, to no great surprise, nonsedating for most depressed patients and activating for a fair number. An effective and safe antidepressant with a good track record in severe depression, bupropion has about the same type and prevalence of side effects as the SSRIs with the notable exception of a relative absence of sexual side effects. As with nefazodone and venlafaxine, divided dosing is necessary.

Pharmacotherapy for depression consists of at least two phases: acute (i.e., the time from beginning treatment until remission) and continuation (i.e., a four- to nine-month period of treatment following remission to protect against relapse). Treatment of recurrent (unipolar) depression also usually includes a third, long-term phase of maintenance pharmacotherapy to prevent recurrence.

At least a 50 percent reduction in depressive symptoms is a minimum standard for a response during acute-phase therapy. If patients have been appropriately diagnosed and are compliant with treatment, about 50 percent to 70 percent will show substantial symptomatic improvement within four to six weeks of beginning pharmacotherapy. People who fail to respond but show no side effects may warrant even longer trials at higher dosages, with appropriate monitoring to ensure safety.

The decision to stop an effective antidepressant after a sustained period of remission is best viewed as a collaborative effort between physician and patient. To help their patients, physicians need to be well-informed about the risks for relapse and recurrence associated with discontinuation of medication. For patients recovering from acute, first episodes of depression, the analogy of a broken leg works quite well, with the withdrawal of medication (i.e., removal of the cast) indicated after a prescribed period for healing. Continuation treatment is recommended for almost all patients for a period ranging from four months to nine months. Ending continuation-phase treatment is not recommended if the patient is experiencing serious, ongoing interpersonal difficulties or has clear-cut residual symptomatology. Further, it is unwise to discontinue antidepressant medication in a patient who has a history of three or more prior depressive episodes.

Maintenance pharmacotherapy typically lasts for at least four to five years. Evidence indicates that it is most effective when an antidepressant dosage is maintained at the level used acutely. The once-popular half-dose strategy appears to be only about half as effective. It is unclear what length of recovery really constitutes a safe period before one might consider withdrawal of medication. In our studies of people who have suffered at least three prior depressive episodes, recurrence rates of greater than 70 percent were observed after discontinuation following three years of maintenance pharmacotherapy. It is helpful to negotiate "contracts" between patients and physicians for discrete periods of maintenance treatment (e.g., one to two years). Renewed discussion of the risks and benefits of maintenance therapy may be undertaken each year. For some people, indefinite (i.e., lifetime) treatment may offer the best protection against recurrent depression.

PSYCHOSURGERY
Damaging the Brain to Save the Mind

J O A N N   E L L I S O N   R O D G E R S

Philosophers tell us that the horizon of knowledge is always out of reach. How far out of reach is the practical question and the source of all dilemmas having to do with treating the sick. Do doctors wait until they really *know*—or know more—before they try this treatment or that? If they wait, will it mean more suffering for a patient? Is suffering tolerable if there are means of relieving it? Are some risks ever worth taking? Are some ever not?

The treatment dilemma posed by psychosurgery—surgery to treat psychiatric disorders—is this: Experts know something about mental illness and about operations that can help some patients; but they don't know enough to completely assure patients, families, each other, or the rest of us that surgery is the best, or proper, course. That it is ever worth the risk.

Perhaps they can *never* know enough. Driving the demand for, and use of, psychosurgery is the belief—some call it the pretension—that the human brain can understand and repair its own mind. And more, that scientists will come to understand the mind and brain better by studying it the way they study it now—anatomically, biochemically, and empirically, by analyzing and observing its parts and the things it does.

Publicly, the subject of psychiatric brain surgery hasn't been discussed since 1978, when the National Commission for the Protection of Human Subjects of Biomedical and Behavioral Research issued a report saying that psychosurgery had a deservedly bad reputation for wretched excess. But the report also documented successes, declared that psychosurgery was not the unmitigated horror its critics

had labeled it, and decreed that—with strict regulations and safeguards—psychosurgery was acceptable for certain cases and that more research and good record-keeping were needed.

As a result, perhaps, psychosurgery—albeit under new names, more refined and more selective than the lobotomies that psychiatrists and neurosurgeons abandoned more than 30 years ago—is still very much around. Actually, it never completely went away.

Although the number of procedures have plunged since the heyday of psychosurgery (50,000 estimated in the United States alone between 1939 and 1960), there are still at least 200 to 300 openly declared psychosurgeries labeled as such each year being performed by a few dozen surgeons here and abroad. Reports are trickling in of more operations being done in South America and the developing world. And if we count the operations that affect the "psyche" but disclaim changes in mood and behavior as primary goals, the total is certainly in the thousands and growing.

Psychosurgery has now greatly evolved. Surgeons no longer destroy large amounts of brain tissue in futile efforts to "cure" schizophrenia and neurosis. Instead, they take pinpoint aim at millimeter-long clusters of cells to stop suicidal depression, disable obsessive-compulsive disorders, cripple anxiety, and smother the uncontrollable rage and aggression that keep sick people in locked wards. They go after destructive behavior that accompanies organic diseases of the body and brain.

The great promise of psychosurgery is not without critics. For some, the abuses of the past remain open sores on the na-

tional conscience. Some see it as Frankenstein-style science. Others dismiss the whole idea as plain goofy—based on oversimplified views of human behavior and emotional chaos. And certain religious groups, such as the Scientologists, brand psychosurgery and all physical treatment of mental illness as assassination attempts on the mind.

Practically nothing has been written to update the general public in the last 10 years about the new operations, their availability, and any ongoing problems they pose. While psychosurgery's past excesses have been forever characterized by Ken Kesey's Randle McMurphy in *One Flew over the Cuckoo's Nest,* the conventional wisdom of that era is now vulnerable to new knowledge and rising demands for help from the mentally ill and their advocates. Moreover, today, as in the past, the need to balance treatment with protection from abuse is especially important for the ill who are homeless, poor, female, children, imprisoned, and minorities: They were historically the guinea pigs of psychosurgery and could become so again. On the other hand, they could become beneficiaries of a therapy that still has promises to keep.

They could be Matthew.

I must tell you that I am very afraid of this man. Even under guard he is unpredictable, very scary. He is like a feral animal, a cat. He raises his arms and dives into people. He could kill.
　　　　　　　—Matthew's neurosurgeon, 1990

The story of Matthew frames much of the reasonable and unreasonable debate over the need for psychosurgery and its potential abuse. Matthew has a social his-

From *Psychology Today,* March/April 1992, pp. 35-39, 78, 84, 86. Excerpted from *Psychosurgery: Damaging the Brain to Save the Mind* by Joann Ellison Rodgers. © 1992 by Joann Ellison Rodgers. Reprinted by permission of the Elaine Markson Literary Agency.

tory of violent behavior and a medical history that makes modern psychosurgery a last—and long delayed—hope. The following excerpts from a letter written on January 4, 1990, to Matthew's lawyer from a neurologist describe the cold, clinical details:

Dear Mr.—

Matthew is a 24 year old, right-handed man who has had severe and uncontrollable seizures since age 11. The cause of the seizures is encephalitis, which is an infection (presumed viral) of the brain. This infection produced scarring which resulted in spontaneously recurrent abnormal electrical discharges. When the electrical discharges build up to a certain level he will have seizures. During his seizures, he will have an aura [warning] of an unpleasant emotion, he will become confused, he will yell, grimace, turn his [head] side to side and will run about.

I have personally observed several of these episodes. He appears very frightening to others during the episodes. On one occasion we had a laboratory technician hide behind the door for many minutes after Matthew slammed into the door during a seizure. If someone is in his path, he will stare at them, then run into them or push them violently out of the way.

We monitored him in our critical care neurology unit with videoelectroencephalography recordings in June of 1986. During that time we could observe his typical range episodes, and correlate them with abnormal electrical activity in the brain. His seizures have occurred as often as 10 times a day.

On October 5, 1987, Matthew had surgery on the right side of his brain, and on November 24, 1987, on the left side of his brain in a structure called the amygdala. This is a structure that is often involved in seizures and in manifestations of violent behavior. Unfortunately, the procedure was of no lasting benefit to Matthew. I believe that Matthew has sufficient brain injury that he cannot control his outbursts of aggression. Some of these are explicitly because of seizures [and] completely beyond his control. Others are not related to seizures, but occur because he has brain damage, delusional thinking, and lacks the normal inhibitory behavior that people must exert in society.

Regrettably, this is likely to be a continuing condition with Matthew.

It is sometimes difficult to tell whether violence is part of a seizure, or whether it is acting out of "bad temper." In Matthew's case, I think all these are [beyond his control].

Matthew's medical situation is unfortunate. We have been unable to manage this satisfactorily with medications and with surgery. I would hope that the court and authorities would view his problems as a medical rather than a criminal issue.

Sincerely ...

Matthew is slight in build, with boyishly silky, slightly long, dark wavy hair; he sports a neatly trimmed beard. On an early June evening in 1990, he has permission for a special visit with his parents and a guest—special because authorities at the high-security hospital for the criminally insane are strict about the number of visits to each inmate per week. Matthew has spent almost a year here, and 16 more years in schools and hospitals for young people with severe neurological and psychiatric disease. Since the beginnning of the summer, the internal review board of a prestigious medical center has been considering his parents' request for neurosurgery to get him out.

We had to put our belongings in a metal locker behind the guard's desk, keeping only a small tape recorder, and passed through an airport-style metal detector. Armed guards escorted us through two sets of locked doors, along a corridor into a room with brown Formica furniture upholstered in bright blue vinyl. Matthew sits in one of the chairs, facing us, wearing khakis, clean white socks, slip-on Keds, a hospital shirt tucked neatly into his beltless pants, and sunglasses. A burly security guard stays for the visit, too—protection against Matthew's unpredictable and violent rages.

Matthew: (Shaking hands.) How do you do ma'am. How about a soundcheck? Sure. (Leaning forward, singing into the tape recorder.) "I just called to say I looove you, I just called to say how much I care."

Visitor: I want to ask you about your feelings, Matthew, about getting a brain operation.

Matthew: Yes. I want to leave here. With violent seizures, I have been put here. They don't really know about them and they think it's just me being bad and acting out. When I was in [a state mental hospital] this lady named Fran told me I was a bad case, and making it up. Yes ma'am, she said it, but I'm not.

Visitor: If doctors said to you, "Matthew there's a chance this could help," you would do this, have an operation on your brain?

Matthew: Yes. (Turning to look at the guard talking loudly on the wall phone.) Can you wait until he is off the phone? I am having trouble concentrating. I'm sorry for the interruption. Please excuse me for saying to wait.

Visitor: When you have your violent seizures, do you remember anything?

Matthew: No, wait, wait, yes. Sometimes. Yeah. Like I was telling my father last night. I don't know how I do it. But—put your fingers over your ear (we all cup our hands over our ears) and for about a second, I hear a muffling sound. You can hear air coming.

Visitor: You mean like putting a seashell over your ear?

Matthew: Yes, yes, yes, exactly, exactly. After that, I get a ringing sound in both ears. One time with a violent seizure, I was in the shower room up at ward 8 and I went into one of the showers, and I went in there and I was hearing the ringing sound. And what happened was this man Rudolph—

Visitor: [Rudolph] works in the hospital?

Matthew: Yeah, and he walked in and I hit him, I forget where, I hit him and he grabbed me and I think we were fighting. (Matthew clenches his fists and works them back and forth to indicate a fight.) And he threw me in seclusion and it's just that I think some of this problem is 50–50, you know, part violent seizures, and they [the attendants] just . . . just (a long pause).

Visitor: They don't know what to do?

Matthew: They don't know if it's a seizure or if like once when I was on [ward] 3, I just want my way. Wanting your way, what I mean by that is, on 3, here I am, and I was mad and when I get mad, first I'm mad, then I'm madder, then madder and madder and so forth. [But] on 8 I wasn't about to blow my top or get mad.

Matthew's mother: Or get out of control?

Matthew: (Smiling and with a chuckle.) Yes, thank you, out of control. What happened was, they said, "Matt, how long would you like to be in your room?" [I guess all the] seclusion rooms were taken or something, I'm not sure. So they put me in my room and I was lying down like this (he leans over in the chair onto his side) and suddenly I went into a seizure like that (he snaps his fingers) and with no ringing in the ear or anything.

Visitor: Sometimes you have a warning and can remember and sometimes you can't.

Matthew: Yes ma'am. And what happened

was I was lying on my bed and I guess I got scared or something else bad and I grabbed the pillow and put it over my face and I started to scream and after that, well, I forgot what happened but nothing positive. I went to a screened window in the room and I was banging on that, and screaming, not from the seizure but just screaming and a lady walked in and said, "Matthew, if you don't stop it I'll take your cigarettes away from you." And so I'm in this seizure.

Matthew's father: No, you said you were not in the seizure. That you are finished with the seizure. Did this happen after the seizure? Can you tell when the seizure is over? That's what you told us before. Your mind is fuzzy and you don't always know what's going on.

Matthew's mother: Can you feel when it's over?

Matthew: Sometimes I can. Sometimes I'm not really conscious. This one I'm talking about was one where I was still in seizure. I will say that when I went to the [screened-in] window, I was banging with my hand, and banged on the two beds and what happened is that I had a feeling like one time that I was looking through this window on 3 and so I (long pause) … I couldn't control what I was doing, but my mind was telling me what to do. Like I— if I was in seizure now I'd look at this wall (he points to a wall next to us) and say let's do that and I would go to the wall and kick it or whatever and that's what it was like at the screened window and I saw that and I thought of things.

Visitor: What things?

Matthew: (Glancing quickly at his parents.) My mother and father know about this. About God. What it is is that I had a feeling that this happened before, that I did that before and, well, what it was then was there was this other window and this man would always tell me to look out the window. He said, "Matt, look what's out there," and I'd say "what, what," and once he said to me, "Matt look out there, look at that," and I said, "No, no I'm not going to look out there because it will happen again."

Visitor: What happened then that you did not want to happen again?

Matthew: I'm not about for that to happen again. What it was, I had this feeling that the person said to me, "You'll see out the window, you'll see what happens when you die." And so I, um, I just had the feeling I was supposed to do this and do that and I was in the seizure but for some reason I, well, like what I said about the wall.

Matthew's mother: Is this the thing where you believed God was out there, out of heaven, and it was your fault that God wasn't in heaven anymore and that's why so many terrible things were happening to you and everyone else and—

Matthew: Yes. Also, I had a feeling I was supposed to bang the window and beds and I was there and I hit the window like this (he demonstrates with his arm) and [a] male staff [member] was called and he said, "Matt, calm down now," and they put me in bed and next thing I knew, they shut the door and took my clothes off.

Visitor: If you could leave here, what would you like to do?

Matthew: You mean a job?

Visitor: Anything.

Matthew: I would like to go home with my parents and see my sisters-in-law, my brothers, and my neighbors. And my grandmother. Whenever I get to two months without acting out, I act out or get a bad seizure and then I have to start over and I can't go home. But I like the things my father and I used to do. We went to [a] park and walked around a lot. I'd like to live in a group with other people, and the Epilepsy Foundation has places and that's where I'd like to go after I'm out of here, yes ma'am.

Matthew's father: After he got encephalitis, everything left. Matthew didn't remember knowing how to count, or say the alphabet, or even how to walk for a long time. Now he can do some things. Matt, you're a survivor. Don't forget that.

Matthew's mother: What mommy says. Say it. You don't belong here.

Matthew: I will get out if I can stay calm, cool, and collected. (Lots of laughter.)

The hour is over. Matthew shakes hands. The guard asks another to escort the visitors out so he can take Matthew back to his ward. Matthew is smiling in the hall. He extends his arms out wide and says something to the visitor in Polish. His father translates: "He says he loves you, and will you marry him?"

****

Matthew's parents live in a middle-class neighborhood in a medium-size, mid-Atlantic city. His father, retired after a nearly fatal heart attack several years ago, worked in a maritime-industry plant as an engineer. His mother, robust and sad, is a full-time homemaker. Their superclean brick row house is pleasantly furnished and crowded with memorabilia of their children; but their memories are overwhelmed by the details of Matthew's sickness, which began with a viral illness during a vacation at the beach when he was 10.

Matthew's mother: The first really awful time was after his initial illness, after we thought he might really get completely well. I'll never forget it. Matt came out of the bedroom shrieking that his hands were growing, that he had to go to the bathroom but the "poopie" was all over and was attached to him by strings, and begging us to cut them. We thought that he was having a nightmare. So his daddy went to lay down with him and soon he fell asleep.

Then at 8 A.M. we heard Matthew [again]. We heard him running. He was only a little boy. It was his first grand mal seizure and it left him delusional, hallucinating, and robot-like walking into walls. He stopped breathing [so] we headed for the hospital. That's when his hospitalizations became multiple and the specialists diagnosed him as having brain damage from a viral infection. That's what they think, though they never really know. And the seizures began in earnest, one after the other, sometimes hundreds a day and violent.

Matthew's father: We had to make sure he was restrained on the number of occasions that he was hospitalized. He would bite his mother's ear. And he would make these inhuman noises. If he ever got a hold of you, he'd grab you like a vice.

Matthew's mother: It's a helplessness you feel every day of Matthew's life. Among other things, it took more than a year for doctors at [the medical center] to finally witness one of the animal rages we were living with and fearing every day. You know. Like when you stop having a toothache when you go to the dentist. He wouldn't have them when we went to the hospital or for a check-up, and it got to the point where no one believed us. We were accused of being hysterical, of exaggerating, of not wanting to care for Matthew.

Matthew's father: One day we went to the seizure clinic for blood tests of his drug levels and we were in the courtyard to smoke and he began to attack me with animal noises, and he burst through the security guards and raced through the seizure clinic. Two doctors grabbed him. He growled and fought. He ripped their clothes. They really got an eyeful. He was well over 18 by then. When this happened, the doctor said to bring him into the intensive care unit to monitor him. Like always, it came from nowhere, out of the blue. They strapped him down and he just tore the cloth strips off. He made huge screams. He flipped his hospital bed upside down and shrieked and shrieked. His mother went into the room to try and calm him. She took her life in her hands.

Matthew's mother: Well, now he is in a hospital for the criminally insane, but he is not a criminal really, and whether or not he is psychotic is open to question. We know the things he does are bad. But his brain is damaged, and no one can predict when he'll get his attacks. Sometimes he gets depressed and obsessed with anything he hears, sees, or talks about for long periods of time.

Matthew's father: I visit him every day they let me, every day.

Matthew's mother: I feel guilty about not going to see him very much. I'm worried about it. If we tell him to get his okay for us to come, then he'll drive himself and us nuts asking about it. And then he might get upset while you're there. The Epilepsy Foundation has a group home. If he got better, they might be able to take him there. I know that. In the institution, I worry about men taking advantage of him. And I worry about what will happen to Matt when we go. His brothers will take care of him. They're very close, but it hurts and it's tough. God it's tough. What is especially heartbreaking is that his anger is not bad, not wrong. Matt knows what he has lost.

****

Less clear is what he might gain from surgery. But on November 20, 1990, two days before Thanksgiving, Matthew, his family, and his doctors get the chance to find out.

Since the 1940s and '50s, neurosurgeons have removed areas of the amygdala and the temporal lobe to stop violent behavior, with variable success. In 1987, surgeons operated on both the right and left amygdala in Matthew, whose temporal-lobe epilepsy apparently damaged circuits involved in the hypothalamus. Located under the thalamus, the hypothalamus receives input from most other parts of the brain and regulates many body activities as well as the hormone-producing pituitary gland, at the base of the brain. Along with the pituitary, the hypothalamus is one of the major routes carrying signals of psychological stress—good and bad—to the heart, lungs, bladder, and other internal organs. The damage to Matthew's hypothalamus left him with an unpredictable, assaultive, dangerous, hair-trigger temper.

He also suffers from obsessive thoughts and behavior.

The amygdalotomies unfortunately did not work. After three years, dozens of rage seizures, and a violent assault on a nurse, surgeons will try again to kill—by cutting out a small part of Matthew's abnormal brain—about a square centimeter of it. He'll have a cingulotomy: an operation designed to dampen motivation, to calm. It is also performed for cancer pain that even narcotics can't help. "I did one on a bone-cancer patient," said the surgeon. "Before the operation he cried in agony all day. After, he was completely relaxed. He read most of the time. He had no more suffering. He had no more emotions, either, nor was he capable of any real mental work. It was drastic. Like a lobotomy. Matthew's will not be that drastic."

Drastic or not, there is nothing left to try. "This kid's brain is totally out of control," says a child neurologist who consulted on Matthew's condition. "When the amygdalotomies failed, his own neurologist wept. He said he didn't know how to face the family. He cried, really cried. There's nothing left now but high-security institutionalization and sedation to the point of near coma. The new surgery is a chance. It's a Hobson's choice for us all," the neurologist added. "Even if it stops the violent rages, we don't know if it will stop the obsessive behavior."

*****

7:15 A.M. In the wide corridor of the medical center's basement neuroradiology suite, Matthew waits on a gurney, held securely in four point restraints. With him are his mother, older brother Jim, and a guard from the state mental hospital. In anticipation of his cingulotomy, he had been transferred from the high-security, prison-style hospital; there is hope that if the surgery succeeds, the halfway house, sheltered workshop training, and independence await. Matthew is nervous but cheerful, wrapped in pastel gowns, his feet and legs in vented stockings, IV line taped securely to his right arm. "I'm not getting my hopes too high this time," his mother says, her eyes on Matthew. "I am," his father says. Matthew is quiet.

Matthew's surgeon walks by in a three-piece suit he'll soon exchange for pale green scrubs. He stops for a minute to talk, holding on all the while to his briefcase. He pats Matthew's foot. "I'll see you soon," he says.

Matthew's family will see neither their son nor the surgeon for the next nine hours.

****

Operating suite 2 really is a suite. The largest of the rooms is the operating room itself; unlike conventional ORs, it houses a modern CT scanner, with its hollow-scooped bed and donut-shaped scanning apparatus. Five freestanding monitors are on site as well, to track drugs and vital signs. Behind the scanner, Vincent Lerie, a radiation technician, and Gerry Beveringen, a scrub nurse, set up three sterile tables for equipment.

Most prominent alongside the usual scissors, knives, sutures, gauze pads, needles, and tubes are the Radio Frequency Lesion Generator and the stereotactic halo. This circular frame holds the patient's head in a fixed position and guarantees millimeter-precise positioning of the brain probe and needle tip that the Lesion Generator will heat to 75 degrees Centigrade. Over the next few hours, Lerie will switch it on 10 separate times to destroy 10 tiny pieces of brain tissue in Matthew's cingulate gyrus, deep in the temporal lobes beneath his cerebral cortex.

The cingulum itself is part of the limbic system (or "primitive" emotional brain) that carries signal-making nerve fibers around the system—including the signals that trigger Matthew's rage-producing seizures. The heated needle will create dead space to act as "firebreaks" in Matthew's brain and hopefully stop transmission of these rage-triggering signals. The stereotactic equipment eliminates the risk of "blind" freehand reaches into the limbic system by automatically lining up points on the computer to make a topographic map of Matthew's brain.

The CT roadmaps guide the surgical probes safely past areas of the cerebral cortex that control sensory and motor functions (including smell and sight, and arm and leg movement) and safely away from the thalamus that is the main relay station taking messages to the higher centers of the cortex.

To compare this cingulotomy to old prefrontal lobotomies is like comparing a Civil War conscript's musket fire to the launch of a Tomahawk missile. The lesions to be made in Matthew's cingulum are anatomically "miles" from the frontal lobe, but the changes—the calming, flattening—they produce will be somewhat similar. That's because the neural fiber pathways work in parallel and bundle together in various spots deep in the brain.

Thousands of psychosurgeries, along with modern technology have brought less of the knife and enough of the desired effect, without the mutilating damage of frontal lobotomy.

Space is crowded in the suite, especially with plans for a half-dozen or more onlookers: radiologists, students, physician assistants. A glass-walled anteroom faces the OR and contains four computer monitors and other equipment. All of it will be used to display and interpret scanner information and pinpoint targets for the team that has planned this sortie into Matthew's limbic system like a military operation.

An adjacent small room holds the computer that operates the scanner, and connecting the areas is a small corridor and cul-de-sac enclosing a "light wall" to read the pictures made of the scans. It also houses a 30-cup, ever-filled coffeepot.

7:50 A.M. Toby Eagle, the nurse anesthetist, and Steve Derrer, the anesthesiologist, bring Matthew in and transfer him to the CT scanner bed where he will stay, anesthetized, throughout the operation. They gently explain the tubes.

"Matt, I'm going to give you some medicine through the tube," Derrer says. "It'll feel hot for a second," adds Eagle. Matthew whimpers for an instant and then is quiet. Eagle puts a nose and mouth mask quickly over his face. "Just a little oxygen," she fibs to him. It's really nitrous oxide, and in just moments, he is asleep. Derrer has injected a cocktail of drugs through the tube—Pentothal, fentanyl, flourane. "Have a good rest, Matt," Eagle says gently. He can't hear her.

7:56 A.M. Eagle passes a breathing tube into Matthew's throat, adds more line. The front part of his hair is shaved from his forehead to about halfway back. They leave the rest, including beard and sideburns. "He cares a lot about his hair," says Gerry. "Most young guys do." Matthew's eyes are taped shut now and the supporting part of the stereotactic frame is placed under his head and shoulders, clamped to the bed that supports him and screwed into his skull with four white screws at the temples.

8:35 A.M. Vince clears everyone out of the room so he can turn on the CT scanner, which hums. The surgeon, Sumio Uematsu, along with the radiologists, neurologists, and technicians, are crammed into the CT monitor room on and off for most of this first hour. At about 9 A.M., Uematsu looks at reconstructed scans that highlight an important

landmark: the telltale butterfly-shaped structure of the corpus callosum. From there, it's only about two centimeters back to the cingulum—the target. He also locates, among the varied shades of white, gray, and black, the cerebral artery he must avoid.

More than 35 scans are done. "It's got to be right, perfect, absolutely right. We need to check and recheck, check and recheck," says Uematsu. He keeps saying this aloud, yet to himself, almost like a prayer or a mantra.

9:30 A.M. A neurologist who has cared for Matthew for many years arrives with a copy of a medical-journal article written by Tom Ballantine, a Massachusetts neurosurgeon who has done more than 600 cingulotomies for chronic pain. In it are detailed photographs of the sites in the brain where Ballantine recommends placing lesions.

Still holding the article, he gazes at Matthew's draped form through the glass. He does not go into the operating room even when this first round of scanning is completed at 10:15. Instead, he leaves the suite to see Matthew's family. He will come and go often during the day.

10:16 A.M. Physician's assistant Debbie Mandelblatt places a white stretch cap on Matthew's skull, and over the cap a clear, stretchable plastic—not unlike thick Saran wrap—and fastens it down like a sausage casing. The wrap holds the scalp skin taut and sterile and isolates the slits the surgeon will cut in it to reach the skull and brain. "We'll make two burr holes, or entries," Uematsu tells onlookers. "The right side first." Two hours and 15 minutes into this operation, the first real surgery is about to happen.

Five separate times the surgical team validates the settings on a mockup before the coordinates are locked down on the stereotactic frame. Now the electrode probe is positioned on every plane: It can be moved in any direction and the target will always be in the center of the probe.

10:30 A.M. Uematsu makes a one-inch cut in the Saran wrap and skull cap, then slices the skin and underlayers of the scalp. He uses a retractor to hold the skin back and stitches it in place. It's quiet in the room as Uematsu picks up a hand drill, and drills the burr hole, beginning slowly and building to a vigorous circular motion with the handle. He drills and drills into the skull. With suction and irrigation, pieces of bone and tissue gush out on the table under Matthew's head, but very little blood. He sleeps peacefully.

10:45 A.M. Drilling stops. Uematsu uses currettes (tiny, sharp, curved knives) to clean out the hole. The top half of the stereotactic frame is fastened over the hole. There is a faint smell of burning as he electrically seals the covering of the brain, or dura. Now it's time to set the electrode needle into the brain. The necessary apparatus, already locked into the right place, is lifted from the mockup frame and placed over the bottom half of the device affixed to Matthew's skull. The surgeon will not need to make any judgments about where to put it. The probe will go through the holder and stop automatically at the target area.

He selects the right-size probe from the stainless-steel tray held by Gerry Beveringen, and sets it aside. The frame is ready, the coordinates have been checked a dozen times.

"No," he says. "We'll scan again." Another cross check. He will inject air into the brain, take more scans and make sure the frame's positioned for exactly the right spot. "Then," Uematsu says, "if we are, I put the needle in."

Vince clears the OR for the scans.

11:30 A.M. It has taken 45 minutes and two injections of air to learn that the black dots of air highlighted in the scanning images are right on target. "Better than textbook, better than perfect," Uematsu exclaims for the first of many times this day. "Now. Now we're ready to go."

The probe is in place, the needle tip resting on the target. Gerry wheels over the Frequency Lesion Generator, irreverently referred to as the "cooking machine." It is the only gallows humor of the day. But it is accurate.

The electrode is hooked up to the source of current. Gerry squirts a clear gel on a tinfoil-covered rigid plate and inserts it under Matthew's back. Then he runs a wire with an alligator clamp to the retractor handles and hooks it up. "Grounding Matthew," he says to no one in particular. "Grounded."

"In case something breaks," Uematsu explains.

11:43 A.M. "Set for seventy-five degrees for ninety seconds," Uematsu orders Gerry. The dials are set.

"Okay," Uematsu says, "cook." He forces a smile. No one returns it.

Through the same hole, Uematsu positions the probe four more times in the same plane to create four other tiny lesions around this first central lesion. Some at 90 seconds, some at 45 seconds. All at 75 degrees Centigrade. "Cook," he orders. "Cook," again. "Cook. Cook." The lesions are less than an eighth of an inch apart, all on the right side. That's Matthew's right, his right hemisphere, his right cingulum. It's close to noon.

The right side is pronounced finished, and a new set of scans is taken to confirm the lesions. "There," says Uematsu quietly, pointing to a perfect circle of black blots. "All there. Perfect. Better than the textbook. Now, ready to do the left side."

12:15 A.M. "Do you know how we learned how long to cook?" Uematsu asks as he makes the second burr hole. "Egg whites. We picked egg whites in 1967, in our first studies, to see how long and how hot to go through egg whites and create a hole of the right diameter that would not close up."

Over the next two hours, five more lesions are placed in the cingulum on the left side of Matthew's brain. The air target studies are again done to verify the placement, then they "cook," the heated tip cutting the brain. Then more scans make sure the lesions are sufficient and in place.

3:40 P.M. Steve Derrer has awakened Matthew and escorted him to the recovery room. Uematsu and others have talked to Matthew's family. "Perfect," Uematsu announces. "Better than the textbook." But they all must wait now, to see if the "textbook" surgery was not just successful in its execution, but also in its goal.

Matthew's neurologist is nervous. There's much that can still go wrong, he says. Brain damage or return of the seizures that might have found an alternative pathway for the abnormal electrical signals.

6 P.M. Matthew wakes fully and talks a "blue streak," but then unexpectedly lapses into a stupor. He apparently is unable to talk, move his limbs or arms. An angry, upset neurologist says, "It's not looking good." They take Matthew back to the OR for an emergency scan. Everything looks okay. The doctors hope the problem is temporary, from swelling that will subside. Matthew's parents are with him all night.

Wednesday, November 28, 11 A.M., eighth floor of the neuroscience wing: Matthew is propped up in bed in room 811, eating seedless red grapes from a plastic bag, half watching a television set suspended from the corner of the ceiling above his bed. His mother is all smiles; his father grinning.

"God, we are happy today," his mother says. "I knew it all the time. He's doing just great." Matthew has no pain, not even a headache, but he is still somewhat stunned and slow to react. Full recovery from the surgery is still days or more away, although he will return to Spring Grove Hospital on Sunday if all goes as planned. After six months without rages, they'll know if the cingulotomy has brought success—peace and the chance for a better life.

This morning, little more than a week after his operation, Matthew remembers names and faces slowly, but he does remember. His arms and legs and toes work. He can talk. "Rodgers," he says after his mother's prompt of a visitor's first name. "Writing a book," he says. A moment later there's a smile, which broadens when his father says quietly, "Perfect. So far, perfect. Better than the textbook."

Over Memorial Day weekend, 1991, six months after Matthew's surgery, his parents are still careful not to trumpet their hope. But all the signs remain positive. Over the holiday, Matthew is spending most of his time on a home visit with his family, and weekend leave from the hospital is now regularly scheduled. Matthew's social worker has begun the process of enrolling him in a special course at the hospital that teaches independent living skills—cooking fundamentals, washing clothes—because paperwork is under way to place him in a community-based group home.

"There have been no rages since his operation," Matt's mother says. "He's still having seizures, but no rage episodes at all. And he seems to have much, much better control of his anger. It doesn't escalate into chaos. He takes the time to calm down when he becomes angry. We think we have a success here, but the doctors—and we—still don't know how long it will last."

The absence of experience is a lingering reminder of the ongoing ignorance surrounding the new psychosurgery—and of the continuing political, medical, and social isolation of patients like Matthew and of his family. There is still a giant wall of timidity surrounding surgical treatment of psychiatric and behavioral disorders that turns away heads and minds. Even in the wake of success, the doctors don't want to go public with their endeavor. Lost in the silence most of all is that there are newer psychosurgical treatments for mental illness that need cheering on. So far, the cheerleaders are mostly the families of patients. And even their cheers are muted, reflecting the cautions and concerns of the medical profession.

"Matt's still scared," his mother says. "We are, too. That suddenly something will happen. When Matt comes on visits, he gets angry with me at times because he senses that I'm still wary of being alone with him. I'm still remembering those rages, his physical strength; how he could hurt others and himself. It hurts Matt now to think that I'm leery of him, that I'm afraid to be alone around him."

Confidence that the scars made in his brain can keep control of his mind will take time to build. Meanwhile, the family cautiously moves ahead.

Epilogue: The week before Christmas, 1991, I talked at length with Matthew's father, the cockeyed optimist who always believed that his son deserved another surgical chance for a life free of rages.

"Everything," he told me, "is looking good. The best news is that Matthew is now living in a low-security area [of the state hospital] and has great freedom. We're working hard to get him into a group home next, and since he's been free of rages for more than a year now, we think this will work out."

"What will Matt do for Christmas?"

"He'll be home with us and the family. It's gonna be a great Christmas."

As we spoke, I sensed some reserve in the father who has seen too much to be sanguine and too little to be cynical. And yet, there was a future to hope for, to plan and to execute for Matthew and his family. A future of relative tranquillity and contentment, this Christmas and next.

Credits/Acknowledgments

Cover design by Charles Vitelli.

1. Perspectives on the Causes and Diagnosis of Abnormal Behavior
Facing overview—© 1998 by Cleo Freelance Photography.
10—*Scientific American* illustration by Ian Worpole. 12—*Scientific American* illustration by Carol Donner.

2. Anxiety Disorders, Mood Disorders, and Suicide
Facing overview—© 1998 by PhotoDisc, Inc. 71—Box with graphics adapted from *Touched with Fire: Manic Depressive Illness and the Artistic Temperament* by Kay Redfield Jamison. © 1993 by Kay Redfield Jamison. Reprinted by permission of The Free Press, a division of Simon & Schuster. 72—*Scientific American* graphics by Lisa Burnett. 73—Graphics adapted from "Contributions to a Pathography of the Musicians: Robert Schumann" by E. Slater and A. Meyer in *Confinia Psychiatrica*, Vol. 2, 1959, pp. 65-94. Reprinted by permission of S. Karger, AG Basel Publishers, Switzerland.

3. Schizophrenia
Facing overview—WHO photo by Jean Mohr.

4. Drug/Alcohol Abuse and Violence
Facing overview—© 1998 by PhotoDisc, Inc.

5. Dissociative Disorders and Memory
Facing overview—© 1998 by PhotoDisc, Inc.

6. Physical Symptoms
Facing overview—© 1998 by PhotoDisc, Inc.

7. Therapy: Psychological Approaches
Facing overview—© 1998 by Cleo Freelance Photography.

8. Biological Therapies
Facing overview—Dushkin/McGraw-Hill photo.

PHOTOCOPY THIS PAGE!!!

ANNUAL EDITIONS ARTICLE REVIEW FORM

■ NAME: _____ DATE: _____

■ TITLE AND NUMBER OF ARTICLE: _____

■ BRIEFLY STATE THE MAIN IDEA OF THIS ARTICLE: _____

_____

■ LIST THREE IMPORTANT FACTS THAT THE AUTHOR USES TO SUPPORT THE MAIN IDEA:

_____

_____

_____

_____

■ WHAT INFORMATION OR IDEAS DISCUSSED IN THIS ARTICLE ARE ALSO DISCUSSED IN YOUR TEXTBOOK OR OTHER READINGS THAT YOU HAVE DONE? LIST THE TEXTBOOK CHAPTERS AND PAGE NUMBERS:

_____

_____

_____

_____

■ LIST ANY EXAMPLES OF BIAS OR FAULTY REASONING THAT YOU FOUND IN THE ARTICLE:

_____

_____

_____

_____

■ LIST ANY NEW TERMS/CONCEPTS THAT WERE DISCUSSED IN THE ARTICLE, AND WRITE A SHORT DEFINITION:

_____

_____

_____

_____

*Your instructor may require you to use this ANNUAL EDITIONS Article Review Form in any number of ways: for articles that are assigned, for extra credit, as a tool to assist in developing assigned papers, or simply for your own reference. Even if it is not required, we encourage you to photocopy and use this page; you will find that reflecting on the articles will greatly enhance the information from your text.

We Want Your Advice

ANNUAL EDITIONS revisions depend on two major opinion sources: one is our Advisory Board, listed in the front of this volume, which works with us in scanning the thousands of articles published in the public press each year; the other is you—the person actually using the book. Please help us and the users of the next edition by completing the prepaid article rating form on this page and returning it to us. Thank you for your help!

ANNUAL EDITIONS: ABNORMAL PSYCHOLOGY 98/99
Article Rating Form

Here is an opportunity for you to have direct input into the next revision of this volume. We would like you to rate each of the 44 articles listed below, using the following scale:

1. **Excellent: should definitely be retained**
2. **Above average: should probably be retained**
3. **Below average: should probably be deleted**
4. **Poor: should definitely be deleted**

Your ratings will play a vital part in the next revision. So please mail this prepaid form to us just as soon as you complete it.
Thanks for your help!

Rating	Article	Rating	Article
	1. Major Disorders of Mind and Brain		22. Health and Behavioral Consequences of Binge Drinking in College: A National Survey of Students at 140 Campuses
	2. Does Psychiatric Disorder Predict Violent Crime among Released Jail Detainees? A Six-Year Longitudinal Study		23. Addicted
	3. Out of the Shadows		24. The Fear of Heroin Is Shooting Up
	4. Is Mental Illness Catching?		25. Predators: The Disturbing World of the Psychopaths among Us
	5. Basic Behavioral Science Research for Mental Health: Vulnerability and Resilience		26. Creating False Memories
	6. Insanity Pleas Fail a Lot of Defendants as Fear of Crime Rises		27. Is There Evidence for Repression? Doubtful
	7. Panic and Panic Disorder in the United States		28. Does Repression Exist? Yes
	8. Making Sense of Mania and Depression		29. Multiple Personality Disorder
	9. Wounds That Never Heal: How Trauma Changes Your Brain		30. Is It Normal Aging—Or Alzheimer's?
	10. Don't Face Stress Alone		31. Hearts and Minds—Part I
	11. Dysthymic Disorder: The Chronic Depression		32. Behavioral Medicine, Clinical Health Psychology, and Cost Offset
	12. Update on Major Depression		33. Dying to Win
	13. Manic-Depressive Illness and Creativity		34. Munchausen Syndrome by Proxy: Case Accounts
	14. Suicide—Part I		35. Mental Health: Does Therapy Help?
	15. Age at Onset in Subtypes of Schizophrenic Disorders		36. A Buyer's Guide to Psychotherapy
	16. Maternal Influenza, Obstetric Complications, and Schizophrenia		37. Patterns of Symptomatic Recovery in Psychotherapy
	17. Is It Nature or Nurture?		38. What You Can Change and What You Cannot Change
	18. The Release of the Mentally Ill from Institutions: A Well-Intentioned Disaster		39. Cognitive-Behavioral Therapy Today
	19. Schizophrenia: A Disorder of Brain Circuitry		40. One Pill Makes You Larger, and One Pill Makes You Small . . .
	20. Thalamic Abnormalities in Schizophrenia Visualized through Magnetic Resonance Image Averaging		41. Prescriptions for Happiness?
	21. The War over Weed		42. Mother's Little Helper
			43. Pharmacotherapy for the Treatment of Depression
			44. Psychosurgery: Damaging the Brain to Save the Mind

(Continued on next page)

ABOUT YOU

Name _____ Date _____

Are you a teacher? ❏ Or a student? ❏

Your school name _____

Department _____

Address _____

City _____ State _____ Zip _____

School telephone # _____

YOUR COMMENTS ARE IMPORTANT TO US!

Please fill in the following information:

For which course did you use this book? _____

Did you use a text with this *ANNUAL EDITION*? ❏ yes ❏ no

What was the title of the text? _____

What are your general reactions to the *Annual Editions* concept?

Have you read any particular articles recently that you think should be included in the next edition?

Are there any articles you feel should be replaced in the next edition? Why?

Are there any World Wide Web sites you feel should be included in the next edition? Please annotate.

May we contact you for editorial input?

May we quote your comments?

No Postage
Necessary
if Mailed
in the
United States

ANNUAL EDITIONS: ABNORMAL PSYCHOLOGY 98/99

BUSINESS REPLY MAIL

First Class   Permit No. 84   Guilford, CT

Postage will be paid by addressee

Dushkin/McGraw·Hill
Sluice Dock
Guilford, CT 06437